Essential Infectious Disease Topics for Primary Care

Current Clinical Practice

Series Editor
Neil S. Skolnik, MD
Abington Memorial Hospital, Jenkintown, PA
Temple University School of Medicine, Philadelphia, PA

Essential Infectious Disease Topics for Primary Care

Edited by

Neil S. Skolnik, MD
Abington Memorial Hospital, Jenkintown, PA
Temple University School of Medicine, Philadelphia, PA

Associate Editor

Ross H. Albert, MD, PhD
Abington Memorial Hospital, Jenkintown, PA

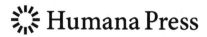 Humana Press

Editor
Neil S. Skolnik
Abington Memorial Hospital
Jenkintown, PA
USA

Associate Editor
Ross H. Albert
Abington Memorial Hospital
Jenkintown, PA
USA

Series Editor
Neil S. Skolnik
Abington Memorial Hospital
Jenkintown, PA
USA

ISBN 978-1-58829-520-0   e-ISBN 978-1-60327-034-2
DOI: 10.1007/978-1-60327-034-2

Library of Congress Control Number: 2007938050

Printed on acid-free paper

9 8 7 6 5 4 3 2 1

springer.com

Preface

It was the best of times, it was the worst of times,
it was the age of wisdom, it was the age of foolishness.

—Charles Dickens
A Tale of Two Cities

One of the major reasons that patients go to the doctor is to seek diagnosis and treatment for infectious diseases. The current approach to infectious disease is influenced by two competing factors: good evidence for how and when to use increasingly powerful antibiotics, and the increasing prevalence of antibiotic resistance, threatening to make those same antibiotics less effective, or even ineffective, in the treatment of disease. These competing issues make the choices of primary care physicians, who prescribe, by far, more antibiotics than any of the other medical specialties, even more important in determining both short- and long-term outcomes for patients who acquire infections.

Patients present to their doctors with illnesses that vary in severity from viral upper respiratory infections that require no treatment to meningitis, in which the correct antibiotic must be chosen and administered quickly to avoid life-threatening consequences. Primary care physicians must be sensitive to individual and social circumstances, as in the treatment of sexually transmitted diseases, and will often treat infectious diseases that have important public health implications, such as in the treatment of latent tuberculosis infections and screening for chlamydia infection.

This book provides an evidence-based approach to the most common and important infectious diseases seen by family doctors and internists. We have emphasized parsimonious use of antibiotics when the evidence shows that antibiotics are helpful, and knowledgeable restraint when an antibiotic is not needed. It is this balance of information and wisdom that will enable primary care physicians to continue to effectively treat patients with infectious diseases.

Essential Infectious Disease Topics for Primary Care is the result of a collaboration between the Departments of Family Medicine at Abington Memorial Hospital and Drexel School of Medicine. Although the two departments have worked together for years in the training of excellent Drexel medical students in the field of Family Medicine, this is the first time they have worked together on an academic project of significant scope. I believe that all involved feel that the collaboration was worthwhile and enjoyable. Ross H. Albert, who graduated from Drexel School of Medicine just 2 years ago with an MD, PhD, agreed to lend his considerable skills to this project, giving enthusiasm, perspective, and a meticulous approach that characterizes all of his work. Thanks are also due to the other members of the department of Family Medicine at Abington Memorial Hospital—Mathew M. Clark, Amy Clouse, Pamela Ann Fenstemacher, Trip Hansen, and John Russell—who have together created an academic family medicine residency program at a community hospital that provides incredibly high-quality training for residents who are interested in the art and science of family medicine. Special thanks to Todd Braun, who gave generously of his time reading selected chapters in manuscript form and gave excellent constructive input. Thanks are due again to the administration of Abington Memorial Hospital, particularly Dick Jones, Meg McGoldrick, Gary Candia, and the chief-of-staff, Jack Kelly, who have given unwavering support to our department and supported our mission of providing excellent care to diverse patients in a practice where attending and resident physicians share in the joys and the responsibilities of patient care.

No plant, no person, and no book grows to its best and fullest without the love and support of family. The highest of thanks goes to my wife, Alison, who is my confidant and keeper of the key to the joy and soul of our household; my son Aaron, who continues to amaze me with his keen eye for detail, his love of nature, and above all his love of fishing; and my daughter Ava, whose beauty, intelligence, and wit are a joy.

Neil S. Skolnik, MD
Associate Director of the Family Medicine Residency Program,
Abington Memorial Hospital,
Jenkintown, PA; and
Professor of Family and Community Medicine,
Temple University School of Medicine, Philadelphia, PA

Contents

Part III   Sexually Transmitted Diseases

Part IV   Skin, Bone, and Joint Infection

Part V   Other Infectious Disease Topics

Contributors

Ross H. Albert, MD, PhD
Family Medicine Residency, Abington Memorial Hospital, Jenkintown, PA

Todd Braun, MD
Chief of Infectious Diseases, Abington Memorial Hospital, Jenkintown, PA

Mathew M. Clark, MD, MA
Associate Director, Family Medicine Residency Program, Abington Memorial
Hospital, Jenkintown, PA; Associate Clinical Professor of Family and Community
Medicine, Temple University School of Medicine, Philadelphia, PA

Tina H. Degnan, MD
Family Medicine Residency, Abington Memorial Hospital, Jenkintown, PA

Andrew Deroo, MD
Department of Surgery Residency, The George Washington University School
of Medicine, Washington, DC

Pamela Ann Fenstemacher, MD, CMD, FAAFP
Associate Director, Family Medicine Residency, Abington Memorial Hospital,
Jenkintown, PA

Janet Fleetwood, PhD
Professor and Vice Chair for Academic Affairs, Department of Family,
Community and Preventive Medicine, Drexel University College of Medicine,
Philadelphia, PA

Michael Gagnon, MD
Family Medicine Residency, Abington Memorial Hospital, Jenkintown, PA

Kelly L. Gannon, DO
Family Medicine Residency, Abington Memorial Hospital, Jenkintown, PA

Rosemary Harris, MD
Assistant Professor, Department of Family, Community and Preventive Medicine,
Drexel University College of Medicine, Philadelphia, PA

Gene Hong, MD, CAQSM
Hamot Chair and Associate Professor, Chief Division of Sports Medicine,
Department of Family, Community and Preventive Medicine, Drexel University
College of Medicine, Philadelphia, PA

Michele Lamoreux, MD
Assistant Professor of Family, Community and Preventive Medicine, Drexel
University College of Medicine, Philadelphia, PA

Nirandra Mahamitra, MD
Family Medicine Residency Program, Drexel University, Philadelphia, PA

Thomas C. McGinley, Jr., MD
Associate Director, Sacred Heart Family Medicine Residency Program,
Allentown, PA

Matthew Mintz, MD
Associate Professor of Medicine, The George Washington University School
of Medicine, Washington, DC

Jennifer Neria, MD, MPH
Family Medicine Residency, VCU-Fairfax Family Practice, Fairfax, VA

Judith A. O'Donnell, MD
Associate Professor of Medicine, Division of Infectious Diseases, Drexel
University College of Medicine and Hospital Epidemiologist, Hahnemann
University Hospital, Philadelphia, PA

John Russell, MD
Associate Director, Family Medicine Residency, Abington Memorial Hospital,
Jenkintown, PA; Associate Clinical Professor of Family and Community Medicine,
Temple University School of Medicine, Philadelphia, PA

Neil S. Skolnik, MD
Associate Director, Family Medicine Residency Program, Abington Memorial
Hospital, Jenkintown, PA; and Professor of Family and Community Medicine,
Temple University School of Medicine, Philadelphia, PA

Megan Werner, MD, MPH
Attending Physician, Westside Health, Wilmington, DE

Anne T. Wiedemann, MD
Attending Physician, Department of Family Medicine and Palliative Care,
Abington Memorial Hospital, Jenkintown, PA

Adrian Wilson, DO
Attending Physician, Westside Health, Wilmington, DE

Steven Zinn, MD
Assistant Professor, Department of Family, Community and Preventive Medicine,
Drexel University College of Medicine, Philadelphia, PA

Part I
Upper Respiratory Tract Infections

Chapter 1
Clinical Guidelines

Community-Acquired Pneumonia

John Russell

Overview and Epidemiology

Lower respiratory tract infections are a major cause of mortality worldwide, the sixth leading cause of death and the most common from infectious disease. In the USA, William Osler referred to pneumonia as "the Old man's friend" and "Captain of the men of death." These spoke to the high lethality that the disease had at the turn of the 20th century. Pneumonia still is the cause of great morbidity and mortality despite advances in antibacterial therapies. Overall, there are 2 to 3 million cases of pneumonia in the USA and approximately a half million hospitalizations. Mortality rates range from < 1% in those treated as outpatients to up to 30% in hospitalized patients. Overall, the incidence of pneumonia is higher during the winter.

Community-acquired pneumonia (CAP) is defined as an acute infectious process of the lower respirator tract in a patient living outside of a nursing care facility or not hospitalized in the last 2 weeks. The "typical" pneumonia has cough, fever, leukocytosis, pleuritic chest pain, and purulent sputum with *Streptococcus pneumoniae* as the prototypical pathogen. The "atypical" pathogens (*Mycoplasma pneumoniae, Chlamydophila pneumonia, Legionella sp.*) have less fever and scant sputum and often have nonpulmonary manifestations.

Patients should have evidence of pneumonia on a chest radiograph by way of an infiltrate or findings on physical exam consistent with pneumonia. There might be diminished breath sounds or localized rales. Because physical exam findings are neither sensitive nor specific, it is recommended that patients receive further testing with chest radiographs, which have higher sensitivity and specificity than physical exam.

The Infectious Diseases Society of America (IDSA) and the American Thoracic Society (ATS) jointly issued clinical guidelines on the care of CAP in immunocompetent adults in 2007[3]. Throughout the guidelines, a grading system is used to categorize the strength of evidence behind various recommendations in the guidelines (Table 1.1).

N.S. Skolnik (ed.), *Essential Infectious Disease Topics for Primary Care.*
© Humana Press, Totowa, NJ

Table 1.1 IDSA/ATS grading system

Category (grade)	
Quality of evidence	Interpretation
I (high)	Evidence from well-conducted, randomized, controlled trials
II (moderate)	≥1 well-designed trial without randomization; might be cohort, patient series, or case-controlled studies
III (low)	Evidence from case studies and expert opinion

Likely Pathogens in CAP

In the most rigorously performed studies on CAP, the yield of a specific pathogen did not exceed 50%. Therefore, the treatment of CAP is empirically based. The most common etiologic agent in outpatients, inpatients, and the critically ill is *S. pneumoniae*. Outpatients also have "atypical" pathogens, such as *M. pneumoniae*, and *C. pneumonia*. Outpatients will also have respiratory viruses and nontypeable *Haemophilus influenzae*.

Hospitalized patients will have all the same pathogens as outpatients but will also have aspiration and *Legionella* species. Those patients in the intensive care unit (ICU) will have all of the aforementioned pathogens as well as gram-negative bacillus.

Chest Radiography

Chest radiography is indicated for all patients with suspected pneumonia (moderate recommendation, level III evidence). The radiograph is essential for establishing a diagnosis and distinguishing pneumonia from acute bronchitis. Physical exam is neither sensitive nor specific in establishing the diagnosis of pneumonia. There may be times when one is unable to obtain a chest radiograph because of limited resources but, because of the lack of clinical accuracy of the physical exam, this practice should be discouraged. The incidence of false negative chest radiograph results can be up to 30% in *Pneumocystis carinii* pneumonia, but this is not true in the case of immunocompetent adults. For patients who are admitted to the hospital with the clinical diagnosis of pneumonia with a negative chest radiograph, it might be reasonable to repeat the radiograph in 24 to 48 hours. The role of chest CT scanning in the setting of negative chest radiographs is not clear. Because lung tumors can cause postobstructive pneumonia, a posttreatment chest radiograph should be obtained in any patient at risk for lung cancer.

Other Diagnostic Testing

For the ambulatory patient who is to be treated as an outpatient, the search for an etiologic agent is optional (moderate recommendation, level III evidence). Testing is rarely done and treatment is empirically based. In addition, patients should have oxygenation status measured by pulse oximetry.

In patients who are being hospitalized for pneumonia, testing to search for an etiology of the pneumonia is optional (moderate recommendation, level I evidence). Patients in the following categories: ICU admissions, failure of outpatient antibiotics, leukopenia, pleural effusions, alcohol abuse, liver disease, cavitary lesions, severe structural/obstructive lung disease, positive antigen testing for legionella or pneumococcus, and asplenia, should have two pretreatment blood cultures obtained as well as expectorated sputum (moderate recommendation, level I evidence). The sputum should be obtained before antibiotic therapy and should only be cultured if a good quality specimen can be obtained (moderate recommendation, level II evidence). Induced sputum should be reserved only for evaluation of *M. tuberculosis* and *P. carinii*.

Patients who are being hospitalized or evaluated for possible hospitalization should have testing including a complete blood count, electrolyte and blood urea nitrogen measurement, liver functions, and oxygen saturation. Patients between 15 and 54 years of age should be considered for HIV testing with proper consent.

Specific Pathogen Testing

S. pneumoniae

A new method of testing for *S. pneumoniae* is a pneumococcal urine antigen assay. It is an immunochromatographic membrane test that detects pneumococcal cell wall polysaccharide. It should yield results in approximately 15 minutes. It can be used in conjunction with sputum Gram's stain and culture for diagnosis. Potentially the urine antigen assay will provide accuracy similar to Gram's stain in a timelier manner.

The testing has been found to have a sensitivity in the 50 to 80% range, with a specificity of approximately 90%. It should be used it the setting of ICU admissions, failure of outpatient antibiotics, leukopenia, pleural effusions, alcohol abuse, liver disease, asplenia, and travel in the last 2 weeks (moderate recommendation, level II evidence).

Legionella Species

Legionella is implicated in 0.5 to 6% of CAP cases. Risk factors for *Legionella* are exposure, increasing age, smoking, and compromised cell-mediated immunity. Epidemiologic risk factors include travel outside of home, exposure to spas, changes in domestic plumbing and comorbid illnesses, including renal failure, liver failure, diabetes, and malignancy. Overall mortality rates are 5 to 25%. A large percentage of hospitalized patients require ICU admission. Testing for *Legionella* is appropriate for any hospitalized patient with a history of alcohol abuse, failure of outpatient antibiotics, travel within the past 2 weeks, pleural effusions, or ICU admissions (moderate recommendation, level II evidence). Testing should be performed via urine antigen assay and culture of respiratory secretions using selective media. The urine test is a rapid assay that detects 80 to 95% of community-acquired cases. It only detects *L. pneumophilia* serogroup 1. The urine antigen test becomes positive on day 1 of illness and remains positive for weeks. In the setting of epidemiologic evidence of disease, treatment should be administered despite negative testing. Patients with positive urine antigen testing are more likely to have positive sputum cultures for *Legionella*.

C. pneumoniae

C. pneumoniae is a common respiratory pathogen. There is no clear "gold standard" for the diagnosis. The IDSA CAP Committee recommends testing methods including serology, culture, polymerase chain reaction (PCR), and tissue diagnostics or immunochemistry. Acceptable ways to obtain the diagnosis for *C. pneumonia* pulmonary infections are the demonstration of a fourfold increase in IgG or a individual IgM titer of at least 1:16 via a microimmunofluorescence assay (MIF), isolation of a tissue culture, or a PCR assay of respiratory secretions. In patient care settings, acute and convalescent titers may not be practical and the clinician should use the timelier PCR or IgM testing.

Viral Pneumonia

Respiratory viruses are a common cause of CAP. They are seen most commonly in the elderly, in patients with chronic obstructive pulmonary disease (COPD) or other comorbidities. The incidence of viral infections in CAP ranges from 4 to 39% in studies. Three-quarters of the viral infections are one of three viruses: respiratory syncytial virus (RSV), influenza, and parainfluenza viruses. There can be secondary bacterial infection in 26 to 77% of hospitalized adult patients with viral pneumonias. The most common pathogen seen is *S. pneumoniae*, but earlier studies found *S. aureus* in one-quarter of cases. Empiric treatment of bacterial superinfection should provide activity against *S. pneumoniae, S. aureus*, and *H. influenzae*.

RSV antigen detection tests are readily available but are insensitive for detecting disease in adults and are not generally recommended. The rapid detection test for influenza is recommended for both epidemiologic and treatment purposes. Tests that can distinguish between influenza A and B are recommended. Treatment within 48 hours of the onset of symptoms with antivirals targeted against influenza is recommended. Influenza A and B can be treated with oseltamivir or zanamivir. Amantadine and rimantadine only treat influenza A, and have been subject to resistance in the past few influenza seasons. Patients with symptoms of uncomplicated influenza longer than 48 hours should not be treated with medications. The drugs can be used to reduce viral shedding in patients hospitalized with CAP.

Site of Treatment Decision

The decision regarding place of treatment is an important step in the management of CAP. In the USA, 75% of the 1 million pneumonia admissions come through emergency care units. The IDSA/ATS recommendation is that the decision on place of treatment is based on three steps: 1) safety and ability for patient to be treated at home, 2) clinical judgment, and 3) the use of severity of illness scores (CURB-65) or prognostic models (Pneumonia Severity Index [PSI]) to determine the safety of outpatient therapy (strong recommendation, level I evidence). For those patients who are appropriate for outpatient management, there can be marked cost savings and increased patient satisfaction.

The CURB-65 is a severity of illness score from the British Thoracic Society based on five criteria: confusion, uremia, respiratory rate, blood pressure, and age older than 65 years. Confusion is based on change from baseline; uremia is designated as a BUN >20 mg/dL; respiratory rate elevation is that >30 breaths per minute; blood pressure is <90 mmHg systolic or <60 mmHg diastolic; and age is older than 65 years. For patients with a score of 0 to 1, outpatient management is acceptable, those with a score of 2 should be admitted to the general medical wards, and scores of 3 or greater should be admitted to intensive care.

The PSI is a validated prognostic model. Patients are classified into one of five risk classes, with class I having the lowest risk and class V the highest risk. Initially, patients are screened for low-risk status based on age younger than 50 years, comorbid illness (cancer, congestive heart failure [CHF], renal disease, liver disease, and cerebrovascular disease), vital signs, and mental status. The patients not assigned to class I are further evaluated by a point system based on age, comorbid illnesses listed previously, physical exam findings, presence of abnormal oxygenation, elevated blood urea nitrogen, acidosis on arterial blood gas, hyponatremia (<130 mmol/L), hyperglycemia (>250 mg/dL), anemia (hematocrit <30%), and presence of pleural effusion. The patient's sex and residence in a nursing facility also are part of the scoring system. Patients in class I to III have an overall low mortality and can be treated safely at home unless there are social factors that prevent the patient safely being treated at home.

Empiric Therapy

In the most diligent of CAP studies, an etiologic agent is only found in 40 to 60% of cases. Clinicians need to treat patients empirically based on certain historical data until a specific pathogen can be found. Treatment can then be tailored to the specific pathogen. For patients admitted through the emergency care unit, antibiotics should be started in the emergency room (level I). For empiric treatment of outpatients, refer to Table 1.2; for empiric treatment of hospitalized patients, refer to Table 1.3.

Table 1.2 Outpatient empiric therapy of CAP

Outpatient characteristics	
Previously healthy	
No recent antibiotics	Macrolide or doxycycline
Recent antibiotics (<3 months), lung disease, liver disease, heart disease, diabetes, alcohol, malignancy, asplenia, immunosuppression	Levofloxacin, moxifloxacin, gemifloxacin alone or Azithromycin, clarithromycin plus high-dose amoxicillin or Azithromycin, clarithromycin plus high-dose amoxicillin–clavulanate
Nursing home (patient not at risk for MDRO)	Ceftriaxone or Levofloxacin, moxifloxacin, or gemifloxacin

Table 1.3 Inpatient empiric therapy of CAP

Inpatient characteristics	
Medical ward	
Not at risk for MDRO	Levofloxacin, moxifloxacin, gemifloxacin (oral only) or azithromycin, clarithromycin plus a β-lactam (ceftriaxone, cefotaxime, ampicillin preferred) could substitute doxycycline for macrolide
At risk for MDRO	Piperacillin–tazobactam, imipenem, meropenem, or cefepime + ciprofloxacin or Levaquin (750) or Piperacillin–tazobactam, imipenem, meropenem, or cefepime + azithromycin and an aminoglycoside or Piperacillin–tazobactam, imipenem, meropenem, or cefepime + levofloxacin or moxifloxacin and an aminoglycoside ±Vancomycin
Intensive care	
Pseudomonas infection is not an issue	A β-lactam plus azithromycin, clarithromycin, or levofloxacin, moxifloxacin, gemifloxacin
Pseudomonas infection is an issue	Piperacillin–tazobactam, imipenem, meropenem, or cefepime + ciprofloxacin or Levaquin (750) or Piperacillin–tazobactam, imipenem, meropenem, or cefepime + azithromycin and an aminoglycoside or Piperacillin–tazobactam, imipenem, meropenem, or cefepime + levofloxacin or moxifloxacin and an aminoglycoside
Pseudomonas infection is an issue but patient has a β-lactam allergy	Aztreonam plus levofloxacin or Aztreonam plus moxifloxacin ± aminoglycoside
MRSA is an issue	Add Vancomycin or linezolid

Patients need coverage for *S. pneumoniae* and *Chlamydia* and *Mycoplasma*. Low-risk patients can receive macrolides or doxycycline whereas higher-risk outpatients need respiratory quinolones or expanded macrolides plus high-dose macrolides. Treatment of nursing home residents is more complicated. They may have forms of healthcare-associated pneumonia (HCAP). Hospital-acquired pneumonia (HAP) is a pneumonia that develops after 48 hours in the hospital. Ventilator-associated pneumonia (VAP) occurs in intubated patients. Nursing home patients often resemble HAP and VAP in pathogens. Patients who do not respond to initial therapy should be considered for multidrug-resistant organisms (MDRO).

Hospitalized patients need treatment with broader-spectrum antibiotic treatment. The extent of the spectrum is based on patients' risk for MDRO. A patient who is at low risk can be treated with a respiratory quinolone or an advanced macrolide plus a β-lactam. If patients are at risk for MDRO, they should be covered with antibiotics that address normal pathogens plus pseudomonas and methicillin-resistant *S. aureus* (MRSA), if indicated. If a specific pathogen is recovered, then the regimen can be tailored to specific pathogens and their individual susceptibilities.

Specific Antibacterial Agents

Macrolides

Macrolides are active against most common pathogens that cause CAP. Data from clinical trials has shown good results against strains with resistance in vitro. The extended spectrum macrolides, azithromycin and clarithromycin, can each be given once daily. Drawbacks are related to resistance and tolerability. Macrolide resistance can occur in 20 to 30% cases of *S. pneumonia*. Resistance can develop during therapy. The resistance occurs more often than in fluoroquinolones or β-lactams. Overall, erythromycin is less well tolerated because of gastrointestinal (GI) side effects. Erythromycin is also less effective against *H. influenzae*.

Ketolides

Ketolides are semisynthetic derivatives of macrolides. They were designed to be effective against macrolide-resistant gram-positive cocci. Telithromycin is a ketolide that may be an alternative to macrolides in CAP. Telithromycin is a once-daily, well-tolerated antibiotic. It is active against *S. pneumoniae*, including macrolide-resistant strains, *H. influenzae, Moraxella catarrhalis*, as well *Legionella, Mycoplasma*, and *Chlamydophila species*.

Amoxicillin

Amoxicillin is the preferred drug of choice for oral treatment of susceptible strains of *S. pneumoniae*. At doses of 3 to 4 g daily, it covers 90 to 95% of strains of pneumococcus. The drawback to using amoxicillin as a treatment is that there is no coverage of atypical pathogens. It is also problematic that very high doses are required for coverage of *S. pneumoniae*.

Amoxicillin–Clavulanate

Compared with amoxicillin, the combination of amoxicillin plus clavulanate has better coverage against anaerobes, *H. influenzae*, and methicillin-sensitive *S. aureus*. Similar to amoxicillin, it has no activity against atypical pathogens. It is more expensive than amoxicillin, and GI symptoms are common.

Cephalosporins

Oral cephalosporins are active against 75 to 85% of *S. pneumoniae* and almost all species of *H. influenzae*. Ceftriaxone and cefotaxime are injectable medications that cover 90 to 95% of *S. pneumoniae* and *H. influenzae* and methicillin-sensitive *S. aureus*. Neither the oral nor the injectable forms of cephalosporins are active against atypical agents.

Doxycycline

Doxycycline is active against 90 to 95% of strains of *S. pneumoniae*, as well as *H. influenzae* and atypical pathogens. It is also active against many agents used in bioterrorism. Despite it being an affordable and well-tolerated medication, it is rarely used to treat CAP in clinical practice.

Fluoroquinolones

As a class, the fluoroquinolones are active against a broad spectrum of agents that cause CAP. This includes more than 98% of strains of *S. pneumoniae* in the USA. Despite its wide spectrum of activity, there are fears of increasing resistance to these medications. They can be given once daily and are very well tolerated. They are overall far more expensive than erythromycin and doxycycline.

Clindamycin

Clindamycin is active against 90% of strains of *S. pneumoniae* but not *H. influenzae* and atypical pathogens. It also has very good activity for anaerobic infections. It is favored for toxic shock caused by pneumonia associated with group A streptococci. It is not active against *H. influenzae* and atypical pathogens. It can cause high rates of diarrhea and *Clostridium difficile* colitis.

Discharge Criteria

Hospitalized patients can be safely changed to oral antibiotics when the patient, with a functioning GI tract, is improving clinically, able to take oral medications, and is hemodynamically stable (strong recommendation, level II evidence). For a patient to be safely discharged from the hospital, they should be clinically stable, have no other active medical problems, and have a safe environment in which to fully recover. Patients do not need to be observed in the hospital after the switch to oral therapy (moderate recommendation, level II evidence). Patients should be treated for at least 5 days of antibiotics.

Special Populations and Circumstances

Pneumonia in Elderly Persons

With 60,000 annual deaths, pneumonia is the sixth leading cause of death in senior citizens. Elderly people that live in extended care facilities are at increased risk of morbidity and mortality from pneumonia. The most common pathogen is *S. pneumoniae* CAP, which is also the most common pathogen in younger patients. The elderly, especially those with comorbidities or those living in extended care facilities, are more likely to have gram-negative bacteria and *S. aureus* as etiologic agents than their younger counterparts. Risk factors besides age that put seniors at increased risk are institutionalization, difficulty swallowing, inability to take oral medications, lung disease, heart disease, immunosuppression, alcoholism, and male sex.

When a elderly person presents with pneumonia, they are likely to have fewer symptoms than younger adults. The fewer number of symptoms are mostly related to a decrease in the febrile response to illness (chills, sweats). Prevention of pneumonia through vaccination against pneumococcus and influenza should be part of the primary care management of senior citizens.

Pneumonia in the Context of Bioterrorism

With the ability to disseminate some infectious agents via an aerosolized route, bioterrorism attacks might present as pneumonia. The agents with the greatest risk of severe respiratory illness are *Bacillus anthracis, Franciella tularensis*, and *Yersinia pestis*. A case of inhaled anthrax would always indicate bioterrorism, whereas pneumonic tularemia or pneumonic plague may or may not be caused by bioterrorism. Clinicians should know the clues to bioterrorism and the mechanism of alerting public health officials in cases of suspected bioterrorism.

In 2001, there were 11 cases of inhalation anthrax from contaminated mail in the USA. Diagnostic features that might distinguish inhalational anthrax from CAP include a widened mediastinum on chest x-ray, hyperdense mediastinal lymph nodes on chest CT scan, and a bloody pleural effusion. Blood cultures were positive in eight of eight untreated patients in 2001. The blood cultures were positive in the first day. Mortality rates are in the 45 to 80% rate. The incubation period was approximately 4 days. The work-up of inhalation anthrax should include a blood culture and a chest CT scan. The most important therapeutic interventions are antibiotic therapy and draining of pleural effusions. Antibiotic treatment should be prolonged because of the potential persistence of spores in animal models. Prophylaxis can be achieved with prolonged courses (60 to 100 days) of doxycycline or ciprofloxacin.

F. tularensis causes < 200 infections per year in the USA. An aerosolized attack with *F. tularensis* is referred to as a "typhoidal" or "pneumonic" tularemia. After an incubation period of 3 to 5 days, the patient might present with nonspecific symptoms of fever, dry cough, malaise, and pleuritic chest pain. The chest x-ray should show pneumonia with mediastinal adenopathy. Cultures of blood, pharynx, and sputum should be obtained and evaluated in a biocontainment level 3 laboratory because of safety concerns.

Standard treatment is streptomycin, but gentamicin is an acceptable alternative. Tetracycline and chloramphenicol have also been used, but with higher failure rates. Ciprofloxacin is not approved for tularemia but has had clinical success in human and animal studies. Treatment should be for 2 weeks. In studies, the mortality rate has been found to be 1.4%.

Y. pestis is an ideal biologic weapon because of its high mortality without treatment and can be transmitted from person to person. Patients might present with high fevers, chills, headache, cough, bloody sputum, leukocytosis, and bilateral pneumonia on chest radiograph. Patients can decompensate quickly to septic shock and death. Patients lack the swollen, tender lymph node or bubo that is characteristic of bubonic plague.

Patients should have blood culture and sputum culture and Gram's stain. The Gram's stain shows safety pin-shaped gram-negative coccobacilli. Healthcare workers should use respiratory precautions until the patient has undergone 48 hours of therapy. Antibiotic treatment would be streptomycin or gentamicin for 10 days. Patients with face-to-face contact or suspected exposure should receive 7 days of prophylaxis with tetracycline or fluoroquinolone.

Update on Performance Indicators

Previous IDSA guidelines recommended starting antibiotics within 8 hours of admission. A more recent Medicare analysis of pneumonia hospitalizations found that earlier treatment with antibiotics improved outcomes. Patients who received antibiotics within 4 hours of arrival to the hospital had a mean length of stay that way 0.4 days shorter than patients who received their antibiotics later. Earlier initiation of antibiotics had a greater impact than antibiotic choice. These factors have led to a change in the IDSA guidelines. Patients hospitalized with CAP should have antibiotics initiated with 4 hours of registration at the hospital.

Patients should also have assessment of oxygenation by pulse oximetry or arterial blood gas measurement within 8 hours of admission. There should also be a documented infiltrate on chest x-ray or other imaging study in all patients except those with decreased immune function that might not be able to mount an inflammatory response (A-I).

In ICU patients with severe enigmatic pneumonia, a target of at least 50% of patients should receive some type of testing for Legionella by either urine antigen testing or culture.

Smoking has a long and heralded connection with respiratory diseases. Smoking is the biggest risk factor for pneumococcal bacteremia in immunocompetent, non-elderly adults. Smoking cessation should be a goal for persons that smoke who are hospitalized with CAP (moderate recommendation; level III evidence).

Prevention

Influenza

All persons older than the age of 50 years or younger patients with risk factors for pneumonia should receive a yearly inactivated influenza vaccine each fall (strong recommendation, level I evidence). Household contacts, aged 5 to 49 years, of patients at risk for influenza may receive the nasally administered live, attenuated influenza vaccine (moderate recommendation, level III evidence). The live, attenuated vaccine should not be used in those with asthma or immunodeficiency. The influenza vaccine should be offered to at-risk patients on hospital discharge, or outpatient encounters in the late fall or early winter. All healthcare workers, in any setting, should receive an annual influenza vaccine (moderate recommendation, level III evidence).

Pneumococcal Vaccine

Pneumococcal polysaccharide vaccine is indicated for all people older than 65 years of age and selected high-risk patients (strong recommendation, level II evidence). High-risk patients include patients with diabetes, cardiovascular disease, lung disease, alcohol abuse, liver disease, cerebrospinal fluid (CSF) leaks, HIV, renal failure, sickle cell disease, nephrotic syndrome, hematologic, malignancies, or those on long-term immunosuppressive medications. Vaccination status should be assessed at all hospital admissions (moderate recommendation, level III evidence). Patients should receive a repeat vaccination in 5 years if they received their first dose younger than 65 years of age. Vaccination can occur on hospital discharge or during outpatient therapy (moderate recommendation, level III evidence).

Selected Reading

1. American Thoracic Society Guidelines for the Management of Community Acquired Pneumonia. Am J Respir Crit Care Med 163:1730–1754; 2001.
2. Guidelines for the Management of Adults with Hospital-Acquired, Ventilator-Associated, and Healthcare-Associated Pneumonia (HCAP). Am J Respir Crit Care Med 171:388–416; 2005.
3. IDSA/ATS Guidelines for Management of CAP in Adults. Clin Inf Dis 44 Supp 2:27–72; 2007.

Chapter 2
Pharyngitis

Adrian Wilson

Introduction

One of the most common chief complaints in a primary care physician's office is sore throat. Although a broad variety of differential diagnoses must be considered, ranging from infectious or inflammatory etiology to traumatic or neoplastic processes, the vast majority of these symptoms derive from either a viral or bacterial source. The physician must narrow the differential, decide which clinical and laboratory data may be helpful, select the most appropriate management plan for the patient's symptoms and disease process, and prevent further complications. This chapter reviews the most common causes of pharyngitis, relevant available clinical information, appropriate laboratory tests, recommended treatment guidelines, possible complications, and general strategies for evaluating patients with acute pharyngitis.

In the 1990s, more than 6.7 million visits with a primary complaint of sore throat were made by adults to physicians' offices, emergency departments, or other primary care providers in the Unites States.[2] Currently, acute pharyngitis accounts for approximately 2% of all primary healthcare visits for adults and 6% for children annually (more than 10 million visits).[7,10] Of these cases, approximately 30% are idiopathic, 30 to 60% have a viral etiology, and 5 to 15% are caused by bacteria.[8] Of the possible bacterial sources, Group A β-hemolytic streptococci (GABHS) is the most frequently isolated pathogen, causing acute pharyngitis in 5 to 15% of adults and 15 to 36% of children in the USA.[4,10] Although this chapter reviews the broad range of causes of pharyngitis, the emphasis is on the diagnosis and treatment of GABHS, because this is the only common cause of sore throat that warrants antibiotic treatment.

In recent years, fear of GABHS infection and its possible complications, and growing expectation of antibiotic prescriptions by patients has resulted in overuse of antibiotics for treatment of acute pharyngitis. Reportedly, 50 to 75% of all cases of pharyngitis are currently treated with antibiotic therapy, approximately 40% of which use broad-spectrum antibiotics or antibiotics that are not indicated.[7,10,14] Spurred by efforts from the Centers for Disease Control and Prevention (CDC) and Infectious Diseases Society of America (IDSA), recent guidelines have been established to decrease the frequency of unnecessary antibiotic use, and to concentrate instead on clinical protocol and appropriate laboratory evaluation.

N.S. Skolnik (ed.), *Essential Infectious Disease Topics for Primary Care.*
© Humana Press, Totowa, NJ

Pathophysiology

Pharyngitis is an inflammation of the pharynx that can lead to a sore throat. Etiologic agents are passed through person-to-person contact, most likely via droplets of nasal secretions or saliva. Symptoms often manifest after an incubation period ranging from 1 to 5 days, and occur most commonly in the winter or early spring. Outbreaks of pharyngitis may occur in households or classrooms, and, infrequently, may be linked to food or animal sources.

The most common bacterial cause of pharyngitis, GABHS, is also known as *Streptococcus pyogenes* and may exist as single, paired, or chained gram-positive cocci. These bacteria possess protein M, a potent virulence factor that inhibits bacterial phagocytosis, as well as a hyaluronic acid capsule that enhances its ability to invade tissues. Multiple exotoxins and two hemolysins (Streptolysin S and Streptolysin O) further enhance the virulence of GABHS. Cocci may be detected on cultures (grown on blood agar), latex agglutination tests, or rapid tests using labeled monoclonal antibodies.

The viruses and other nonstreptococcal bacteria that also can cause pharyngitis are discussed in greater detail below, in the "Differential Diagnosis" section.

Clinical Presentation

History

Pharyngitis can present with sudden onset of sore throat, fever, headache, tender anterior cervical lymphadenopathy or lymphadenitis, and, occasionally, abdominal pain, nausea, vomiting, fatigue, or rash. When GABHS is the etiologic agent, fevers are often >38.5 °C (101.3 °F), tonsillar exudates are common, and patients may experience fevers, chills, and myalgias.[8] Children may sometimes present with atypical symptoms such as abdominal pain and emesis, regardless of the cause of their pharyngitis.

Physical Exam

On examination, the typical findings of acute pharyngitis may include an erythematous and swollen pharynx, tonsillar hypertrophy and inflammation (with or without tonsillar exudates), fever, edematous uvula, petechial rash along the palate, and tender anterior cervical lymphadenopathy. Occasionally, a scarlatiniform rash may be present, often seen in association with a GABHS infection.

Clinical Guidelines

Given the above historical and physical findings, a number of clinical tools have been established to help determine whether GABHS is the likely causative pathogen. The most widely accepted of these tools is the Centor Clinical Prediction Rules for the diagnosis of GABHS in adults, which uses the presence (or absence) of four main criteria (see Table 2.1).[4,12]

If the patient has none or one of these symptoms, suspicion for GABHS is very low and no further testing or treatment is necessary. If the patient meets two, three, or four of the criteria, a diagnostic laboratory test is indicated. Some physicians will begin antibiotic therapy presumptively for patients with severe symptoms who meet three or four of the Centor criteria, and may not send a diagnostic test in addition to testing. The absence of three or four criteria has a negative predictive value near 80%.[4,14] The Centor Clinical Prediction Rules are endorsed by the IDSA and listed currently among the CDC recommendations online at: www.cdc/gov/drugresistance/community/files/ads/Acute_Pharyngitis.pdf.

Ultimately, the usefulness of clinical prediction rules depends on the prevalence of disease in a given community. In a GABHS-dense population, a higher score on a GABHS prediction tool would convey a higher probability of actually having a bacterial infection than in regions where overall prevalence was lower.[4]

Laboratory Evaluation

There is significant debate surrounding the selection of which laboratory tests are necessary to establish the correct diagnosis and ensure the appropriate treatment course for pharyngitis. Aside from influenza and new-onset HIV, the viral causes of pharyngitis only require supportive care and do not necessitate extensive testing. Of the bacterial causes, only GABHS has an indication for antibiotic therapy. Therefore, the majority of laboratory diagnostics for pharyngitis concentrate on the presence or absence of GABHS.

The gold standard of pharyngitis testing remains the throat culture, collected by swabbing the pharynx and peritonsillar region, and growing the sample on a sheep's blood agar plate. Under ideal circumstances, and often using two samples, the sensitivity and specificity of such cultures reaches 97% and 99%, respectively.[17] In most offices, however, those numbers vary widely, with a sensitivity between 30

Table 2.1 Centor Clinical Prediction Rules

1. Fever (by history or exam)
2. Tender anterior cervical lymphadenopathy
3. Presence of tonsillar exudates
4. Absence of cough
• Presence of 0–1 of the above—no further testing indicated
• Presence of 2–4 of the above—GABHS testing indicated

and 90% and a specificity from 75 to 99%.[8] Some false positive results can be expected with culture results because up to 20% of the US population may be chronic, asymptomatic GABHS carriers.

Another class of available tests are the rapid antigen detection (RAD) tests, which use enzyme or acid extraction from throat swabs, followed by latex agglutination, coagglutination, or enzyme-linked immunoabsorbent assay (ELISA) procedures to isolate GABHS antigen–antibody complexes.[3] Although older models were not as reliable and variation still exists, newer techniques show a sensitivity ranging from 76 to 97% and a specificity >95%.[8,17] Most modern RAD tests produce results within 10 minutes or less.

Serology may be collected for presence or absence of streptococcal antibody titers, but this information will not influence the immediate treatment of the patient's pharyngitis symptoms. Serum titers of deoxyribonuclease B, hyaluronidase, streptokinase, nicotinic acid, and antistreptolysin O (ASO) may rise quickly during acute streptococcal infection (a positive ASO result reflects a fourfold increase), and will peak within 2 to 3 weeks. This information is necessary to support a diagnosis of rheumatic fever, but treatment for pharyngitis needs to begin before the return of serology laboratory results.

Both the American Academy of Pediatrics (AAP) and the American Heart Association consider a positive RAD test definitive evidence for presence of GABHS and indication for antibiotic therapy.[8] The AAP also contends that when GABHS is strongly suspected, a negative RAD test should be followed up with a confirmatory throat culture.[7,8] In an adult patient, clinical suspicion should guide decisions regarding whether further confirmation of a negative RAD test is needed.

Differential Diagnosis

The differential diagnosis for sore throat symptoms is extensive. The most common viral pathogens causing pharyngitis include rhinovirus, coronavirus, adenovirus, herpes simplex virus (HSV), parainfluenza virus, influenza virus, Epstein–Barr Virus (EBV), and human immunodeficiency virus (HIV). Rhinoviruses and coronaviruses comprise more than 25% of viral cases. Acute influenza and HIV are the only viruses for which treatments with antiviral agents may improve symptoms. Otherwise, supportive treatment options are indicated for sore throat symptoms.

As discussed above in the pathophysiology section, the most common bacterial cause of pharyngitis is GABHS, occurring in 5 to 30% of cases. However, there are several other bacterial causes, including Group C streptococci, *Neisseria gonorrhorea*, *Corynebacterium diphtheriae*, *Mycoplasma pneumoniae*, *Chlamydia pneumoniae*, and *Arcanobacterium haemolyticus*.[3] Clinical presentation and associated signs and symptoms are important for differentiating these bacterial infections.

The patients' clinical history and physical examination findings can help distinguish among the several viral, bacterial, and other causes of pharyngitis. Viral infections often include cough, coryza, conjunctivitis, fatigue, hoarseness, generalized body aches, abdominal pain, or diarrhea as additional symptoms. Patients with Epstein–Barr

Virus (EBV) often have severe pharyngitis with tonsillar exudates, but also complain of fatigue, body aches, and systemic complaints. EBV is also associated with posterior cervical lymph adenopathy, splenomegaly, and a classic maculopapular rash that develops if patients receive penicillin-derived antibiotics. A patient presenting with primary HIV may complain of sore throat as well as several other flu-like symptoms, but they are likely to have HIV risk factors in their history (e.g., unprotected intercourse, multiple sexual partners, previous blood transfusion, and intravenous drug use).

Bacterial infections also have particular defining characteristics. *Chlamydia pneumoniae* or *Mycoplasma pneumoniae* can cause lower respiratory symptoms that are more severe, such as bronchitis, pneumonitis, or pneumonia, in addition to pharyngitis. *Arcanobacterium haemolyticum*, formerly known as *Corynebacterium haemolyticum*, is seen more frequently in teenagers and young adults, and may be accompanied by a scarlatiniform rash. The clinical significance of an *A. haemolyticum* infection remains uncertain. Reported cases of *Corynebacterium diphtheriae* are very rare because of childhood vaccinations, but patients with this variety of pharyngitis will frequently complain of hoarseness and stridor caused by circulation of the diphtheria exotoxin, and may also experience cervical adenitis and edema. The defining characteristic of this bacteria is the development of a firmly adherent, gray, inflammatory pseudomembrane across the oropharynx. Group C streptococci also may cause pharyngitis, but would ultimately be distinguished by a RAD test or throat culture.

In addition to the more common viral and bacterial causes of pharyngitis, a number of other causes of sore throat exist. These include Kawasaki disease, trauma or exertional irritation, neoplastic processes, abscess (such as Ludwig's angina, parapharyngeal or retropharyngeal, and peritonsillar), thyroiditis, gastroesophageal reflux disease (GERD), or allergy-related postnasal drip.[18] Pharyngitis secondary to GERD or allergies would likely accompany symptoms of dyspepsia or nasal congestion with postnasal drip, respectively. Trauma or throat strain caused by overuse (shouting, for example) should be elicited via the patient's history of symptom onset. Neoplastic processes can be more subtle, but may have accompanying weight loss, night sweats, fatigue, or dysphagia. An abscess would likely cause higher fevers, more discomfort, and persistent symptoms despite typical first-line antibiotic treatment. Airway compromise, hoarseness, or neck swelling may accompany abscesses depending on their location. Kawasaki disease is most common in children younger than 3 years of age, and is defined by a number of well-documented features, including pharyngeal erythema, strawberry tongue, nonpurulent conjunctivitis, fever, cervical lymphadenopathy, cracked red lips, and erythema and swelling of the hands and feet with desquamation of periungual regions several days after symptom onset.

Treatment

Therapeutic goals for treating pharyngitis include amelioration of symptoms, decrease in contagion and transmission, prevention of complications, and, to some extent, satisfying the patient's personal goals in the physician–patient interaction.

For the vast majority of pharyngitis cases, supportive therapy purely for symptom control is the most appropriate strategy. A typical viral pharyngitis should resolve within 5 to 10 days, if not sooner. For GABHS pharyngitis, if antibacterial therapy is begun within 3 days of symptom onset, the duration of fever and pain may be shortened by approximately 1 day.[4] The primary purpose of using antibiotics in GABHS pharyngitis is to avoid the development of further complications (discussed in the section below). Children with GABHS should be kept home from school until 24 hours after the initiation of antibiotic therapy.

Supportive therapy for pharyngitis includes appropriately dosed analgesic and antipyretic medicines, proper oral hydration, and rest. Acetaminophen or ibuprofen are indicated for all ages for both pain and fever control, whereas aspirin should be avoided in the pediatric population because it can increase the risk of injury to hepatic and renal structures (Reye's Syndrome).[13] Warm salt water gargles (1/4 teaspoon of salt with 8 ounces of water), soft foods, cool beverages, and frozen desserts can sooth irritated oropharyngeal tissues. Over-the-counter lozenges, sore throat drops, and throat sprays are also available to keep the affected area moisturized or anesthetized. For severe symptoms, viscous lidocaine preparations (e.g., "Magic Mouthwash"), stronger pain medicines or narcotics, or alternative modalities can be tried.

For GABHS, the above supportive measures should be combined with antibiotic therapy. Recommendations for treatment of GABHS pharyngitis have changed very little in the past decade. The CDC, the AAP, and the IDSA all agree that penicillin is the first-line agent to treat GABHS in children and adults.[4,10,16] Treatment should continue for 10 days to eradicate the bacteria from the pharynx (dosing regimens are indicated in Table 2.2). Penicillin-allergic patients should be treated with erythromycin or a first-generation cephalosporin. Preferred antibiotics for recurrent GABHS infection or initial treatment failure include clindamycin, amoxicillin–clavulanic acid, and penicillin G.

Complications

For patients with acute pharyngitis, complications can develop when a bacterial source of infection is not managed properly. Most notably, GABHS is associated with suppurative complications, such as cervical lymphadenitis, peritonsillar or retropharyngeal abscess, mastoiditis, sinusitis, otitis media, bacteremia, endocarditis, and meningitis, as well as nonsuppurative complications, such as poststreptococcal glomerulonephritis and rheumatic fever.[8] Suppurative complications develop as bacteria spreads from pharyngeal mucosal layers to deeper tissue, either directly or via hematogenous or lymphatic routes. Nonsuppurative complications are reflective of streptococcal toxins, streptolysins, and inflammatory processes involving antibodies targeted at the bacteria. GABHS is also linked to scarlet fever, myositis, impetigo, erysipelas or cellulitis, necrotizing fasciitis, and streptococcal toxic shock syndrome.

Peritonsillar and retropharyngeal abscesses form in < 1% of patients complaining of sore throat who are treated with antibiotics. The overall incidence would be

Table 2.2 Dosing regimens for GAHBS

Dosing strategies, initial treatment of GAHBS

1. Penicillin VK (every 250 mg of penicillin VK = 400,000 U of penicillin)

    Children <12 years of age: 25–50 mg/kg/day orally divided three to four times daily for 10 days (maximum, 3 g/day)

    Children >12 years of age: 250–500 mg orally three or four times daily for 10 days (maximum, 3 g/day)

    Adults: 250 mg orally three or four times daily or 500 mg orally twice daily for 10 days

2. Penicillin G

    Children: 0.3–0.6 million units intramuscularly (IM) once for children lighter than 27 kg, or 0.9 million units IM once for children heavier than 27 kg

    Adults: 0.6–1.2 million units IM once

3. Erythromycin stearate

    Children: 30–50 mg/kg/day orally divided three to four times daily for 10 days

    Adults: 250–500 mg orally three to four times daily for 10 days

4. Erythromycin ethyl succinate

    Children: 30–50 mg/kg/day orally divided three to four times daily for 10 days

    Adults: 400 mg orally four times daily for 10 days

5. Cephalexin

    Children: 25–50 mg/kg/day orally divided twice daily for 10–14 days (maximum, 4 g/day)

    Adults: 500 mg orally twice daily for 10–14 days

6. Cefadroxil

    Children: 30 mg/kg/day orally divided twice daily for 10 days (maximum, 2 g/day)

    Adults: 1–2 g orally divided once or twice daily for 10 days

7. Amoxicillin

    Children >3 months: 25–45 mg/kg/day orally divided twice daily or 20–40 mg/kg/day orally divided three times daily for 10 days

    Adults: 500–875 mg orally twice daily for 10 days

Dosing strategies, recurrent infection or treatment failure

1. Clindamycin

    Children: 20–30 mg/kg/day orally divided three times daily for 10 days (maximum, 1.8 g/day)

    Adults: 150 mg orally four times daily or 300 mg orally twice daily for 10 days

2. Amoxicillin–clavulanic acid

    Children >3 months old, but < 40 kg: 25–45 mg/kg/day orally divided twice daily or 20–40 mg/kg/day divided three times daily for 10 days

    Children > 40 kg: dosing similar to adults

    Adults: 500–875 mg orally twice daily for 10 days

3. Penicillin G

    Dosing identical to initial treatment options

even less, but patients do not always present for evaluation until complications have begun.[4] Signs and symptoms related to abscess formation include a more ill-appearing patient with a "hot potato" voice, deviation of the uvula or uneven palate, and occasionally a visible fluctuant peritonsillar mass. Surgical drainage, airway management, and broader-spectrum antibiotic coverage is sometimes necessary to manage these problems effectively.

Poststreptococcal glomerulonephritis is thought to result from a reaction between circulating antibody complexes that may inappropriately bind laminin, type IV collagen, and certain proteoglycans found in the kidneys. Patients can present after a recent streptococcal illness, with hematuria, edema, and an elevated ASO titer.

There is no evidence to suggest that antibiotic therapy decreases the incidence of this complication, and it occurs very infrequently.

Rheumatic fever tends to affect genetically predisposed individuals after a GABHS infection, and occurs in <1 in 100,000 cases of GABHS pharyngitis in the United States and other developed countries.[12,17] Symptoms may present within weeks and are thought to be caused by cross reactivity between antistreptococcal antibodies and sarcolemmal muscle and kidney antigens. The resultant inflammatory process can damage heart muscle and valves (especially, mitral valves), connective tissue, joints, and the central nervous system. Rheumatic fever is a clinical diagnosis made using the Jones Criteria, where either two major or one major and one minor criterion are fulfilled. Major criteria include carditis, migratory polyarthritis, Sydenham's chorea, subcutaneous nodules, and erythema marginatum. Minor criteria include fever, arthralgia, elevated acute phase reactants, and a prolonged PR interval on EKG. Treatment involves GABHS antibiotic coverage for any subsequent pharyngitis attacks and therapy for all clinical manifestations.

Scarlet fever presents as a characteristic erythematous, blanchable "sandpaper-like" rash formed by tiny papules, and is caused by streptococcal pyrogenic exotoxins A, B, and C. Along with typical pharyngitis symptoms, the scarlatiniform rash begins on day 2 or 3 of illness on the trunk and spreads to the extremities, sparing the palms and soles. Patients may also present with circumoral pallor, strawberry tongue, and Pastia's lines, an accentuation of the rash within skin creases. Desquamation of the palms and soles sometimes follows resolution of the scarlet fever rash on day 6 to 9 of illness.

Suggestions for Evaluation and Management

When evaluating a patient with pharyngitis and outlining a treatment plan, the initial goals of sore throat management must be kept in mind:

1. First, the differential must be addressed through history and physical exam.
2. Second, based on the above assessment, the physician must determine which laboratory tests, if any, should be carried out to ensure the proper diagnosis. The Centor Criteria is an effective clinical tool that may help guide this decision. Offering a RAD test or throat culture to those patients with two, three, or four of these criteria will help delineate which patients may need antibiotic treatment. Whether or not a second RAD or throat culture is to be used as back up to initial testing should depend on the level of clinical suspicion and prevalence of GABHS in the region. Differences in individual clinical routines will dictate whether empiric treatment is used for patients with three or four Centor Criteria, or if treatment is based on subsequent laboratory test results. Physicians must be mindful of the growing problem of antibacterial resistance in this country—patients who only fulfill one of the Centor Criteria do not need further testing and should not be given antibiotics.

3. Third, the patient's symptoms should be alleviated. The entire range of supportive therapies, including analgesic and antipyretic medicines, oral hydration, and rest, should be considered for every patient whose symptoms warrant them. These modalities are inexpensive, easy to use, and provide an appreciable degree of comfort relief.

4. Fourth, physicians need to be vigilant for possible complications. If a patient has GABHS pharyngitis, a full 10-day course of PCN or other appropriate antibiotic must be completed to eradicate the bacteria from the pharynx and prevent rheumatic fever. One must be suspicious of symptoms that worsen or persist beyond clinical expectations.

5. Last, physicians should ensure that patients understand the medical course of their illness, and are satisfied with the assessment and treatment plan.

References

1. Bisno AL. Acute pharyngitis. The New England Journal of Medicine. 2001;18:344(3):205–211.
2. Bisno AL. Diagnosing strep throat in the adult patient: do clinical criteria really suffice? Annals of Internal Medicine. 2003;139(2):150–151.
3. Bourbeau PB. Role of the microbiology laboratory in diagnosis and management of pharyngitis. Journal of Clinical Microbiology. 2003;41(8):3467–3472.
4. Cooper RJ, Hoffman JR, Bartlett JG, et al. Principles of appropriate antibiotic use for acute pharyngitis in adults: background. Annals of Internal Medicine. 2001;134(6):509–517.
5. Eaton CA. What clinical features are useful in diagnosing strep throat? The Journal of Family Practice. 2001;50(3):201.
6. Ebell MH. Strep throat. American Family Physician. 2003; 68(5):937–938.
7. Gieseker KE, Roe MH, MacKenzie T, Todd JK. Evaluating the American Academy of Pediatrics diagnostic standard for Streptococcus pyogenes pharyngitis: backup culture versus repeat rapid antigen testing. Pediatrics. 2003;111(6 pt 1):e666–670.
8. Hayes CS, Williamson JR. Management of group A beta-hemolytic streptococcal pharyngitis. American Family Physician. 2001;63 (8):1557–1564.
9. Humair, JP, Revaz, SA, Bovier P, Stalder H. Management of acute pharyngitis in adults: reliability of rapid streptococcal tests and clinical findings. Archives of Internal Medicine. 2006;166(6):640–644.
10. Linder JA, Bates DW, Lee G, Finkelstein JA. Antibiotic treatment of children with sore throat. JAMA. 2005;294(18):2315–2322.
11. McIsaac WJ, Kellner JD, Aufricht P, et al. Empirical validation of guidelines for the management of pharyngitis in children and adults. JAMA. 2004;291(13):1587–1595.
12. Merrill B, Kelsberg G, Jankowski TA, Danis P. What is the most effective diagnostic evaluation of streptococcal pharyngitis? The Journal of Family Practice. 2004;53(9):734, 737–738, 740.
13. Neuner JM, Hamel MB, Phillips RS, et al. Diagnosis and management of adults with pharyngitis. A cost-effective analysis. Annals of Internal Medicine. 2003;139(2):113–122.
14. Ressel G. Principles of Appropriate Antibiotic Use: Part IV. Acute Pharyngitis. American Family Physician. 2001;64(5):870, 875.
15. Schroeder BM. Diagnosis and management of group A streptococcal pharyngitis. American Family Physician. 2003;67(4):880, 883–884.

16. Snow V, Mottur-Pilson C, Cooper RJ, Hoffman JR. Principles of appropriate antibiotic use for acute pharyngitis in adults. Annals of Internal Medicine. 2001;134 (6):506–508.
17. Vincent MT, Celestin N, Hussain AN. Pharyngitis. American Family Physician. 2004;69(6): 1465–1470.
18. www.guideline.gov/summary/summary.aspx?doc_id=7324. National Guideline Clearinghouse: Institute for Clinical Systems Improvement (ICSI). Acute pharyngitis. 2005 May:33.
19. Zwart S, Rovers MM, de Melker RA, Hoes AW. Penicillin for acute sore throat in children: randomized, double blind trial. British Medical Journal. 2003;327(7427):1324.

Chapter 3
Treatment and Management of Acute Otitis Media

Ross H. Albert and Neil S. Skolnik

Otitis media is among the most commonly diagnosed diseases in children presenting to physicians' offices.[1] It accounts for millions of dollars of healthcare costs annually, and accounts for more than half of all pediatric antibiotic prescriptions annually.[2] The management of otitis media in the primary care setting has become more complicated in recent years, despite the introduction of vaccines that have decreased complications of the disease. Rising healthcare costs, increasing antibiotic resistance, and changing parental expectations all play a role in the process. In 2004, The American Academy of Pediatrics (AAP) and American Academy of Family Physicians (AAFP) released guidelines for the diagnosis and treatment of otitis media to attempt to simplify disease management.[3] This chapter addresses epidemiology, risk factors, and pathogenesis of acute otitis media (AOM), and focuses on the diagnosis and treatment strategies currently recommended in the 2004 AAP/AAFP guidelines.

Epidemiology and Risk Factors

AOM occurs most frequently in infants and young children, with its highest incidence between the ages of 6 and 24 months old. Studies have suggested that between 60 and 80% of infants have at least one episode of AOM by 1 year of age. AOM is far less frequent in school age children and even less frequent in adolescents.[4] The overall incidence of AOM is very high, increasing significantly during the last 20 years.[5]

Various risk factors have been identified for AOM, in addition to young age, as described above. This is important, because the AAP/AAFP guidelines suggest that risk factor modification might play a role in the treatment strategy of AOM. Attendance at daycare has been shown to be a risk factor for otitis media in children. One study showed a >fivefold increase in otitis media compared with children not attending daycare.[6] Exposure to tobacco smoke also increases risk for AOM.[7] Although pacifier use and supine bottle feeding seem to increase risk, breast feeding has been shown to be protective against AOM.[8]

N.S. Skolnik (ed.), *Essential Infectious Disease Topics for Primary Care.*
© Humana Press, Totowa, NJ

Bacteriology and Vaccine Effects

Otitis media is primarily caused by bacteria, although up to 15% of cases are caused by viruses. The development of otitis media is a sequential process—initially, an upper respiratory tract infection or other insult causes inflammation of the mucosa of the nasopharynx and eustachian tubes; the eustachian tubes become obstructed, causing an accumulation of secretions in the middle ear; finally, bacteria and viruses that colonize the upper respiratory tract accumulate and proliferate in the effusion, leading to symptomatic disease.[9]

The majority of bacterial AOM is caused by three bacterial species—*Streptococcus pneumoniae, Haemophilus influenzae*, and *Moraxella catarrhalis*. Before the introduction of vaccines targeted at these bacteria, AOM had more often lead to serious complications such as sepsis and meningitis. After the introduction of vaccines targeted against *Haemophilus* and *Streptococcus*, however, these complications became far less common. It was hypothesized that the introduction of the pneumococcal PCV7 vaccine and the conjugate *H. influenza* type b (Hib) would reduce the incidence of otitis media, because the majority of infections were caused by the targeted pathogens. Although it is difficult to determine whether otitis media itself has decreased in incidence, one recent study showed that outpatient visits for otitis media have decreased as much as 20% since the PCV7 vaccine's introduction.[10] *Haemophilus* strains causing otitis have shifted away from the more invasive type b strains to "nontypable" strains, not included in the Hib vaccine. The incidence of *Moraxella*-induced AOM has increased somewhat since the vaccines' introduction, although this has not been associated with an increased severity of infection.[11]

Diagnosis of AOM

The 2004 AAFP and AAP guidelines provided criteria for the diagnosis of AOM. These were introduced in part because of the poor specificity and sensitivity of most historical clues and physical exam findings. One study showed that fever, earache, and increased crying were present in 90% of patients with AOM; however, these symptoms were also present in 72% of patients with other diagnoses.[12] Although ear pain is a reasonable indicator of AOM, lack of ear pain does not exclude the disease, especially in patients younger than the age of 2 years old. Studies suggest that between 30 to 40% of patients younger than 2 years old presented with AOM with no ear complaints.[13]

The 2004 AAP/AAFP guidelines define specific historical and physical exam findings necessary for the diagnosis of AOM. These are summarized in Table 3.1. They stress the importance of accurate diagnosis in the effective treatment of AOM. The patient must have history of acute disease, the presence of effusion, and signs and symptoms of middle ear inflammation. The acuity of onset is critical in defining AOM. Otitis media with effusion is a nonacute process in which fluid can accumulate behind the tympanic membrane without fever or pain. The presence of middle ear effusion is detected by otoscopy. Bulging of the tympanic membrane with loss or

Table 3.1 Definition of AOM

Accurate diagnosis of AOM requires all three of:
1. Acute onset of signs and symptoms of middle ear effusion and inflammation

2. The presence of middle ear effusion demonstrated by:
    • Decreased mobility of tympanic membrane by pneumatic otoscopy
    • Bulging tympanic membrane
    • Air fluid level behind the tympanic membrane
    • Otorrhea

3. Signs and symptoms of middle ear inflammation demonstrated by:
    • Erythema of the tympanic membrane
    • Otalgia, severe enough to interfere with normal daily activity or sleep

Modified from Diagnosis and Management of Acute Otitis Media, Clinical Practice Guideline, AAP/AAFP, 2004 (3).

change of normal landmarks, or an air fluid level may be seen. The most sensitive method for detecting effusion is by pneumatic otoscopy (i.e., the use of an insufflator to blow air and mobilize the tympanic membrane). The mobility of the tympanic membrane is the key to the differentiation of the presence or absence of effusion. Signs of inflammation are defined by otalgia (ear pain) or erythema of the tympanic membrane. There is some controversy over defining AOM as having pain or erythema, studies have shown that an erythematous tympanic membrane is insufficient to accurately diagnose AOM.[14] Tympanocentesis and myringotomy, which had been used more frequently in the past, are now rarely needed. If bacterial isolates are needed for culture and sensitivity of resistant infections, these techniques may still be used.

Treatment of Otitis Media

The management of AOM has two main components—pain control and antibiotic therapy. The AAP/AAFP guidelines stress that pain control is critical for effective treatment. Pain control addresses both patient comfort and parental concerns. The guidelines do not endorse any one method, but note that the safety of oral and topical analgesics such as acetaminophen and otic preparations likely outweighs any minor risks for their use. From a practical perspective, a focus on pain control attends to patients' immediate symptoms, and redirects attention away from immediate antibiotic therapy, which may be unnecessary in this process, which often resolves without antimicrobial treatment.

Observation Versus Immediate Treatment for AOM

An important change in the paradigm for the treatment of otitis media is the current option to initially observe select patients for 48 to 72 hours without antibiotic treatment. This strategy has come from two key observations—the first is that antibiotic resistance is rapidly increasing because of antibiotic overuse; the second observation is that the majority of AOM will resolve spontaneously if left untreated.[15] This watchful waiting strategy is only acceptable for select patients: "This option should be limited to otherwise healthy children 6 months to 2 years of age with nonsevere illness at presentation and an uncertain diagnosis and to children 2 years of age and older without severe symptoms at presentation or with an uncertain diagnosis." The patients' risk for complications must also be considered. Because otitis media can put children at risk for speech, language, and learning problems, high-risk children should not simply be observed. The at-risk children include those with preexisting hearing deficits, with speech or language delay, with certain pervasive developmental disorders, and with other developmental delays.

Watchful waiting also takes into consideration surgical treatment as an option for the treatment of AOM. Data suggesting that tympanostomy tubes do not prevent or change speech or language delay further supports a watchful waiting strategy in low risk children.[18]

One practical approach to the observation of otitis without initial treatment, which has been validated in controlled studies, is the use of "wait and see prescriptions" (WASPs) or "safety net prescriptions" (SNAPs).[16, 17] These help address parental anticipation of an antibiotic prescription and physician scheduling and time constraints in reevaluation of patients. Using the WASP or SNAP strategy, in patients without risk factors, high fevers, or other diagnoses, a parent may be given a prescription for an antibiotic with instructions to not fill the prescription until the appropriate time of observation has been tried. This technique results in lower antibiotic use in otitis media, with equivalent results in patient outcomes.

Antibiotic Treatment of Otitis Media

When antibiotic treatment is necessary, the appropriate choice of antibiotics is essential for effective treatment of AOM. AAFP and AAP guidelines advanced from the 1996 CDC AOM guidelines are based on current data, which showed increasing numbers of *S. pneumoniae* species expressing β-lactamase.[11] The 1996 CDC guidelines had suggested that amoxicillin at 40 to 45 mg/kg/day was appropriate for initial treatment. High-dose amoxicillin was only recommended with certain risk factors or with failed initial treatment.

The 2004 AAFP/AAP guidelines suggest initial treatment for AOM with 80 to 90 mg/kg/day, or "high-dose" amoxicillin, regardless of risk factors or clinical course. New to these guidelines is that amoxicillin–clavulonic acid be used if amoxicillin therapy fails, or if the patient presents with high fever or severe otalgia (see Fig. 3.1). This is because of the high level of β-lactamase producing strains of *S. pneumoniae*. For patients with non-type 1 allergy (i.e., not anaphylaxis), cephalosporins are recommended as appropriate second-line therapies. Among these cephalosporins is a recommendation for 1 or 3 days (depending on course of disease) of once-daily intramuscular or intravenous ceftriaxone for patients unable to tolerate oral medications.

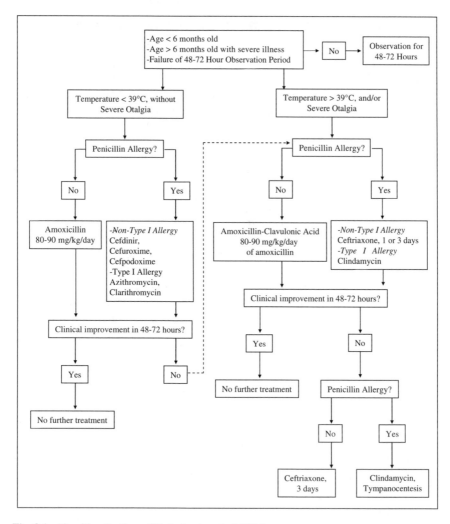

Fig. 3.1 Algorithm for the antibiotic treatment of AOM.

This short course of therapy allows outpatient or emergency room treatment of patients who might otherwise require hospitalization for intravenous antibiotics. For patients with true type 1 allergies to amoxicillin or cephalosporins, azithromycin and clarithromycin are recommended for use. However, studies suggest that azithromycin is minimally effective against *Haemophilus* species. Clindamycin is suggested as second- or third-line treatment against species resistant to cephalosporins and β-lactamase inhibitors. Trimethoprim–sulfamethoxazole, currently used for the treatment of penicillin-resistant *Staphyloccocus* in other disease processes, is not part of a treatment regimen for otitis media.

Tympanostomy Tubes, Tympanostomy, and Adenoidectomy

Tympanostomy tubes have long been a part of recurrent AOM treatment. The rationale for tympanostomy tubes is two fold—first, the tubes act as a conduit for the drainage of the middle ear space; second, the tubes help to equalize pressures between the middle ear and the outside environment.

The theoretical benefits of tympanostomy tubes are clear—they are effective at initially clearing the effusions from the middle ear and, thus, allowing decreased middle ear inflammation and improved hearing in those with hearing loss. However, the usefulness of tympanostomy tubes has been challenged by more data, which showed that those benefits seem transient. Multiple studies have shown no change in outcome in hearing and in long-term development as time continues.[18]

Studies have also addressed combined tympanostomy and adenoidectomy for the prevention of recurrent AOM. One study suggested that tympanostomy and adenoidectomy was more effective at decreasing recurrent otitis media than tympanostomy alone in children ages 4 to 8 years old.[19] In children younger than 4 years old, however, the combined procedure does not seem to confer any added benefit over tympanostomy alone.[20] With the decreasing incidence of otitis media as children age, and the benefit of the combined procedure only seen in older children, it seems that tympanostomy and adenoidectomy should only be performed in rare cases, and only when a repeat tympanostomy procedure is required.

Summary and Recommendations

AOM is extremely common in the outpatient setting. It is primarily a pediatric illness, occurring less frequently as patients become older. Otitis media is typically caused by bacteria, though some have viral etiologies. *S. pneumoniae, H. influenzae*, and *M. catarrhalis* are the predominant bacteria causing AOM. Vaccination against *S. pneumoniae* and *H. influenzae* in the Hib and PCV7 vaccines have decreased serious complications of AOM significantly.

The 2004 AAP/AAFP guidelines for AOM set forth diagnostic criteria and treatment strategies for the illness. Acute onset of illness, presence of middle ear effusion, and middle ear inflammation are needed for the accurate diagnosis of AOM. Pneumatic otoscopy is the most sensitive method to detect middle ear effusion and inflammation. Initial treatment of AOM includes effective pain control and assessment of antibiotic necessity. The 2004 guidelines suggest a period of observation for a subset of children without fever or other severe symptoms before antibiotic therapy. It is in these observed patients that SNAPs might be used. When antibiotics are to be used, "high-dose" amoxicillin is the first-line treatment for AOM, with amoxicillin–clavulonic acid as second-line therapy; cephalosporins or azithromycin and clarithromycin can be used for those with non-type 1 and type 1 allergies, respectively, to amoxicillin as alternative medications.

References

1. Dowell SF, Schwartz B, Phillips WR. Appropriate use of antibiotics for URIs in children: Part I. Otitis media and acute sinusitis. The Pediatric URI Consensus Team. Am Fam Physician. 1998 Oct 1;58(5):1113–1118, 1123.
2. Berman S, Byrns PJ, Bondy J, Smith PJ, Lezotte D. Otitis media-related antibiotic prescribing patterns, outcomes, and expenditures in a pediatric medicaid population. Pediatrics. 1997 Oct;100(4):585–592.
3. American Academy of Pediatrics Subcommittee on Management of Acute Otitis Media. Diagnosis and management of acute otitis media. Pediatrics. 2004 May;113(5):1451–1465.
4. Teele DW, Klein JO, Rosner B. Epidemiology of otitis media during the first seven years of life in children in greater Boston: a prospective, cohort study. J Infect Dis. 1989 Jul;160(1):83–94.
5. Lanphear BP, Byrd RS, Auinger P, Hall CB. Increasing prevalence of recurrent otitis media among children in the United States. Pediatrics. 1997 Mar;99(3):E1.
6. Rovers MM, Zielhuis GA, Ingels K, van der Wilt GJ. Day-care and otitis media in young children: a critical overview. Eur J Pediatr. 1999 Jan;158(1):1–6.
7. Arcavi L, Benowitz NL. Cigarette smoking and infection. Arch Intern Med. 2004 Nov 8;164(20):2206–2216.
8. Uhari M, Mantysaari K, Niemela M. A meta-analytic review of the risk factors for acute otitis media. Clin Infect Dis. 1996 Jun;22(6):1079–1083.
9. Rovers MM, Schilder AG, Zielhuis GA, Rosenfeld RM. Otitis media. Lancet. 2004 Feb 7;363(9407):465–473.
10. Grijalva CG, Poehling KA, Nuorti JP, Zhu Y, Martin SW, Edwards KM, Griffin MR. National impact of universal childhood immunization with pneumococcal conjugate vaccine on outpatient medical care visits in the United States. Pediatrics. 2006 Sep;118(3):865–873.
11. Bluestone CD, Stephenson JS, Martin LM. Ten-year review of otitis media pathogens. Pediatr Infect Dis J. 1992 Aug;11(8 Suppl):S7–11.
12. Niemela M, Uhari M, Jounio-Ervasti K, Luotonen J, Alho OP, Vierimaa E. Lack of specific symptomatology in children with acute otitis media. Pediatr Infect Dis J. 1994 Sep;13(9):765–768.
13. Kontiokari T, Koivunen P, Niemela M, Pokka T, Uhari M. Symptoms of acute otitis media. Pediatr Infect Dis J. 1998 Aug;17(8):676–679.
14. Pellman H. Thoughts on the American Academy of Pediatrics/American Academy of Family Physicians clinical practice guideline on acute otitis media: a different perspective. Pediatrics. 2005 May;115(5):1443–1444.
15. Rosenfeld RM, Kay D. Natural history of untreated otitis media. Laryngoscope. 2003 Oct;113(10):1645–1657.
16. Spiro DM, Tay KY, Arnold DH, Dziura JD, Baker MD, Shapiro ED. Wait-and-see prescription for the treatment of acute otitis media: a randomized controlled trial. JAMA. 2006 Sep 13;296(10):1235–1241.
17. Siegel RM, Kiely M, Bien JP, Joseph EC, Davis JB, Mendel SG, Pestian JP, DeWitt TG. Treatment of otitis media with observation and a safety-net antibiotic prescription. Pediatrics. 2003 Sep;112(3 Pt 1):527–531.
18. Paradise JL, Feldman HM, Campbell TF, Dollaghan CA, Colborn DK, Bernard BS, Rockette HE, Janosky JE, Pitcairn DL, Sabo DL, Kurs-Lasky M, Smith CG. Effect of early or delayed insertion of tympanostomy tubes for persistent otitis media on developmental outcomes at the age of three years. N Engl J Med. 2001 Apr 19;344(16):1179–1187.
19. Coyte PC, Croxford R, McIsaac W, Feldman W, Friedberg J. The role of adjuvant adenoidectomy and tonsillectomy in the outcome of the insertion of tympanostomy tubes. N Engl J Med. 2001 Apr 19;344(16):1188–1195.
20. Hammaren-Malmi S, Saxen H, Tarkkanen J, Mattila PS. Adenoidectomy does not significantly reduce the incidence of otitis media in conjunction with the insertion of tympanostomy tubes in children who are younger than 4 years: a randomized trial. Pediatrics. 2005 Jul;116(1):185–189.

Chapter 4
Management of Chronic Obstructive Pulmonary Disease Exacerbations and Acute Bronchitis

Michael Gagnon

Chronic Obstructive Pulmonary Disease

Chronic obstructive pulmonary disease (COPD) affects approximately 14 million Americans and is currently the fourth leading cause of death in the United States. It is currently the only leading cause of death with an increasing mortality rate, and healthcare costs associated with the disease are estimated at 32 billion dollars per year. Between 1980 and the year 2000, the mortality rate for women with COPD tripled whereas the rate for men increased 13%.[1]

Pathogenesis

COPD is a disease that encompasses both chronic bronchitis and emphysema and is associated with chronic inflammation of the small airways and destruction of alveoli. Inflammation is mediated by neutrophils that release protease enzymes, resulting in the eventual destruction of alveoli.[2] Chronic inflammation causes fibrosis, which, in the lung, leads to airway constriction. The excess mucus associated with COPD then gets trapped in the narrowed airways, causing air trapping and bronchospasm. Occlusion of terminal bronchioles can result in the death of the distal alveoli. The narrowed airways, hyperinflation, and reduced gas exchange abilities caused by alveoli destruction results in respiratory failure. Chronic hypoxia results in an increased pulmonary vascular resistance and can eventually lead to pulmonary hypertension and right heart failure.

Risk Factors

The most important risk factor associated with the development of COPD is cigarette smoking. The irreversible damage done to lung tissue through smoking causes an acceleration of the normal age-related decline in lung function. Smokers are more than ten times more likely than nonsmokers to die of COPD. Other risk factors for the development of COPD are family history of COPD, middle to old age, as well as environmental pollutants, including second-hand smoke. Genetic disorders, such as α-1-antitrypsin deficiency can also lead to early onset emphysema and COPD.

Diagnosis

The diagnosis of COPD needs to be considered in any patient with a chronic cough, sputum production, and a history of exposure to cigarette smoking. Dyspnea is a key feature of COPD, however, it may not be present until later in the disease. The objective diagnosis of COPD is made by spirometry, and postbronchodilator spirometry values are the mainstay for classification of the disease (see Table 4.1). Postbronchodilator spirometry confirms irreversible lung disease consistent with COPD.

The diagnosis of an acute exacerbation of COPD is based largely on changing symptoms in an individual with known COPD. An increased volume, purulence, or tenacity of sputum associated with increased dyspnea are common characteristics of COPD exacerbations. Commonly, patients will also have increased cough, wheeze, and fever. Dyspnea is the most consistent complaint associated with exacerbations. Other symptoms include malaise, fatigue, and a reduction in exercise capacity. For those patients with underlying severe COPD, a reduced level of consciousness is an indicator of a severe exacerbation. Exacerbations can mimic several other illnesses, including pneumonia, congestive heart failure, pneumothorax, pleural effusion, pulmonary embolism, and an arrhythmia.

To help elicit the severity of an exacerbation, the time duration of symptoms, as well as the volume and purulence of sputum should be ascertained. The degree of

Table 4.1 Classification of COPD

Stage	Spirometry	Symptoms
Stage 0 (at risk)	Normal spirometry	Chronic symptoms; cough, sputum
Stage I (mild COPD)	$FEV_1/FVC < 70\%$ $FEV_1 > 80\%$ predicted	Chronic symptoms of cough and sputum production may or may not be present
Stage II (moderate COPD)	$FEV_1/FVC < 70\%$ $50\% > FEV_1 < 80\%$ predicted	Chronic symptoms of cough and sputum production may or may not be present
Stage III (severe COPD)	$FEV_1/FVC > 70\%$ $30\% < FEV_1 v< 50\%$ predicted	Chronic symptoms of cough and sputum production may or may not be present
Stage IV (very severe COPD)	$FEV_1/FVC < 70\%$ $FEV_1 < 30\%$ predicted or $FEV_1 < 50\%$ with chronic respiratory failure	

Adapted from[3].

breathlessness associated with coughing is also an important indicator of severity, as is a history of hospitalizations, including admissions to the intensive care unit.

Inpatient Versus Outpatient Management

The diagnosis of an exacerbation, although largely a clinical one, can be aided by specific tests that help ascertain the severity of illness and, thereby, guide management. In the office setting, a peak expiratory flow (PEF) rate can be measured easily. A value $<100 L/min$ is generally considered to indicate a severe exacerbation. If spirometry is available in the office, a forced expiratory volume in 1 second (FEV_1) of $<1.00 L$ or $<40\%$ of predicted value also corresponds with a severe exacerbation. Severe exacerbations are best managed in the inpatient setting, at times requiring admission to the intensive care unit with positive pressure ventilation.

Arterial blood gas (ABG) analysis is an important tool in the hospital setting. When performed, results should be compared with the patient's baseline ABG values because patients with long-standing COPD may have underlying abnormalities even when "well." In general, a $PaO_2 < 60 mmHg$ and/or a $SaO_2 < 90\%$ with or without a $PaCO_2 > 50 mmHg$ while breathing room air is consistent with respiratory failure. Furthermore, a $PaO_2 < 50 mmHg$ with a $PCO_2 > 70 mmHg$ and a pH <7.30 is indicative of a life-threatening exacerbation and needs prompt critical care management.

The decision to manage an exacerbation at home or in the hospital is not always as obvious as this, however, and encompasses several factors, including underlying disease severity.

Those with severe underlying disease having an exacerbation are much more likely to require hospital-level care than those with mild disease. Other indications for hospital-based treatment of exacerbations include poor home support, older age, and significant comorbid illness. The onset of new symptoms, such as dyspnea at rest, or new signs, such as cyanosis or peripheral edema, would also indicate a need for hospital-based care. Furthermore, if there is diagnostic uncertainty, an emergency room visit to exclude other causes for the symptoms or signs is warranted. Table 4.2 shows a summary of recommended indications for hospital-based treatment.

Table 4.2 Criteria for inpatient management

- Severe underlying disease
- Significant comorbid illness
- Older age (>70 years)
- Onset of new severe symptoms, such as dyspnea at rest or new signs, such a peripheral edema or cyanosis
  - Diagnostic uncertainty
  - Worsening hypercapnea or hypoxemia change in mental status
  - Poor home support

Management

Supplemental Oxygen

Although giving oxygen to a dyspneic, hypoxic patient should be an intuitive response, many physicians worry about the risk of hypercapnea and the possibility of reducing respiratory drive as a result of giving too much oxygen to a patient with chronic disease. Prevention of hypoxia initially outweighs concerns for hypercapnea, and regulated oxygen delivery with appropriate oxygen saturation goals can reduce the incidence of hypercapnea. Venturi masks are the preferred mode of choice when selecting an oxygen supplementation device because the amount of oxygen delivery can be controlled. An ABG can be done approximately half an hour after initiation of therapy to check for an insidious rise in arterial carbon dioxide levels. An oxygen saturation of 90 to 92% and a PaO_2 of 60 to 65 mmHg gives good oxygen saturation and is less likely to lead to hypercapnea. Values much $>$ a PaO_2 of 60 mmHg give little added benefit and increase the risk of CO_2 retention.

Bronchodilator Therapy

Bronchodilator therapy is recommended by the GOLD guidelines, and has been shown to be beneficial in exacerbations of COPD. Patients should increase the dose and or frequency of current bronchodilator therapy initially to every four hours.

The current GOLD[3] guidelines suggest that a β-2-agonist be initiated first and, if there is not a significant response, an anticholinergic medication should be added quickly thereafter. The guidelines, although stating that β-2-agonists should be used first, do so because of a larger body of evidence supporting their efficacy. The guidelines go on to state that there is no evidence to show a difference in efficacy between the different classes of short-acting bronchodilators. The use of combination therapy is still controversial because there is little evidence to support its use. Bronchodilators have been shown to increase the FEV_1 and forced vital capacity (FVC) by 15 to 29%.

The possibility of adding methylxanthine medications, such as intravenous aminophylline or oral theophylline, to patients with severe exacerbations can be considered. The evidence for use of these medications is inconsistent and generally only exhibits modest improvements in lung function, with an increased rate of adverse events. If these medications are going to be used, it is recommended that serum theophylline levels be monitored.

Corticosteroid Therapy

Corticosteroid therapy is proven to reduce symptoms and improve both gas exchange and airflow in randomized control trials. Steroid therapy for acute COPD exacerbations has also been proven to reduce treatment failures at 30 and 90 days as well as to reduce length of hospital stay. Significant improvements in FEV_1 have been shown on day 1 of therapy, however, this difference was no longer significant after 2 weeks of therapy. The optimal dose and duration of corticosteroid therapy is still unknown and the length of steroid taper is left to the judgement of the clinician. There is evidence that 10 to 14 days of therapy beginning with 30 to 40 mg of prednisolone daily is an appropriate compromise between efficacy and safety, however, the strength of the recommendation is weak and based only on expert consensus opinion.[3,4] There is strong evidence that 10 days of therapy improves FEV_1 and FVC and has more rapid resolution of symptoms than 3 days of treatment, however, there was no difference in recurrence rate at 6 months between the two therapies.[5]

Antibiotics

Bacterial infections are common cause of COPD exacerbations, and the use of antibiotics expedite improvement. Antibiotic therapy is shown to be most useful in patients with severe exacerbations. Patients with increased volume or purulence of sputum as well as with dyspnea are more likely to benefit from antibiotics than those without these three symptoms. Meta-analysis, however, supports the use of antibiotic therapy in patients with purulent sputum plus either increased volume of sputum or dyspnea.[6] Antibiotic therapy has been shown to shorten symptom duration as well as improve PEF rates during a COPD exacerbation. Patients with severe exacerbations requiring mechanical ventilation have also been shown to benefit from the use of antibiotic therapy.

The most common bacterial causes of mild exacerbations of COPD are *Streptococcus pneumoniae, Moraxella catarrhalis*, and *Haemophilus influenza*. Studies have shown a correlation between the type of bacterial infection and the underlying disease severity. Those patients with mild disease tend to have *S. pneumoniae*-predominant infections. As the COPD advances and patients' FEV_1 is reduced, the bacterial infections are more likely to include organisms such as *M. catarrhalis, H. influenza*, and, in severe underlying disease, *Pseudomonas aeruginosa*. Patients with very severe COPD (stage IV), frequent use of antibiotics, and recent hospitalizations are at increased risk for pseudomonal infections.

When choosing an antibiotic, the underlying disease severity, frequency of previous antibiotic use, as well as the severity of the exacerbation must be considered. For patients with both mild disease and mild exacerbations not requiring hospitalization, *S. pneumoniae, M. catarrhalis*, and *H. influenza*, as well as *Chlamydia pneumoniae* and viruses are most often the causative agents. For those patients with more severe disease (stages II–IV) with moderate to severe exacerbations requiring hospitalization for treatment, the same organisms must be considered, however, the Enterobacteriaceae, including *Klebsiella pneumoniae* and *Escherichia coli* also play a role. Patients with the most severe disease and severe exacerbations may have any of the organisms previously described. The risk of a pseudomonal infection must also be assessed in these individuals, and appropriate antibiotic coverage should be selected. The optimal length of antibiotic treatment has not been determined, however, it is recommended that patients be treated for 3 to 10 days once starting antibiotics. Table 4.3 is an overview of antibiotic choices associated with exacerbation severity and probable pathogens.

Sputum Gram's stain is generally not beneficial and sputum cultures can be reserved for those patients who fail first-line therapy.

Noninvasive Positive Pressure Ventilation

Noninvasive mechanical ventilation has been shown repeatedly to improve outcomes in patients with COPD exacerbations. It is given as a combination of continuous positive airway pressure (CPAP) and pressure support ventilation (PSV). It has been shown to increase blood pH and to reduce pCO_2 and treatment time, as well as to reduce the severity of breathlessness within the first 4 hours of treatment. Hospital stays are decreased with the use of noninvasive positive pressure ventilation (NIPPV), and the rate of mortality and intubation is markedly reduced as well. One-year mortality rates have been shown to be less in those receiving NIPPV than in those receiving either conventional mechanical ventilation or maximal medical therapy alone. The following are indications for the use of NIPPV:

- Paradoxical abdominal motion associated with moderate to severe dyspnea
- Acidosis (pH < 7.35) in the moderate to severe range as well as hypercapnea $PaCO_2$ >6.0 kPa, 45 mmHg.
- Respiratory rate >25 minute

Patients need to be followed closely and monitored for improvement in their ABG values in a high-dependency unit or intensive care unit setting.

There are several contraindications for the use of NIPPV, including respiratory arrest, cardiovascular instability (hypotension, arrhythmias, and myocardial infarction), impaired mental status, inability to cooperate, somnolence, high aspiration risk because of copious or viscous secretions as well as recent gastroesophageal surgery, craniofacial trauma/fixed nasopharyngeal abnormality, burns, and extreme obesity.

Noninvasive ventilation can be deemed successful when pH improves, dyspnea is relieved, the exacerbation is alleviated without the need for intubation, and the patient is able to leave the hospital.

Invasive Ventilation

Patients should be considered for invasive ventilation if they meet one or more of the following criteria:

- Patients with severe dyspnea, use of accessary muscles and paradoxical abdominal motion
- Impending respiratory failure and life-threatening acid–base disturbances, i.e.:
  acidosis (pH < 7.25)
  hypercapnea ($PaCO_2$) >60 mmHg, 8.0 kPa

Table 4.3 Antibiotic treatment in COPD exacerbation

Patient group[a]	Initial oral treatment	Alternative treatments	Parenteral treatment	Common pathogens
Mild COPD (stage I) Patients not requiring hospitalization >1 cardinal symptom	• β-Lactam (ampicillin/amoxicillin[c]) • Tetracycline • Trimethoprim/sulfamethoxazole	• β-Lactam/β-lactam inhibitor (co-amoxiclav) • Macrolide (azithromycin, clarithromycin, roxithromycin) • Cephalosporins (2nd or 3rd generation)		H. influenzae S. pneumoniae M. catarrhalis C. pneumoniae[b] viruses
Moderate to Severe COPD (Stages II–IV) Patients requiring admission to the hospital without risk factors for P. aeruginosa	• β-Lactam/β-lactam inhibitor (co-amoxiclav)	• Fluoroquinol one (gatifloxacin, gemifloxacin, levofloxacin, moxifloxacin)	• β-Lactam/β-lactam inhibitor (co-amoxiclav, ampicillin–sulbactam) • Cephalosporin (2nd or 3rd generation) • Fluoroquinolone (gatifloxacin, levofloxacin, moxifloxacin)	All in first group plus: • Enterobacteriaceae (K. pneumoniae, E. coli)
Moderate to very Severe COPD (stages II–IV) Patients requiring hospitalization with risk factors for P. aeruginosa	• Fluoroquinolones (ciprofloxacin, levofloxacin, high dose)		Fluoroquinolones (ciprofloxacin, levofloxacin, high dose) β-Lactam with P. aeruginosa activity	All of above plus: P. aeruginosa

[a]Management within groups is not absolute and must be considered on an individual basis, incorporating risk factor assessment for each patient. Risk for a more severe exacerbation includes frequent exacerbations, recent use of steroids or antibiotics, and comorbid disease.

[b]Chlamydia pneumonia has not been confirmed as a cause of exacerbation in some areas (e.g., United Kingdom).

[c]In countries with a high rates of S. pneumonia resistance to penicillin and β-lactam resistance by M. catarrhalis and H. influenza, opinions differs regarding the usefulness of high doses of amoxicillin or co-amoxiclav as first-line agents.

39

- Respiratory frequency > 35 breaths per minute
- Respiratory arrest
- Impaired mental status, somnolence
- NIPPV failure or contraindications
- Cardiovascular complications, including hypotension, shock, or heart failure
- Other complications, including metabolic abnormalities, sepsis, pneumonia, pulmonary embolism, barotrauma, and massive pleural effusion

Other Beneficial Treatments

Adequate nutrition has also proven to be helpful in COPD exacerbations. Patients too dyspneic to eat may require short-term tube feeding and fluid administration. The immobilized patient will benefit from subcutaneous heparin to reduce the risk of thromboembolic disease while recovering. Chest percussion, either mechanical or manual, may benefit patients producing large quantities of sputum (> 25 mL/day), or those with lobar atelectasis.

Discharge Planning

Patients recovering from an acute COPD exacerbation will require close follow up and very often require home care. To be discharged from the hospital, patients should not require bronchodilator treatments more often than every 4 hours. Clinical stability should be apparent for 12 to 24 hours before discharge, and the patient's ABG analysis should be stable as well. COPD sufferers should be able to sleep and eat without severe dyspnea, and previously mobile patients should be able to walk unassisted across a room. If the patient requires home oxygen, arrangements need to be made, and the patient and/or caregiver educated to understand the correct use of the oxygen and all of the current medications.

Approximately 4 to 6 weeks after discharge from the hospital, the patient should be reevaluated regarding the need for home oxygen, inhaler technique, and overall ability to cope with the disease. Outpatient pulmonary rehabilitation soon after discharge has been shown to improve exercise capacity and overall health status at 3 months out of hospital.

As in the day-to-day management of COPD, the management of an exacerbation requires close follow up and the intervention of a multidisciplinary team to help guide the patient back to health.

Acute Bronchitis

Acute bronchitis is defined as an acute respiratory illness with a predominant cough. The cough may or may not be productive. Up to 5% of adults in North America report an episode of acute bronchitis in the past year, approximately 90% of which will be evaluated by their physician. This makes acute bronchitis one of the top ten acute office visits in primary care.

Evaluation

The evaluation of acute bronchitis involves excluding pneumonia and other more serious causes of cough. The patients' comorbidities play an important role in the clinician's ability to confidently diagnose acute bronchitis. In patients with underlying congestive heart failure, COPD, or immunocompromised states, the level of suspicion for other entities must be high. However, in the immunocompetent patient with a cough of <2 to 3 weeks duration and otherwise normal vital signs, the diagnosis of acute bronchitis can often be made with confidence. Studies have concluded that a normal physical examination including normal breath sounds, the absence of rales, focal consolidation, or egophony, as well as stable vital signs (normal temperature $< 38\,^{\circ}\mathrm{C}$, respiratory rate < 24 breaths per minute, and heart rate < 100 /minute) all but eliminates the need for a chest x-ray to exclude pneumonia.[7]

Etiology

More than 90% of all cases of acute bronchitis are caused by nonbacterial sources. The prominent viruses implicated in acute bronchitis infecting the lower respiratory tract include influenza A and B as well as respiratory syncytial virus and parainfluenza. Adenovirus and rhinovirus cause infections of the upper respiratory tract. It is thought that up to 5 to 10% of all acute bronchitis can be caused by bacterial organisms such as *Mycoplasma pneumoniae, C. pneumoniae,* and *Bordetella pertussis*. These are generally associated with a more chronic persistent cough. There is little or no evidence that the common organisms associated with pneumonia (*S. pneumoniae, M. catarrhalis*, and *H. influenza*) cause acute bronchitis in immunocompetent patients.

Management

Studies have revealed no reduction in the duration of symptoms associated with antibiotic treatment and, therefore, they are not recommended for treatment regardless of the duration of cough. If there is high clinical suspicion for pertussis in a patient with a prolonged cough (> 2–3 weeks), patients should tested and treated to reduce transmission rates. The most common proven pathogen associated with acute uncomplicated bronchitis is influenza. Newer antiviral agents will help with symptomatology associated with influenza, however, they need to be taken within 48 hours of the onset of symptoms to be effective. Clinical suspicion in the midst of an outbreak must be high.

Symptomatic treatments include the use of albuterol metered-dose inhalers with spacer devices for those patients with a bronchospastic component to their cough. If limited to patients with wheeze or bronchial hyperresponsiveness, β-2-agonists are effective in reducing the length and severity of cough associated with acute bronchitis. The use of anticough agents, such as dextromethorphan and codeine, have a modest effect on the duration and severity of cough in patients with acute bronchitis and a cough of 2 to 3 weeks duration. Other methods for reducing cough frequency and severity include reducing dust and pollen exposure, as well as the use of humidifiers, although these have very limited evidence (but are generally low cost and very low-risk forms of treatment).

The most important management aspect of acute bronchitis for patient satisfaction seems to be communication. Many patients will arrive at their primary care physician's office with a persistent cough, expecting antibiotics. This is likely because of preconceived notions exacerbated by past primary care physicians treating acute bronchitis with antibiotics. The following points may assist with the sometimes difficult discussion regarding why antibiotics are not being prescribed.

- Give the patient realistic expectations regarding the duration of the cough (10–14 days after the office visit)
- Refer to the symptoms as a "chest cold" rather than bronchitis because this term is less associated with a need for antibiotic therapy
- Personalize the risk for the patient associated with the use of antibiotics (i.e., yeast infections, gastrointestinal upset, risk of *C. difficile*, rare but serious reactions)
- Discuss the overuse of antibiotics and the development of resistant strains of bacteria[7]

These points may improve overall patient satisfaction with the appointment, while administering appropriate therapy for their illness.

References

1. Mannino DM, Homa DM, Akinbami LJ, Ford ES, Redd SC. Chronic obstructive pulmonary disease surveillance—United States, 1971–2000. MMWR Surveill Summ 2002;51:1–16.
2. Barnes PJ. Mechanisms in COPD; Differences from Asthma. Chest 2000;117(suppl 2):105–145.
3. Global Initiative for Chronic Obstructive Lung disease (GOLD), World Health Organization (WHO), National Heart, Lung and Blood Institute (NHLBI). Global strategy for the diagnosis, management and prevention of chronic obstructive pulmonary disease. Bethesda (MD): Global Initiative for Chronic Obstructive Lung disease, World Health Organization, National Heart, Lung and Blood Institute. 2005;115p.
4. American Thoracic Society (ATS), European Respiratory Society (ERS) position paper on COPD. ATS/ERS Task Force, Eur Respir J 2004;23:932.
5. Sayiner A, Aytemur ZA, Cirit M, Unsal I. Systemic glucocorticoids in severe exacerbations of COPD. Chest 2001;119:726–730.

6. McCrory DC, Brown C, Gelfand SE, Bach PB. Management of exacerbations of COPD: a summary and appraisal of the published evidence. Chest 2001;119:1190–1209.
7. Gonzales R, Bartlett JG, Besser RE, Cooper RJ, Hicker Jm, Hoffman JR, Sande MA. Principles of appropriate antibiotic use for treatment of uncomplicated acute bronchitis: Background. Ann Intern Med 2001;134:521–529.

Chapter 5
Latent Tuberculosis Infection

Testing and Treatment

Pamela Ann Fenstemacher

Introduction

During the early 1900s, one out of every five Americans developed active tuberculosis (TB). Despite a decline to the lowest incidence of TB ever seen in the United States, there are still approximately 15 million people infected in this country alone. Each year, TB claims the lives of more than 3 million people and newly infects 8 million more throughout the world. The first effective efforts to combat TB began in England in the early 1800s, when decreasing crowding and improving ventilation in housing led to an improvement in TB mortality. In the late 1800s, when the attenuated bacille Calmette–Guérin (BCG) vaccine was developed and introduced, TB mortality declined even more dramatically where the vaccine was used. The discovery of streptomycin in 1944 followed by effective treatment regimes to cure people of TB led not only to a continued decline in the mortality from TB, but led to the first decline in the worldwide incidence of TB as well.

The first recommendation for treating latent *Mycobacterium tuberculosis* infection (LTBI) in the general population was given by the American Thoracic Society in 1965; however, even when these recommendations were broadened and more people were being treated, the morbidity from TB never dramatically fell in the United States as was projected. Controversy erupted less then 10 years later, when the hepatotoxicity of isoniazid (INH) began to be recognized in the early 1970s and it became less certain who would benefit from being treated for LTBI. During a decline of local TB control programs in the late 1980s, there was a resurgence of TB in the United States. This resurgence was also contributed to by the human immunodeficiency virus (HIV) epidemic, the immigration of large numbers of persons from countries with a high prevalence of TB, and the rise of multidrug-resistant mycobacterial organisms. In response to this increasing threat, the CDC developed a strategic plan in 1989 that gave the responsibility for detection and treatment of LTBI in high-risk groups to public health agencies that were encouraged by the CDC in 1995 to begin assisting local providers with TB screening programs appropriate for their communities. Neighborhood health centers, jails, homeless shelters, and methadone and syringe/needle-exchange programs are all examples of community-based social service organizations with high-risk populations that were recommended for targeted testing. When public health control measures were again emphasized, the overall incidence of TB declined to an all-time low of 7.4 cases/100,000 general population in 1997.

Despite the significant public health efforts for TB reduction, many high-risk groups, such as foreign-born persons living in the United States, continue to have rising rates of TB infection. Usually these infections are brought with the person from their country of origin and may have a multidrug-resistant rate in excess of 20%. Although the decline in the overall incidence of TB in the United States is encouraging, global efforts may be needed to eliminate disease in potential reservoir groups.[1]

Pathophysiology

TB is spread through the air by suspended droplets produced when an infected person sneezes or coughs. After infection, the organisms grow and reproduce for 2 to 12 weeks until cell-mediated immunity mounts and stops the progression of illness. Although a minority of people exposed to infected droplets develops active TB disease, most TB infections are asymptomatic and remain latent. The majority of TB infections are radiologically silent as well. Individuals with LTBI, but no active disease, are not infectious. Because there is often little immune response at first, the purified protein derivative (PPD) tuberculin does not immediately turn positive. The PPD response is a delayed-type hypersensitivity reaction that may also be seen in various non-TB *Mycobacterium* or with vaccination from *M. bovis*.

Risk of Active TB

Ten percent of individuals who are infected with TB and who do not receive preventive treatment will eventually develop active disease. The greatest risk for developing active disease is concentrated in the first 1 to 2 years after infection, when the rate of developing active disease among people whose skin test has converted from negative to positive is approximately 1 to 2% per year, compared with 0.1 to 0.2% per year in subsequent years. Children younger than 5 years of age with skin test conversion are not only at high risk for recent conversion, but are also at especially high risk of progressing to active TB and disseminating the disease. The risk of developing active TB is also high in adolescents and young adults.

Persons with illnesses that cause relative immunosuppression have a greater likelihood of developing active disease as well. Rates of progression to active TB among HIV-infected persons are high, especially with concurrent injection drug use. Injection drug users without HIV are also at increased risk for progression to active TB. Immunosuppression induced by immunosuppressive agents or prolonged therapy with steroids needed for solid organ transplant or other disease states, and neoplasms (e.g., lung cancer, lymphoma, and leukemia), especially carcinoma of head or neck, also place a person at increased risk of activating TB. Other clinical conditions associated with a high risk of progression to active TB include fibrotic lesions on chest x-rays (presumed from previous untreated TB), silicosis, diabetes (especially if poorly controlled), and chronic renal failure on hemodialysis. When a person is underweight by 15% or more, or has had gastrectomey with weight loss and malabsorption or a jejunoileal bypass, they are also known to be at greater risk of developing active TB.

Screening for TB

Screening should only be done in groups considered at high risk for exposure to TB. Groups of persons at increased risk for recently being infected with TB include close contacts of persons with infectious pulmonary TB, persons with a conversion of their skin test in the past 2 years, and persons who have recently emigrated from a country with a high endemic rate, especially if they are children younger than 5 years of age. Other people at high risk for acquiring a recent TB infection are homeless persons, injection drug users, and persons with HIV infection because of high rates of TB transmission. Anyone who works or resides in an institutional setting (e.g., homeless shelters, correctional facilities, nursing homes, and residential homes for patients with AIDS) is also at ongoing risk for developing TB infection, but the risk of transmission varies greatly among institutions and their sites (Table 5.1).

Diagnosis of Active TB

The identification and treatment of persons who have active TB remains the first priority in controlling the spread of the disease.[2] Eliciting a history of exposure and screening appropriate high-risk groups are critical because patients with active TB

Table 5.1 Groups at high risk of TB exposure

- Homeless
- HIV infected
- Injection drug users
- Healthcare workers
- Recent immigrants from countries with high TB endemic rates (within 5 years), or who frequently travel to counties with a high prevalence of disease
- Contacts of people with infectious pulmonary TB

Residents and employees of congregate settings:
- Correctional facilities
- Nursing homes
- Homeless shelters
- Residential homes (especially if for AIDS)

may be minimally symptomatic or asymptomatic until the disease is far advanced. Most people with active TB have pulmonary TB characterized by cough and systemic signs of fever, anorexia, chills, weight loss, weakness, night sweats, and general malaise. Infants and children may have minimal symptoms of active disease until dissemination occurs. Of note, patients with coexisting HIV have a higher incidence of nonpulmonary TB. In a recent decision analysis involving patients hospitalized because of suspected TB,[5] strong predictors of active disease included upper-zone disease on the chest radiograph, fever, night sweats, and weight loss, along with a CD4 count of < 200 cells/mm (0.2×10^9 cells/L) in HIV-infected patients.[3]

When TB is extrapulmonary, symptoms often manifest from the infected body part, such as altered mental status with central nervous system involvement, back pain with spinal disease, and abdominal pain seen in peritoneal disease. Extrapulmonary TB is most often pleural, followed, in turn, by lymphatic, then bone and joint disease, genitourinary tract, miliary disease, meningitis, and, finally, to the least frequently seen, TB peritonitis.

Testing For TB

It has been recommended that a "decision to test is a decision to treat" if the test is positive. Although a PPD test should always be performed if active disease is suspected, it may be negative in 10 to 25% of patients with active TB.[4] Tuberculin testing should be concentrated on those people who are at high risk of developing active TB, which includes those who have had recent exposure to TB and those who belong to at least one high-risk group. Routine screening of other persons, including children not belonging to a high-risk group for administrative purposes, such as school entrance is discouraged because it wastes resources and generates false-positive test results.

Two tests are available for the detection of LTBI and TB infection. The first, and most commonly used, is the PPD test. The PPD test places 0.1 ml of 5 tuberculin units (TU) of PPD of TB intradermally on the dorsal surface of the forearm, producing a wheal. If administration does not produce a wheal, another test dose can be administered a few centimeters away from the first dose. TB infection produces a delayed-type hypersensitivity reaction to the tuberculins in the PPD. The hypersensitivity reaction begins 5 hours after injection with PPD and reaches a maximum at 48 to 72 hours. The tuberculin skin test (TST) should be read 48 to 72 hours after the test is placed, and the transverse diameter of induration should be recorded in millimeters (see Criteria for a Positive Test, below). Tests read after 72 hours may underestimate the size of induration.

The second method for screening for TB infection is the in vitro QuantiFERON®-TB Gold test (QFT-G; manufactured by Cellestis Limited, Carnegie, Victoria, Australia). The QFT-G enzyme-linked immunosorbent assay (ELISA) test received final approval from the US Food and Drug Administration (FDA) in 2005 and is an aid in diagnosing *M. tuberculosis* infections; it detects the release of interferon-γ (IFN-γ) in fresh heparinized whole blood from sensitized persons. These antigens impart greater specificity than is possible with tests using PPD as the TB antigen. In direct comparisons, the sensitivity of QFT-G was statistically similar to that of the TST for detecting infection in persons with untreated culture-confirmed TB. The performance of QFT-G in certain populations targeted by TB control programs in the United States for finding LTBI continues to be studied.

Positive Test Criterion

Because patients with active TB often have poor nutritional status and severe medical illness, the TST can have a false-negative rate up to 25%, which prevents it from being used to exclude the possibility of active TB. To maximize the sensitivity and specificity of the TST for detecting LTBI in asymptomatic individuals, three cut-off levels have been recommended for defining a positive test. The TST levels depend on the risk of an individual having been exposed to TB and are defined below in Table 5.2. For individuals who receive annual testing, an increase in reaction size of > 10 mm within a 2-year period is considered a skin test conversion consistent with recent infection with TB. No available method can distinguish tuberculin reactions caused by vaccination with BCG from those caused by TB; therefore, "it is usually prudent to consider a positive reaction as indicating infection." The BCG vaccine is not likely to cause a reaction of at least 20 mm of induration.

Table 5.2 Criteria for a positive PPD test

Reaction > 5 mm is a positive test
- HIV+ persons
- Recent contacts of TB patients
- Patients with fibrotic changes on chest x-ray consistent with previous TB
- Patients with organ transplants or otherwise immunosuppressed

Reaction > 10 mm is a positive test
- Recent immigrants (within the last 5 years) from high-prevalence countries
- Injection drug users
- Residents and employees of high-risk settings (prisons, nursing homes, hospitals, homeless shelters)
- *Mycobacteria* lab personnel
- Persons with clinical conditions that place them at high risk: silicosis, diabetes mellitus, chronic renal failure, some hematologic disorders (leukemias and lymphomas); other specific malignancies (cancer of head, neck, or lung); weight loss of > 10% of ideal body weight, gastrectomy, jejunoileal bypass
- Children younger than 4 years or infants, children, and adolescents exposed to adults at high risk

Reaction > 15 mm is a positive test
- Persons with no risk factors for TB

Anergy testing is not recommended for several reasons, including because selective nonreactivity to TST can occur, and mumps reactivity may remain after loss of PPD reactivity.

Over time, individuals who have been exposed to TB may have the size of the skin test diminish or even disappear. In these individuals, the initial TST may be negative, but a repeat may then be positive. This is called the "booster effect" and is not a skin test conversion. People who will likely be tested annually, such as health care workers or individuals living in institutions, should have a two-step test; individuals who have a negative initial TST receive a second PPD 1 to 3 weeks later. The results of the second test are considered to reflect the person's true tuberculin status, and should be used in decisions regarding treatment.[6]

QFT-G testing is also indicated for diagnosing infection with *M. tuberculosis*, including both active TB and LTBI. The test can be positive, negative, or indeterminate. QFT-G sensitivity for LTBI might be <that of the TST. QFT-G, as with the TST, cannot differentiate infection associated with TB disease from LTBI. Similar to any other diagnostic test, the predictive value of QFT-G results depends on the prevalence of *M. tuberculosis* infection in the population being tested. The performance of QFT-G, in particular, its sensitivity and its rate of indeterminate results, have not been established in persons who, because of impaired immune function, are at increased risk for *M. tuberculosis* infection progressing to TB disease.

QFT-G can be used in all circumstances in which the TST is used, including contact investigations, evaluation of recent immigrants who have had BCG vaccination, and TB screening of healthcare workers and others undergoing serial evaluation for *M. tuberculosis* infection. QFT-G usually can be used in place of (and not in addition to) the TST. The indeterminate QFT-G result does not provide useful information regarding the likelihood of *M. tuberculosis* infection, and the optimal follow-up of persons with indeterminate QFT-G results has not yet been determined. The options are to repeat QFT-G with a newly obtained blood specimen, administer a TST, or do neither. For persons with an increased likelihood of *M. tuberculosis* infection who have an indeterminate QFT-G result, administration of a second test, either QFT-G or TST, might be prudent. For persons who are unlikely to have *M. tuberculosis* infection, no further tests are necessary after an indeterminate QFT-G result.[7]

Other Diagnostic Tests

Chest Radiograph

Results of the chest radiograph are usually normal in persons with LTBI, although it may show abnormalities suggestive of a previous TB infection. A chest radiograph should be obtained for all patients with LTBI, and whenever pulmonary TB is suspected. A chest radiograph of a TB-infected patient may show one of many abnormalities, including atelectasis, parenchymal consolidation, lymphadenopathy, a pleural effusion, and a miliary pattern. Although lower-lobe involvement may be somewhat more common, any lung lobe may be affected. When TB reactivates, it usually has upper-lobe involvement with cavitating lesions in approximately 50% of patients. In HIV-infected patients, atypical radiographic findings and accompanying extrapulmonary disease occur more commonly as the CD4 counts becomes progressively lower.

Acid-Fast Bacilli Testing

In patients suspected of having active pulmonary TB, three to six sputum specimens should be collected on different days. Acid-fast bacillus (AFB) testing is positive in 50 to 80% of patients with positive TB cultures. In patients who cannot produce sputum, bronchoscopy should be considered.

Sputum Examination for AFB

A sputum culture is not indicated for most patients with a positive PPD being considered for treatment for LTBI. However, a person with a chest x-ray consistent with previous healed TB infection (with the exception of calcified pulmonary nodules) or any patient with suspected active disease should have three consecutive sputum samples obtained on three consecutive days for acid-fast smears and culture. HIV-infected persons with respiratory symptoms should also have sputum cultures done. Because AFB smears are usually complete within 24 hours, they are especially useful in the early detection of active pulmonary TB, however, the overall sensitivity of three acid-fast smears for identifying active TB is only approximately 70%. In immunosuppressed patients, such as those infected with HIV, *M. avium-intracellulare* (an AFB as well) is a frequent colonizer of the respiratory tract. The specificity of acid-fast smears in one study of HIV-positive patients decreased from the usual 99% or more to 52% because of this organism.

Sputum Culture

Although sputum cultures continue to be the gold standard for the diagnosis of active TB (with cultures being slightly more than 80% sensitive and more than 98% specific for active disease) their use is limited when making early treatment decisions. *M. tuberculosis* culture may require 10 to 14 days for identification, and antibiotic sensitivity studies often take 15 to 30 days. Culture is able to detect as few as 10 bacteria/ml, compared with an AFB stain, which needs 5,000 to 10,000 bacteria/ml to detect TB. Culture is also needed to determine species identifications and drug susceptibility any organisms.

Rapid Sputum Testing

Nucleic acid amplification testing, which amplifies and detects *M. tuberculosis* ribosomal RNA or DNA, currently has approximately the same sensitivity and specificity as AFB testing, but is a technique that is expected to evolve rapidly over the next few years. Rapid sputum tests may prove to be useful adjuncts in the early stages of patient evaluation when early treatment and patient management decisions are uncertain or when clinical suspicion does not correlate with the acid-fast smear or culture results.

Testing in Children

Respiratory smears and cultures are less likely to detect disease in children than in adults. Early morning gastric washings, obtained with instillation of 20 to 50 ml of chilled sterile water through a sterile stomach tube, are more likely to yield a diagnosis than bronchoscopy in children. The diagnostic testing for extrapulmonary TB should vary depending on where the disease is suspected to be located.

Treatment of LTBI

Treatment for LTBI should not be undertaken until active TB is excluded. In situations in which there is a positive PPD and a significant chance of active disease, multidrug treatment for active disease can be started until active TB has been excluded and negative sputum cultures have been obtained. Therefore, all persons with a positive PPD need a chest x-ray to exclude active TB. If the chest x-ray is negative for active TB and the person does not have symptoms of active TB, then they are candidates for treatment of LTBI. The standard treatment recommendation for LTBI is INH administered daily for 9 months. It has been determined that 9 months of treatment provides substantially more effect than a 6-month course of treatment, and treatment for 12 months provides minimal additional effect.

Rifampin and pyrazinamide (RIF-PZA) were also a preferred treatment for LTBI until 2001, when it became apparent that the risk of drug-induced liver injury was >had previously been thought. Since 2001, RIF-PZA is no longer recommended for persons with liver disease or with INH-associated liver injury. It is recommended that the 2-month RIF-PZA treatment regimen for LTBI only be used with caution, especially in patients concurrently taking other medications associated with liver injury or in patients with excessive alcohol use. Because the concern of liver injury is so great, it was recommended that no more than a 2-week supply of RIF-PZA should be dispensed at a time and that patients receive close monitoring for liver injury.

Rifampin is contraindicated or should be used with caution in patients with HIV receiving protease inhibitors or nonnucleoside reverse transcriptase inhibitors

Table 5.3 Treatment of LTBI

Drug	Dosage for adults	Monitoring	Choice	Adverse reactions	Special considerations
INH	5 mg/kg/day to a maximum of 300 mg daily for 9 months	Monthly clinical monitoring; baseline LFTs in selected cases, including HIV infection, pregnancy, history of liver disease, or alcoholism, and repeat LFTs if baseline results are abnormal or if patient is pregnant, postpartum, at high risk for liver disease, or has symptoms of an adverse reaction to INH	Preferred	Hepatitis, hepatic enzyme elevation, rash, peripheral neuropathy, mild CNS effects. Alcohol use and previous history of liver disease increase the risk of INH-induced hepatitis	For pediatric dosing, please see the literature; pyridoxine (vitamin B6) 25–50 mg/day might prevent peripheral neuropathy and CNS effects
INH	15 mg/kg/dose to a maximum of 900 mg twice weekly for 9 months		Alternative		Directly observed therapy (DOT) must be used; pyridoxine 25–50 mg/day might prevent peripheral neuropathy and CNS effects
INH	5 mg/kg/day to a maximum of 300 mg daily for 6 months		Alternative		Not indicated for HIV-infected persons or those with fibrotic lesions on chest x-ray, or children; pyridoxine 25–50 mg/day might prevent peripheral neuropathy and CNS effects
INH	15 mg/kg/dose to a maximum of 900 mg twice weekly for 6 months		Alternative		DOT must be used; pyridoxine 25–50 mg/day might prevent peripheral neuropathy and CNS effects

(continued)

53

Table 5.3 (continued)

Drug	Dosage for adults	Monitoring	Choice	Adverse reactions	Special considerations
Rifampin plus pyrazinamide	Rifampin 10 mg/kg/day to maximum of 600 mg/ day plus pyrazinamide, 15–20 mg/kg/day to maximum of 2.0 g daily for 2 months	Clinical monitoring at weeks 2, 4, and 8 when given with pyrazinamide; baseline CBC, platelets, and LFTs in selected cases (see below)	Should generally not be offered to HIV+ or HIV– persons with LTBI	As with rifampin below and with pyrazinamide: GI upset, hepatitis, rash, arthralgias, gout	May also be offered to persons who are contacts of INH-resistant, rifampin-susceptible TB; see precautions described above for HIV patients, check for other drug–drug interactions; rifampin can permanently discolor soft contact lenses
Rifampin	10 mg/kg/day to maximum of 600 mg daily for 4 months	As above, selected cases include HIV infection, pregnancy, history of liver disease or alcoholism; repeat tests if baseline results are abnormal or if patient has symptoms of adverse reactions	Alternative	Hepatitis, thrombocytopenia, flu-like symptoms, orange coloring to body fluids, rash	For persons who cannot tolerate pyrazinamide, see above
Rifampin plus pyrazinamide	Twice weekly dosing of Rifampin 10 mg/kg/ dose to maximum of 600 mg/dose plus weekly dosing 50 mg/ kg/dose pyrazinamide to maximum of 4.0 g per dose, for 2–3 months	As above	Second alternative if other Rifampin dosing cannot be used Should generally not be offered to persons with LTBI	As with rifampin below and with pyrazinamide: GI upset, hepatitis, rash, arthralgias, gout	DOT must be used, see above

LFT, liver function test; CBC, complete blood count.

(consider rifabutin). Because rifampin decreases the level of many drugs, including methadone, Coumadin, oral contraceptives, oral hypoglycemic agents, digitalis, and anticonvulsants, it is important to monitor drug levels and carefully check for drug–drug interactions when using this drug. Rifampin turns secretions and urine orange and will also permanently discolor soft contact lenses.

Special Considerations

The ISDA Guideline gives special consideration to persons with fibrotic lesions on chest x-ray, pregnant and lactating women, and persons infected with HIV. If a person has a fibrotic lesion on chest x-ray, three treatment regimens are recommended by the Infectious Diseases Society of America (IDSA) guidelines: INH daily for 9 months; 2 months of rifampin plus pyrazinamide; or 4 months of rifampin. Persons with chest x-ray results consistent with healed primary TB (such as calcified solitary pulmonary nodules, calcified hilar lymph nodes, or apical pleural capping) are not at increased risk of TB when compared with those with normal chest x-ray results, and their need for treatment should be determined by their other risk factors and size of the PPD reaction.

The need to treat LTBI in pregnancy is controversial. Some evidence suggests that women in pregnancy and in the early postpartum period may have a higher incidence of INH-induced hepatitis. Therefore, the risk of progression to active disease must be weighed against the risk of INH-induced hepatitis. Because INH is not teratogenic, women at high risk of progression to active disease (particularly HIV-infected pregnant women or women who have been recently infected) should not have treatment of latent infection delayed because of pregnancy, even during the first trimester. Clinical as well as laboratory monitoring for hepatitis should be performed while taking INH, and pyridoxine supplementation should be given as well. Breastfeeding is not contraindicated for women taking INH, but the infant should receive pyridoxine supplementation.

Treatment of HIV infected patients is similar to that of non-HIV infected patients, except that a 6-month regimen of INH is not acceptable, and, often, rifampin cannot be used in patients on protease inhibitors or nonnucleoside reverse transcriptase inhibitors. In some cases, rifabutin can be substituted for rifampin. Consult the IDSA guidelines for details.[8]

References

1. The Identification and Management of Tuberculosis AFP; May 1, 2001;61(Vol 9).
2. Diagnostic Standards and Classification of Tuberculosis in Adults and Children. Am J Respir Crit Care Med 2000;161:1376–1395.
3. Targeted Tuberculin Testing and Treatment of Latent Tuberculosis Infection. Joint Statement of the American Thoracic Society and the Centers for Disease Control and Prevention. Am J Respir Crit Care Med 2000;161:S221-247; MMWR Aug. 31, 2001;50:733.

4. Essential components of a tuberculosis prevention and control program. Recommendations of the Advisory Council for the Elimination of Tuberculosis. MMWR 1995;44:1–16.
5. El-Sohl A, Mylotte J, Sherif S, Serghani J, Grant BJ. Validity of a decision tree for predicting active pulmonary tuberculosis. Am J Respir Crit Care Med 1997;155:1711-6 [Published erratum appears in Am J Respir Crit Care Med 1997;156:2028.]
6. Huebner RE, Schein MF, Bass JB. The tuberculin skin test. Clin Infect Dis 1993;17:968–75.
7. Guidelines for Using the QuantiFERON®-TB Gold Test for Detecting *Mycobacterium tuberculosis* Infection, US. MMWR December 16, 2005;54:49.
8. Update: Adverse Event Data and Revised American Thoracic Society/CDC Recommendations Against the Use of Rifampin and Pyrazinamide for Treatment of Latent Tuberculosis Infection—US, 2003. MMWR 52(31);735-739.

Chapter 6
Acute Sinusitis

Megan Werner and Mathew M. Clark

Introduction

Sinusitis is defined as inflammation or infection of the mucosa of at least one of the paranasal sinuses. Acute sinusitis lasts 4 weeks or less, subacute sinusitis lasts 4 to 12 weeks, and chronic sinusitis lasts more than 12 weeks. This discussion focuses on the diagnosis and treatment of acute sinusitis in adults and children.

Acute sinusitis is one of the 10 most common conditions treated by primary care providers during office visits, affecting more than 30 million individuals each year in the United States. Although 70 to 80% of patients with sinusitis will be symptom-free by 2 weeks, with or without antibiotics, sinusitis is the fifth most common diagnosis for which practitioners prescribe antibiotics, accounting for 12% of all antibiotics prescribed. Furthermore, there has been a trend toward the prescribing of inappropriately broad-spectrum antibiotics for this condition, contributing to the emergence and spread of antibiotic-resistant bacteria in this country and elsewhere. Accordingly, the need for a clear diagnosis, coupled with effective treatment that emphasizes the judicious use of antibiotics, is clear.

Pathophysiology

There are four pairs of paranasal sinuses. The ethmoid and maxillary sinuses form during gestation and are present at birth. The sphenoid sinuses develop around 5 to 7 years of age, and the frontal sinuses appear at 7 to 8 years of age and are completely developed by adolescence. All of the sinuses drain into the nasal passage via several ostia, roughly 1 to 3 mm in diameter. These narrow ostia are prone to obstruction from edema and inflammatory changes, which then result in the buildup of fluid and pressure in the sinuses. The obstruction may also provide an opportunity for secondary bacterial pathogens to thrive and cause acute bacterial sinusitis, generally after 7 to 10 days of obstruction.

Acute sinusitis can be caused by viral infections, bacterial infections, fungal infections, or allergic inflammation. Viral infections are far more common than

N.S. Skolnik (ed.), *Essential Infectious Disease Topics for Primary Care.*
© Humana Press, Totowa, NJ

Table 6.1 Microbiology of acute sinusitis

S. pneumonia	30–40%
H. influenza	20–30%
Moraxella catarrhalis	12–20%
S. pyogenes	3–5%
Gram-negative bacteria	< 3%
Anaerobes, fungi	rare

bacterial infections, and fungal infections are rare. Many different viruses can cause viral sinusitis. The bacterial pathogens most commonly involved in sinusitis are very similar to those seen in acute otitis media (Table 6.1).

Several factors predispose individuals to acute bacterial sinusitis. The two most common are acute viral upper respiratory infections, which precede approximately three-quarters of cases of acute bacterial sinusitis, and allergic inflammation or rhinitis, which precedes approximately 20% of cases. In addition, anatomic variations or immune deficiencies can help to favor the growth of pathogenic bacteria in the sinuses.

Epidemiology

Approximately 16% of adults each year are diagnosed with sinusitis, and it is estimated that another 20% have symptoms of sinusitis but do not seek medical care. Sinusitis is more commonly seen in the fall, winter, and spring months, as are the predisposing conditions of viral upper respiratory infections and allergic rhinitis. Children have six to eight viral upper respiratory infections each year, including viral sinusitis; approximately 5 to 10% of these infections are complicated by a secondary acute bacterial infection.

Clinical Presentation and Differential Diagnosis

The clinical presentation of acute sinusitis may include purulent nasal discharge, nasal congestion, facial pain or pressure, headaches, and postnasal drip. Less commonly seen are fever, tooth pain, hyposmia or anosmia, halitosis, cough, or ear pain or pressure. Symptoms generally last several days, with bacterial infections usually causing more severe symptoms that last longer than do those associated with viral infections. The most challenging aspect of differential diagnosis involves distinguishing between sinusitis associated with a viral infection and sinusitis that involves a bacterial pathogen. Other, less common, sources of these symptoms that could be considered include allergic rhinitis, dental disease, and neoplasm.

Diagnosis

Because the clinical presentation of acute sinusitis shares many clinical features with other causes of upper respiratory symptoms, differentiating between acute sinusitis and other conditions as well as between bacterial and viral sinusitis can be challenging. Despite considerable overlap, differences in clinical findings have been suggested as a way to help differentiate bacterial from viral infections. No single clinical finding can be used to accurately diagnose acute bacterial sinusitis, but various sets of signs and symptoms have been proposed to help clinicians identify those infections more likely to require antibiotic treatment. These recommendations are based on expert interpretation of available data and have not been validated in clinical trials (Table 6.2). In one consensus statement, the Centers for Disease Control and Prevention (CDC), along with several physician specialty organizations, concluded that the four signs and symptoms most helpful in identifying acute bacterial sinusitis are:

- Purulent nasal discharge
- Maxillary facial or tooth pain, especially if unilateral
- Unilateral maxillary sinus tenderness
- Worsening symptoms after initial improvement (biphasic or "double sickening" pattern)

Table 6.2 Summary of acute sinusitis decision tools

Joint recommendations by the CDC, AAFP, ACP-ASIM, IDSA[a]	Recommendations by the Task Force on Rhinosinusitis	
Clinical findings:	Major findings:	Minor findings:
Purulent nasal discharge	Facial pain or pressure	Headache
Maxillary facial or tooth pain, especially unilateral	Facial congestion or fullness	Halitosis
	Nasal obstruction	Fatigue
Unilateral maxillary sinus tenderness		Dental pain
Worsening symptoms after initial improvement	Nasal purulence or discolored postnasal discharge	Cough
	Hyposmia or anosmia	Ear pain, pressure or fullness
	Fever	
Interpretation:	Interpretation:	
Presence of these symptoms makes ABRS more likely	ABRS if ≥2 major findings **OR** 1 major finding and ≥2 minor findings	

[a]CDC: Centers for Disease Control and Prevention, AAFP, American Academy of Family Practice; ACP-ASIM, American College of Physicians–American Society of Internal Medicine; IDSA, Infectious Diseases Society of America; ABRS, acute bacterial rhinosinusitis.

In children, clinical findings that reliably differentiate viral from bacterial upper respiratory infections are difficult to identify. The classic symptoms seen in acute bacterial sinusitis in adults, headache and facial pain, are often absent in children, whereas fever is common in children with viral infections. Findings in children are often nonspecific, such as rhinorrhea, nasal congestion or obstruction, fever, purulent anterior or posterior nasal discharge, snoring, mouth breathing, feeding problems, halitosis, cough, and hyponasal speech. Cough and nasal discharge are the most common symptoms. Acute bacterial sinusitis is more likely in children if the symptoms are severe, including multiple consecutive days of high fever and a moderately ill appearance.

Timing of symptoms has also been proposed as way to differentiate viral upper respiratory infections from acute bacterial sinusitis. Symptoms from a viral infection can last from 1 day to 5 weeks, although most patients feel improved or well after 7 to 10 days. Sixty percent of sinus aspirate cultures from patients with symptoms for at least 10 days grow bacteria. Therefore, various groups have proposed cutoffs of 7 to 14 days, after which, acute bacterial sinusitis should be considered in an adult with typical symptoms. In children, upper respiratory symptoms from viral infections generally have peaked and begun to resolve by the tenth day of illness, therefore, the recommendation is that acute bacterial sinusitis be considered in children with persistent, typical symptoms for at least 10 days that have not begun to improve.

Physical exam usually adds little to the differentiation between the types of acute sinusitis, because patients with viral, bacterial, and, in some cases, allergic sinusitis will have similar physical exam findings. If present, unilateral facial tenderness can help indicate a bacterial infection, as indicated in the decision tools listed above. In children, periorbital swelling is suggestive of ethmoid sinusitis.

The value of diagnostic imaging in the evaluation of acute sinusitis is limited. Because plain radiographs usually do not add further information to a careful clinical evaluation, they are not recommended in the evaluation of uncomplicated sinusitis. Computed tomography (CT) is also not recommended for the evaluation of acute uncomplicated sinusitis. In a study of individuals with upper respiratory tract symptoms of 2 to 3 days duration, most (>85%) had abnormalities of one or more paranasal sinuses on CT. After 2 weeks, during which time no subjects received antibiotics, the abnormalities improved or resolved in 80% of subjects. Almost 100% of children who underwent CT for reasons other than sinus disease and who had an upper respiratory tract infection during the preceding 2 weeks had abnormalities noted in their sinuses. However, CT scans are recommended for those with severe or persistent infections that do not respond to treatment, those with frequent recurrent infections, or those in whom surgery is contemplated because of its role in defining the anatomy of the sinuses as well as any abnormalities that may contribute to the disease.

Intranasal cultures and nasal mucus smears are not helpful in diagnosing acute sinusitis or in differentiating the cause of the symptoms, nor are routine laboratory tests such as a complete blood count (CBC) or erythrocyte sedimentation rate (ESR). The gold standard diagnostic procedure is sinus aspiration and culture, although there is rarely a role for this painful and invasive technique.

In the vast majority of cases, the diagnosis of acute sinusitis and the determination of whether it is bacterial in origin are made clinically. Based on the available research and guidelines, it is reasonable to consider the diagnosis of acute sinusitis in those with the symptoms listed above, and to consider a bacterial origin if the symptoms last more than 7 to 10 days, are severe, or initially improve and then worsen after 5 to 7 days.

Treatment

Treatment of acute sinusitis depends primarily on the etiology of the disease. Treatment options include medications that decrease the general symptoms, such as decongestants and nasal saline, as well as those that treat a specific cause, such as antihistamines in allergic disease or antibiotics in acute bacterial sinusitis.

If acute bacterial sinusitis is diagnosed based on the criteria discussed above, antibiotics are recommended for adults and children to achieve more rapid clinical improvement and cure. Randomized, double-blinded, placebo-controlled trials have been performed in adults and children comparing antibiotic treatment with placebo in subjects with clinical and radiographic diagnoses of acute bacterial sinusitis. These trials consistently have shown that there is a small but statistically significant decrease in symptoms at 10 to 14 days after starting treatment with antibiotics versus placebo. It should be noted, however, that most subjects receiving placebo recovered without antibiotics. The goal of treatment is to decrease symptoms, prevent serious complications and sequelae such as osteomyelitis or orbital abscess, and prevent permanent mucosal damage. Therefore, treatment of suspected acute bacterial sinusitis should include antibiotics if symptoms are moderate to severe or if symptoms persist despite symptomatic treatment.

Antibiotic choice depends on the age of the patient and the presence or absence of risk factors for antibiotic resistance. All antibiotics have been shown to be approximately equally effective in clinical trials, with all those listed below demonstrating resolution of symptoms in more than 85% of subjects. Further studies have shown that narrow-spectrum agents, such as amoxicillin, are as effective as newer, broad-spectrum agents are as a first-line treatment. Although amoxicillin has only partial coverage of *Haemophilus influenzae*, it is a reasonable first-line agent because many infections caused by organisms with in vitro resistance still will improve with treatment. Doxycycline and TMP-SMX can be used as alternatives in penicillin-allergic patients, but they can have failure rates up to 25% because of incomplete coverage of *H. influenzae* and *Streptococcus pneumoniae*. In most areas, resistance to TMP-SMX is too high to consider it a second-line agent if amoxicillin fails to produce improvement. Erythromycin, tetracycline, and second-generation cephalosporins with less activity against *H. influenzae* (cefaclor, cefprozil, loracarbef) should not be used.

First-line agents are used in individuals with no recent antibiotic use or other risk factors for increased likelihood of antibiotic resistance. Second-line agents are used in individuals who do not improve with a first-line agent or who have any of the following risk factors for resistance: antibiotic use in the past month, high levels of resistance in the community, failure of a prophylactic agent, smoking, child in day-care, frontal or sphenoidal sinusitis, or complicated sinusitis. The American Academy of Pediatrics and the Clinical Advisory Committee on Pediatric and Adult Sinusitis recommend similar algorithms for choosing antibiotics (Table 6.3).

Duration

The optimal duration of therapy has not been determined through systematic controlled trials, but most clinical trials use a course of antibiotics lasting 10 to 14 days. The results of some trials of shorter courses of antibiotics are promising, but more data is needed before shorter courses become routinely accepted. Another proposed approach is to treat patients with antibiotics until they become symptom free, then for an additional 7 days. This recommendation strives to balance appropriate minimum length of treatment with avoiding prolonged treatment in asymptomatic individuals who are unlikely to be compliant.

Other Treatments

Other treatments that target symptoms can be used for viral or bacterial sinusitis. Because most upper respiratory infections will resolve without antibiotics, these ancillary medications are the mainstay of treatment for most cases of acute sinusitis. Oral decongestants are likely to be helpful in relieving symptoms and can be

Table 6.3 Antibiotic choice in acute bacterial sinusitis

First line:	Amoxicillin	
Second line:	children and adults:	high-dose amoxicillin–clavulanate, cefuroxime, cefpodoxime, cefdinir
	Adults:	fluoroquinolones with adequate *S. pneumonia* coverage, such as levofloxacin, moxifloxacin, gatifloxacin

Options for penicillin-allergic patients:
    Children or adults: cefuroxime, cefpodoxime or cefdinir (if penicillin reaction was not a type I hypersensitivity reaction), clindamycin, clarithromycin or azithromycin, TMP-SMX, doxycycline in older children
    Adults: fluoroquinolones, as above

Options for individuals unable to tolerate oral antibiotics:
    Children or adults: ceftriaxone or cefotaxime
    Adults: fluoroquinolones as above

Combination therapies, used after failure of a second-line agent:
    High-dose amoxicillin or clindamycin plus a third-generation cephalosporin or rifampin

used throughout the course of the disease, although no randomized clinical trials have been conducted specifically to evaluate the effects of decongestants in sinusitis. Care should be taken in patients with glaucoma, ischemic heart disease, and benign prostatic hypertrophy, but decongestants generally do not raise blood pressure substantially in individuals with stable hypertension. Topical decongestants may also help to relieve symptoms in adult patients, but the reduction in mucosal blood flow may increase inflammation, creating more congestion as the medication effects wear off. Topical decongestants should not be used for more than 3 days because of the risk of rebound vasodilation and worsening congestion. These medications are likely to be less effective in children. One clinical trial compared a combination of a topical decongestant and oral antihistamine to placebo in children with acute presumed bacterial sinusitis; all children in this study also received amoxicillin. Subjects in both groups improved quickly; no differences were noted in clinical or radiographic resolution between the two groups.

Nasal Steroids

Nasal steroids have received attention for their role in treating the symptoms of acute sinusitis. In a recent study of mometasone, treatment with 200 mg twice daily (double the usual dose) significantly reduced the duration of symptoms compared with amoxicillin alone or placebo. In children, studies have shown a modest benefit on the symptoms of acute sinusitis from nasal steroids as well, particularly during the second week of treatment and beyond.

Multiple other treatment options have been proposed, but there is little evidence available in adults or children to evaluate their effectiveness. Antihistamines are effective in treating allergic sinusitis and may help relieve symptoms in a patient with acute sinusitis with predisposing allergic rhinitis, but are not recommended for most cases of acute viral or bacterial sinusitis, because they can dry secretions and inhibit mucus clearance. Topical anticholinergics, such as nasal ipratropium, may help to decrease rhinorrhea, but this treatment has only been evaluated in subjects with viral upper respiratory tract infections and not in acute bacterial sinusitis. Saline nasal sprays have also been shown to reduce rhinorrhea in patients with rhinitis, but have never been studied in acute bacterial sinusitis. There is no evidence that echinacea, vitamin C, zinc salt preparations, or mist help to improve sinusitis symptoms.

Summary

Acute sinusitis is a common clinical condition in adults and children, with multiple etiologies. The symptoms of acute sinusitis overlap considerably with other upper respiratory conditions. Because there are no simple diagnostic tests available with sufficient sensitivity and specificity to be useful in routine clinical practice, acute sinusitis is usually diagnosed clinically based on the constellation of signs and symptoms. The determination of the etiology of the sinusitis is also a clinical decision (Table 6.2). Once a diagnosis is made and a presumed etiology identified, many treatment options are available, including antihistamines for allergic rhinosinusitis, antibiotics for bacterial sinusitis (Table 6.3), and nasal steroids and decongestants for all types of acute sinusitis. Narrow-spectrum antibiotics, such as amoxicillin, are recommended as initial treatment in uncomplicated bacterial sinusitis. Most cases of acute sinusitis are uncomplicated and will resolve no matter the treatment. In some cases, however, symptoms do not resolve despite a prolonged course of treatment or they recur several times within a year. In these cases, referral to a specialist is warranted. In the event of complications such as periorbital cellulitis, intracranial abscess, or meningitis, prompt treatment of the complication and evaluation by a specialist is critical.

Suggested Reading

American Academy of Pediatrics. Subcommittee on Management of Sinusitis and Committee on Quality Improvement. Clinical practice guideline: management of sinusitis. Pediatrics 2001;108:798–808.

Barlan IB, et al. Intranasal budesonide spray as an adjunct to oral antibiotic therapy for acute sinusitis in children. Annals of Allergy, Asthma and Immunology 1997;78:598–601.

Brook I, et al. Medical management of acute bacterial sinusitis: recommendations of a clinical advisory committee on pediatric and adult sinusitis. Annals of Otology, Rhinology and Laryngology Supplement 2000 May;182:2–20.

Dolor RJ, et al. Comparison of cefuroxime with or without intranasal fluticasone spray as an adjunct to oral antibiotic therapy for sinusitis. The CAFFS Trial: a randomized controlled trial. JAMA 2001;286:3097–3105.

Gwaltney JM Jr, et al. Computed tomographic study of the common cold. New England Journal of Medicine 1994;330:25–30.

Meltzer EO, et al. Treating acute rhinosinusitis: comparing efficacy and safety of mometasone furoate nasal spray, amoxicillin and placebo. Journal of Allergy and Clinical Immunology 2005;116:1289–1295.

McCormick DP, et al. A double-blind, placebo-controlled trial of decongestant-antihistamine for the treatment of sinusitis in children. Clinical Pediatrics 1996;35:457–60.

Scheid DC, Hamm RM. Acute bacterial rhinosinusitis in adults: part I. Evaluation. American Family Physician 2004;70:1685–1692.

Scheid DC, Hamm RM. Acute bacterial rhinosinusitis in adults: part II. Treatment. American Family Physician 2004;70:1697–1704.

Snow V, et al. Principles of appropriate antibiotic use for acute sinusitis in adults. Annals of Internal Medicine 2001;134:495–497.

Part II
Gastrointestinal Infections

Chapter 7
Gastroenteritis

Andrew Deroo and Matthew Mintz

Introduction

Gastroenteritis is an acute diarrheal disease that affects both children and adults throughout the developed and developing world. In developing countries, acute diarrheal illnesses remain one of the major causes of long-term morbidity and mortality, because, for the majority of the population, access to clean water and safe food sources are limited. Even in developed countries, gastroenteritis remains a major cause of morbidity and accounts for a large portion of the overall economic cost of healthcare.

Diarrhea is defined as three or more episodes of loose stool during a 24-hour time period, or any episode of bloody stooling. Furthermore, diarrhea can be characterized as either acute or chronic. Acute diarrhea is usually defined as diarrhea lasting for shorter than 14 days, whereas chronic diarrhea is usually defined as diarrhea lasting longer than 1 month.

Various studies have been undertaken to define the exact incidence of gastroenteritis worldwide and in the United States since the early 1980s. These studies have failed to show consistent estimates because of differences in data collection, analysis, and presentation. Data from three published prospective community-based studies suggest that nearly 100 million Americans will experience gastroenteritis each year. Other studies estimate the number of Americans affected to be much higher, ranging from 211 million to 375 million, with an economic burden of 1.8 million hospital admissions and 23 billion dollars annually in medical care costs and lost productivity. Regardless of the exact number of cases, gastroenteritis is one of the most common diagnoses in primary care offices.

Pathophysiology

Gastroenteritis can be caused by bacteria, viruses, and parasites (see Tables 7.1–7.3), as well as noninfectious causes. Gastroenteritis can manifest as both inflammatory diarrhea and watery, noninflammatory diarrhea. The infectious pathogens are

N.S. Skolnik (ed.), *Essential Infectious Disease Topics for Primary Care.*
© Humana Press, Totowa, NJ

Table 7.1 Bacterial causes of gastroenteritis: foodborne illnesses (bacterial)

Etiology	Incubation period	Signs and symptoms	Duration of illness	Associated foods	Laboratory testing	Treatment
Bacillus anthracis	2 days to weeks	Nausea, vomiting, malaise, bloody diarrhea, acute abdominal pain.	Weeks	Insufficiently cooked contaminated meat.	Blood	Penicillin is the first choice for naturally acquired GI anthrax. Ciprofloxacin is a second option.
Bacillus cereus (diarrheal toxin)	10–16 hours	Abdominal cramps, watery diarrhea, nausea.	24–48 hours	Meats, stews, gravies, vanilla sauce.	Testing not necessary, self-limiting (consider testing food and stool for toxin in outbreaks).	Supportive care, self-limiting.
Bacillus cereus (preformed enterotoxin)	1–6 hours	Sudden onset of severe nausea and vomiting. Diarrhea may be present.	24 hours	Improperly refrigerated cooked and fried rice, meats.	Normally a clinical diagnosis. Clinical laboratories do not routinely identify this organism. If indicated, send stool and food specimens to reference laboratory for culture and toxin identification.	Supportive care.
Brucella abortus, *B. melitensis*, and *B. suis*	7–21 days	Fever, chills, sweating, weakness, headache, muscle and joint pain, diarrhea, bloody stools during acute phase	Weeks	Raw milk, goat cheese made from unpasteurized milk, contaminated meats.	Blood culture and positive serology.	Acute: Rifampin and doxycycline daily for ≥6 weeks. Infections with complications require combination therapy with rifampin, tetracycline and an aminoglycoside.

Table 7.1 (continued)

Etiology	Incubation period	Signs and symptoms	Duration of illness	Associated foods	Laboratory testing	Treatment
Campylobacter jejuni	2–5 days	Diarrhea, cramps, fever, and vomiting; diarrhea may be bloody.	2–10 days	Raw and under-cooked poultry, unpasteurized milk, contaminated water.	Routine stool culture; *Campylobacter* requires special media and incubation at 42°C to grow.	Supportive care. For severe cases, antibiotics such as erythromycin and quinolones may be indicated early in the diarrheal disease. Guillain–Barré syndrome can be a sequela.
Clostridium botulinum children and adults (preformed toxin)	12–72 hours	Vomiting, diarrhea, blurred vision diplopia, dysphagia, and descending muscle weakness.	Variable (from days to months). Can be complicated by respiratory failure and death.	Home-canned foods with a low acid content, improperly canned commercial foods, home-canned or fermented fish, herb-infused oils, baked potatoes in aluminum foil, cheese sauce, bottled garlic, foods held warm for extended periods of time (e.g., in a warm oven).	Stool, serum, and food can be tested for toxin. Stool and food can also be cultured for the organism. These tests can be performed at some State Health Department Laboratories and the CDC.	Supportive care. Botulinum antitoxin is helpful if given early in the course of the illness. Call 404-639-2206 or 404-639-3753 workdays, 404-639-2888 weekends and evenings.

(continued)

69

Table 7.1 (continued)

Etiology	Incubation period	Signs and symptoms	Duration of illness	Associated foods	Laboratory testing	Treatment
Clostridium botulinum infants	3–30 days	In infants <12 months, lethargy, weakness, poor feedings, constipation, hypotonia, poor head control poor gag and suck.	Variable	Honey, home-canned vegetables and fruits	Stool, serum, and food can be tested for toxin. Stool and food can also be cultured for the organism. These tests can be performed at some State Health Department Laboratories and the CDC.	Supportive care. Botulism immune globulin can be obtained from the Infant Botulism Prevention Program, Health and Human Services, California (510-540-2646). Botulinum antitoxin is generally not recommended for infants.
Clostridium perfringens toxin	8–16 hours	Watery diarrhea, nausea, abdominal cramps; fever is rare.	24–48 hours	Meats, poultry, gravy, dried or pre-cooked foods	Stools can be tested for enterotoxin and cultured organism. Because *Clostridium perfringens* can normally be found in stool, quantitative cultures must be done.	Supportive care. Antibiotics not indicated.
Enterohemorrhagic *Escherichia coli* (EHEC) including *E. coli* O157:	1–8 days	Severe diarrhea that is often bloody, abdominal pain and vomiting. Usually, little or	5–10 days	Undercooked beef, unpasteurized milk and juice, raw fruits and vegetables (e.g.,	Stool culture; *E. coli* O157:H7 requires special media to grow. If *E. coli* O157:H7 is suspected, specific testing must be requested.	Supportive care, monitor renal function, hemoglobin, and platelets closely. Studies indicate that antibiotics may

Table 7.1 (continued)

Etiology	Incubation period	Signs and symptoms	Duration of illness	Associated foods	Laboratory testing	Treatment
H7 and other Shigatoxin-producing *E. coli* (STEC).		no fever is present. More common in children <4 years.		sprouts), salami, salad dressing, and contaminated water.	Shiga toxin testing may be done using commercial kits; positive isolates should be forwarded to public health laboratories for confirmation and serotyping.	be harmful. *E. coli* O157:H7 infection is also associated with HUS, which can cause lifelong complications.
Enterotoxigenic *E. coli* (ETEC)	1–3 days	Watery diarrhea, abdominal cramps, some vomiting.	3 to >7 days	Water of food contaminated with human feces.	Stool culture. ETEC requires special laboratory techniques for identification. If suspected, must request specific testing.	Supportive care. Antibiotics are rarely needed expect in severe cases. Recommended antibiotics include TMP-SMX and quinolones.
Listeria monocytogenes	9–48 hours for gastrointestinal symptoms, 2–6 weeks for invasive disease	Fever, muscle aches, and nausea or diarrhea.	Variable	Fresh soft cheeses, unpasteurized milk, inadequately pasteurized milk, ready-to-eat deli meats, hot dogs.	Blood or cerebrospinal fluid cultures.	Supportive care and antibiotics; Intravenous ampicillin, penicillin, or TMP-SMX are recommended for invasive disease.

(continued)

Table 7.1 (continued)

Etiology	Incubation period	Signs and symptoms	Duration of illness	Associated foods	Laboratory testing	Treatment
	At birth and infancy.	Pregnant women may have mild flu-like illness, and infection can lead to premature delivery or stillbirth. Elderly or immunocompromised patients may have bacteremia or meningitis. Infants infected from mother at risk for sepsis or meningitis.			Asymptomatic fecal carriage occurs; therefore, stool culture usually not helpful. Antibody to listerolysin O may be helpful to identify outbreak retrospectively.	
Salmonella spp.	1–3 days	Diarrhea, fever, abdominal cramps, vomiting. *S. typhi* and *S. paratyphi* produce typhoid with insidious onset characterized by fever, headache, constipation, malaise, chills, and myalgia; diarrhea is uncommon, and vomiting is usually not severe	4–7 days	Contaminated eggs, poultry, unpasteurized milk or juice, cheese, contaminated raw fruits and vegetables (alfalfa sprouts, melons). *S. typhi* epidemics are often related to fecal contamination or water supplies or street-vended foods.	Routine stool cultures.	Supportive care. Other than for *S. typhi*, antibiotics are not indicated unless there is extraintestinal spread, or the risk of extraintestinal spread, of the infection. Consider ampicillin, gentamicin, TMP-SMX, or quinolones if indicated. A vaccine exists for *S. typhi*.

Table 7.1 (continued)

Etiology	Incubation period	Signs and symptoms	Duration of illness	Associated foods	Laboratory testing	Treatment
Shigella spp.	24–48 hours	Abdominal cramps, fever, and diarrhea. Stools may contain blood and mucus.	4–7 days	Food or water contaminated with fecal material. Usually person-to-person spread, fecal–oral transmission. Ready-to-eat foods touched by infected food workers, raw vegetables, egg salads.	Routine stool cultures.	Supportive care. TMP/SMX recommended in the USA if organism is susceptible; nalidixic acid or other quinolones may be indicated if organism is resistant, especially in developing countries.
Staphylococcus aureus (preformed enterotoxin)	1–6 hours	Sudden onset of severe nausea and vomiting. Abdominal cramps. Diarrhea and fever may be present.	24–48 hours	Unrefrigerated or improperly refrigerated meats, potato and egg salads, cream pastries.	Normally a clinical diagnosis. Stool, vomitus, and food can be tested for toxin and cultured, if indicated.	Supportive care.
Vibrio cholerae (toxin)	24–72 hours	Profuse watery diarrhea and vomiting, which can lead to sever dehydration and death within hours.	3–7 days. Causes life-threatening dehydration.	Contaminated water, fish, shellfish, street-vended food.	Stool culture; *Vibrio cholerae* requires special media to grow. If *V. cholerae* is suspected, must request specific testing.	Supportive care with aggressive oral and intravenous rehydration. In cases of confirmed cholera, tetracycline, or doxycycline, is recommended for adults, and TMP-SMX for children (<8 years).

(continued)

Table 7.1 (continued)

Etiology	Incubation period	Signs and symptoms	Duration of illness	Associated foods	Laboratory testing	Treatment
Vibrio parahaemo-lyticus	2–48 hours	Watery diarrhea, abdominal cramps, nausea, vomiting.	2–5 days	Undercooked or raw seafood, such as fish, shellfish.	Stool culture. *Vibrio parahaemolyticus* requires special media to grow. If *V. parahaemolyticus* is suspected, must request specific testing.	Supportive care. Antibiotics are recommended in severe cases; tetracycline, doxycycline, gentamicin, and cefotaxime.
Vibrio vulnificus	1–7 days	Vomiting, diarrhea, abdominal pain, bacteremia, and wound infections. More common in the immunocompromised or in patients with chronic liver disease (presenting with bullous skin lesions).	2–8 days; can be fatal in patients with liver disease and the immunocompromised.	Undercooked or raw shellfish, especially oysters; other contaminated seafood, and open wounds exposed to sea water.	Stool, wound, or blood cultures. *Vibrio vulnificus* requires special media to grow. If *V. vulnificus* is suspected, must request specific testing.	Supportive care and antibiotics; tetracycline, doxycycline, and ceftazidime are recommended.
Yersinia enterocolytica and *Y. pseudo-tuberculosis*	24–48 hours	Appendicitis-like symptoms (diarrhea and vomiting, fever, and abdominal pain) occur primarily in older children and young adults. May have a scarlatiniform rash with *Y. pseudo-tuberculosis*	1–3 weeks	Undercooked pork, unpasteurized milk, contaminated water. Infection has occurred in infants whose caregivers handled chitterlings, tofu.	Stool, vomitus or blood culture. *Yersinia* requires special media to grow. If suspected, must request specific testing. Serology is available in research and reference laboratories.	Supportive care, usually self-limiting. If septicemia or other invasive disease occurs, antibiotic therapy with gentamicin or cefotaxime (doxycycline and ciprofloxacin also effective).

Please call the state health department for more information on specific foodborne illnesses. These telephone numbers are available at: http://www2.cdc.gov/mmwr/international/relres.html. See the reverse side for information hotlines and list of notifiable diseases.

74

Table 7.2 Viral causes of Gastroenteritis: Foodborne illnesses (Viral)

Etiology	Incubation period	Signs and symptoms	Duration of illness	Associated foods	Laboratory testing	Treatment
Hepatitis A	30 days average (15–50 days)	Diarrhea; dark urine; jaundice; and flu-like symptoms, (i.e., fever, headache, nausea, and abdominal pain).	Variable, 2 weeks to 3 months	Shellfish harvested from contaminated waters, raw produce, undercooked foods and cooked foods that are not reheated after contact with infected food handler.	Increase in ALT, bilirubin. Positive IgM and anti-hepatitis A antibodies.	Supportive care. Prevention with immunization.
Norwalk-like viruses	24–48 hours	Nausea, vomiting, watery, large-volume diarrhea; fever rare.	24–60 hours	Poorly cooked shellfish; ready-to-eat foods touched by infected food workers; salads, sandwiches, ice, cookies, fruit.	Clinical diagnosis, negative bacterial cultures, >fourfold increase in antibody titers of Norwalk antibodies, acute and convalescent, special viral assays in reference lab. Stool is negative for WBCs.	Supportive care. Bismuth sulfate.
Rotavirus	1–3 days	Vomiting, watery diarrhea, low-grade fever. Temporary lactose intolerance may occur. Infants and children, elderly, and immunocompromised are especially vulnerable.	4–8 days	Fecally contaminated foods. Ready-to-eat foods touched by infected food workers (salads, fruits).	Identification of virus in stool via immunoassay.	Supportive care. Severe diarrhea may require fluid and electrolyte replacement.

(continued)

Table 7.2 (continued)

Etiology	Incubation period	Signs and symptoms	Duration of illness	Associated foods	Laboratory testing	Treatment
Other viral agents (astroviruses, caliciviruses, adenoviruses, parvoviruses).	10–70 hours	Nausea, vomiting, diarrhea, malaise, abdominal pain, headache, fever.	2–9 days	Fecally contaminated foods. Ready-to-eat foods touched by infected food workers. Some shellfish.	Identification of the virus in early acute stool samples. Serology.	Supportive care, usually mild, self-limiting.

Please call the state health department for more information on specific foodborne illnesses. These telephone numbers are available at: http://www2.cdc.gov/mmwr/international/relres.html. See the reverse side for information hotlines and list of notifiable diseases. ALT, alanine aminotransferase; WBC, white blood count.

Table 7.3 Parasitic causes of Gastroenteritis: Foodborne illnesses (Parasitic)

Etiology	Incubation period	Signs and symptoms	Duration of illness	Associated foods	Laboratory testing	Treatment
Cryptosporidium parvum	7 days average (2–28 days)	Cramping, abdominal pain, watery diarrhea; fever and vomiting may be present and may be relapsing.	Days to weeks	Contaminated water supply, vegetables, fruits, unpasteurized milk.	Must be specifically requested. May need to examine water or food.	Supportive care, self-limited. If severe consider paromomycin for 7 days.
Cyclospora cayetanensis	1–11 days	Fatigue, protracted diarrhea, often relapsing.	May be protracted (several weeks to several months).	Imported berries, contaminated water, lettuce.	Request specific examination of the stool for *Cyclospora*. May need to examine water or food.	TMP-SMX for 7 days.
Entamoeba histolytica	2–3 days to 1–4 weeks	Bloody diarrhea, frequent bowel movements (looks like *Shigella*), lower abdominal pain.	Months	Fecal–oral; may contaminate water and food.	Examination of stool for cysts and parasites—at least 3 samples. Serology for long-term infections.	Metronidazole and iodoquinol.
Giardia lamblia	1–4 weeks	Acute or chronic diarrhea, flatulence, bloating.	Weeks	Drinking water, other food sources.	Examination of stool for ova and parasites—at least 3 samples.	Metronidazole

(continued)

Table 7.3 (continued)

Etiology	Incubation period	Signs and symptoms	Duration of illness	Associated foods	Laboratory testing	Treatment
Toxoplasma gondii	6–10 days	Generally asymptomatic, 20% may develop cervical lymphadenopathy and/or a flu-like illness. In immunocompromised patients; central nervous system (CNS) disease, myocarditis, or pneumonitis is often seen.	Months	Accidental ingestion of contaminated substances (e.g., putting hands in mouth after gardening or cleaning a cat litter box); raw or partly cooked pork, lamb, or venison.	Isolation of parasites from blood or other body fluids; observation of parasites in patient specimens, such as bronchoalveolar lavage material or lymph node biopsy. Detection of organisms is rare, but serology can be a useful adjunct in diagnosing toxoplasmosis. Toxoplasma-specific IgM antibodies should be confirmed by a reference laboratory. However, IgM antibodies may persist for 6–18 months and, thus, may be falsely positive.	Asymptomatic healthy, but infected, persons do not require treatment. Spiramycin or pyrimethamine plus sulfadiazine may be used for immunocompromised persons or pregnant women, in specific cases.

usually transmitted by fecal–oral contact but can also be transmitted by the ingestion of contaminated food or water or via human–human contact. Once ingested, the pathogen enters the lower gastrointestinal (GI) tract and adheres to and colonizes the mucosal lining and produces diarrhea through several different mechanisms.

Bacteria can cause diarrhea through three mechanisms. First, pathogens can secrete an enterotoxin, which, through a series of biochemical responses at the intestinal cellular level, results in an increase in intestinal secretions. This type of diarrhea is usually noninflammatory in nature. Common bacterial pathogens that secrete enterotoxins include *Staphylococcus aureus, Bacillus cereus*, and *Clostridium botulinum*.

The second mechanism by which a bacterial pathogen can cause diarrhea is through the production of cytotoxic mediators. These cytotoxins cause disruption in the integrity of the mucosal lining, preventing adequate mucosal absorption of fluids and electrolytes. This is the mechanism of diarrhea for most bacteria that cause gastroenteritis.

A third mechanism by which a bacterial pathogen can cause diarrhea involves the production of invasins. Commonly known invasin-producing bacteria include enterohemorrhagic *Escherichia coli* and *Shigella*, which produce enterotoxin and the shiga-like enterotoxin. These invasins initiate an energy-dependent endocytosis of the infective pathogen that ultimately leads to tissue invasion by the organism and destruction of the mucosal layer of the intestines. This ultimately results in bloody diarrhea.

Viral pathogenesis in acute diarrheal illness has also been extensively studied. It is thought that viruses, such as rotavirus, do not produce the same virulence factors as bacteria, but cause a disruption in the intestinal mucosal lining, which interferes with the mucosa's ability to absorb fluids. This results in a watery, nonbloody diarrhea.

Protozoan pathogenesis of gastroenteritis is very similar to that of bacterial and viral pathogens. Attachment of the protozoan to the intestinal mucosa and the production of cytotoxins lead to mucosal atrophy and impaired absorption of fluids from the bowel lumen. This is the mechanism by which *Giardia* infection causes a watery diarrhea. On the other hand, *Entamoeba histolytica* colonizes the small intestines and invades the mucosal lining much like enterohemorrhagic *E. Coli* and *Shigella*. This invasion leads to destruction of the mucosal lining and a bloody diarrhea.

Clinical Presentation

History

Acute diarrheal illness can have a wide range of presentations. A patient may present with a slow onset of vomiting and watery diarrhea without other constitutional symptoms, or might present acutely with fevers, vomiting, diarrhea, severe abdominal pain, tenesmus, and bloody diarrhea. The different clinical presentations of gastro-enteritis often help lead practitioners to the underlying etiologic agent. Therefore, a detailed patient history is essential, because it will help define subsequent treatment plans, depending on the causative agent.

A detailed history should include the quantity and quality of the diarrhea (bloody or nonbloody) and duration of time during which the diarrhea has been occurring. Specific examples with different rates of onset and duration include *Giardia*, which can cause a chronic watery diarrhea, and *S. aureus*, which often causes a rapidly occurring, short course of diarrhea. A history of bloody versus nonbloody diarrhea is also helpful in the identification of causative pathogens. Common causes of an inflammatory, bloody diarrhea include enterohemorrhagic and enteroinvasive *E. coli, Shigella, Salmonella, Campylobacter*, and *Entamoeba histolytica*. Common causes of nonbloody diarrhea include rotavirus, Norwalk virus, enteric adenovirus, enterotoxigenic *E. coli, Vibrio cholera, Giardia*, and *Cryptosporidium*.

It is also important to determine whether the patient has had any sick contacts, including contact with sick children or elderly, nursing home patients. These are two common populations that often transmit pathogens via fecal–oral contact in the developed world. Further elucidation of other sick contacts, including sick family members and coworkers with similar symptoms is important, as is a history of consumption of commercially prepared food if there is concern for a foodborne outbreak.

A history of recent travel to any developing nation should also be elicited. Although most incidences of traveler's diarrhea result in a brief course of diarrhea shortly after arrival to the country, a protracted, chronic course can also occur. Finally, it is important to note any recent hospitalizations or antibiotic use by the patient, because *Clostridium difficile* colitis remains a common cause of diarrhea.

Physical Exam

The most important part of assessing a patient with gastroenteritis is determining the patient's hydration status and looking for signs of a systemic response to inflammation, such as a fever. Signs of dehydration include tachycardia and orthostatic hypotension. An increase in the pulse by ten beats per minute, or a drop in systolic blood pressure by 10 mmHg with postural change is highly suggestive of intravascular volume depletion. Other commonly used methods for determining hydration status, such as assessment of skin turgor and mucous membranes, are poor indicators and deemed unreliable.

A thorough abdominal exam should also be carried out, including assessment of tenderness to palpation, distention, and signs of peritoneal inflammation, which are not specific to gastroenteritis, but can help exclude other abdominal causes of vomiting and diarrhea. A rectal exam should also be done to assess for blood or tenderness. Similar to the abdominal exam, no findings of the rectal exam are specific for gastroenteritis.

Laboratory Tests

In most clinical practices, stool samples for ova and parasites, fecal leukocytes, and stool cultures remain the mainstay of laboratory diagnosis, despite evidence that these tests are not cost effective and are rarely needed. Multiple studies have revealed that the yield for stool cultures is very low, at 1.5 to 5.6% and that the estimated cost per positive results exceeds $1,000. These studies do have a role, however, when the diarrhea is chronic in nature or the patient has signs of an inflammatory diarrhea such as fever and bloody stools. In these patients, the yield of laboratory studies greatly increases.

Stool samples for *C. difficile* toxin may be considered in hospitalized patients with diarrhea, especially immunocompromised patients and those who have had recent antibiotic therapy. A nosocomial *C. difficile* infection can add $2,000 to $5,000 to the cost of a hospital stay, and can prove to be fatal to immunocompromised or debilitated patients. Tests for the *C. difficile* toxin have a range of sensitivity from 34 to 100% and a specificity of 88 to 100%.

Differential Diagnosis

The differential diagnosis for diarrhea is very extensive. Of utmost importance is distinguishing from acute versus chronic diarrhea, infectious versus noninfectious causes of diarrhea, and bloody versus nonbloody diarrhea (Table 7.4). Noninfectious causes of diarrhea seen in the primary care setting include lactose intolerance, alcohol-induced gastritis, pancreatic insufficiency, celiac disease, lower or upper GI bleeds, inflammatory bowel disease, and irritable bowel syndrome (IBS). The differential can often be narrowed down through a thorough history and physical exam.

Alcohol-induced gastritis often is associated with vomiting and is seen in alcoholics or those who consume a large quantity of alcohol in a short period of time. Diarrhea may or may not be associated with the presentation of this disease. Diarrhea caused by pancreatic insufficiency is also associated with alcohol use but is usually seen in chronic alcoholics, or those with a history of chronic pancreatitis. Damage to the pancreas leads to a decrease in its secretory functioning. A lack of

Table 7.4 Differential diagnosis of acute and chronic diarrhea

Acute
Alcoholic gastritis
Infectious gastroenteritis
Lactose intolerance
Upper/lower GI bleed
Chronic
Celiac disease
Infectious gastroenteritis
IBS
Pancreatic insufficiency

pancreatic enzymes leads to fat malabsorption and an osmotic diarrhea. Patients will often describe their diarrhea as foul smelling, with mucousy, floating stools.

Celiac disease and lactose intolerance are usually associated with a more chronic diarrheal illness associated with the ingestion of certain foods. In celiac disease, episodes of diarrhea will be associated with ingestion of foods containing gliaden. In lactose intolerance, patients will experience diarrhea and increased gas production with the ingestion of foods high in dairy content. These types of diarrhea can be distinguished from acute gastroenteritis by their chronic nature and their association with the ingestion of specific foods.

Inflammatory bowel disease, Crohn's disease, and ulcerative colitis may present either acutely with severe abdominal pain and bloody diarrhea, or more insidiously, with chronic diarrhea. Family history, extraintestinal manifestations, and lack of known exposure are potential clues. The diagnosis is made with colonoscopy and biopsy.

Lower or upper GI bleeds can also lead to diarrhea by the cathartic effect of blood. Common causes of upper GI bleeds include gastric or duodenal ulcers, gastritis, and esophageal varices. In addition to bloody diarrhea or melena, patients with upper GI bleeds will have hematemesis as a presenting problem, distinguishing these causes of diarrhea from infectious gastroenteritis. Furthermore, the underlying etiology of the upper GI bleed will also cause other associated symptoms, or become apparent though clues in the patient's history, which will help lead to the diagnosis. For example, gastric ulcers are often associated with increased pain with the ingestion of food, and esophageal varices are associated with cirrhosis in chronic alcoholics or those with a history of chronic hepatitis. Lower GI bleeds are commonly caused by diverticulosis, arteriovenous malformations, and cancer. Similar to upper GI bleeds, lower GI bleeds can be distinguished from acute gastroenteritis with bloody diarrhea by other associated symptoms or findings in the history and physical exam.

Finally, IBS can cause episodes of diarrhea mimicking infectious, nonbloody diarrhea. IBS, however, is often associated with a chronic course and intermittent symptoms. Patients will often have change in bowel function associated with stressful events and will often have periods of constipation and bloating between episodes of diarrhea.

Treatment

The mainstay in treatment for acute gastroenteritis is supportive care, because 50% of cases of gastroenteritis are self-limiting and last for <3 days. The most important element of supportive care consists of appropriate fluid and electrolyte replacement. Of course, all outbreaks should be reported directly to the health department.

Most causes of acute gastroenteritis are caused by viruses to which antibiotics have no effect. Another critical consideration is that the institution of empiric antibiotics can increase the symptoms of diarrhea caused by *C. difficile* and prolong the fecal shedding of *Salmonella*. Thus, antibiotic therapy is often reserved for those patients with chronic diarrhea and a history of travel (Fig. 7.1).

Empiric antibiotics, however, may play a role in certain populations. The elderly, the immunocompromised, and patients with other chronic diseases are at increased risk of complications from gastroenteritis, and empiric treatment may be warranted.

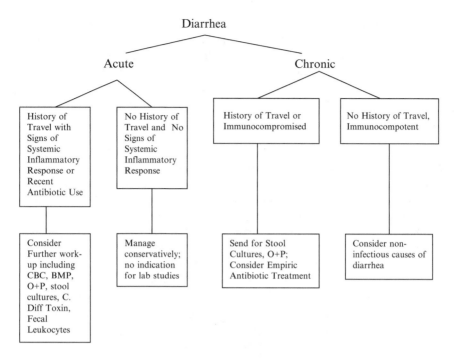

Fig. 7.1 Management of acute and chronic diarrhea. Hx, history; O+P,; CBC, complete blood count; C. diff, *C. difficile.*

According to the Infectious Diseases Society of America, approach to deciding which particular antibiotic treatment to select start with differentiating traveler's/ community-acquired, nosocomial, and persistent diarrhea. If community acquired or acquired from traveling, cultures should be done for *Shigella, Salmonella, Campylobacter, E. coli* 0157, and *C. difficile* toxins. A quinolone or trimethoprim–sulfamethoxazole for children should be used initially, although quinolones should be used for suspected shigellosis and macrolides if resistant *Campylobacter* is suspected. In addition, seafood exposure suggests *Vibrio*, for which doxycycline is effective. For nosocomial diarrhea, patients with a documented infection with *C. difficile* should be treated with oral metronidazole. Treatment for persistent diarrhea will depend on test results and immune status of the patient. *Giardia* is treated with metronidazole. *Cryptosporidium*, if severe, is treated with paromomycin. *Cyclospora* and *Isospora* species are treated with trimethoprim–sulfamethoxazole

Complications

The most common complications associated with gastroenteritis are hemolytic–uremic syndrome (HUS) and Reiter's arthritis. HUS is associated with microangiopathic hemolytic anemia, thrombocytopenia, and renal failure. It has been seen most commonly in patients infected with enterohemorrhagic *E. coli* 0157:H7 infections, with a reported incidence of 3 to 5% in those patients. Reiter's arthritis is a seronegative, polyarticular arthritis often associated with *Campylobacter* infections. Patients can present with a polyarticular arthritis and uveitis.

Conclusions

Gastroenteritis is highly prevalent both locally and abroad, accounting for significant morbidity and substantial cost. Gastroenteritis is can be caused by bacteria, viruses, parasites, or the toxic substance they produce, and is transmitted via the fecal–oral route or by contaminated food. Approach to the patient includes a very thorough history to include time of onset, presence of bloody diarrhea, exposure to sick contacts or contaminated food, and recent travel. Dehydration, which requires prompt attention, must be assessed on physical exam. Laboratory testing must be used judiciously because it can be expensive and often unnecessary. Because most diarrhea is caused by viral agents, and even bacterial causes can be self-limited and symptoms can be exacerbated by antibiotics, supportive care alone is usually the mainstay. However, empiric therapy can be initiated under certain circumstances, especially if patients are severely ill or have a compromised immune system.

Suggested Reading

Cheng A, McDonald J, Thielman N. Infectious diarrhea in developed and developing countries. *Journal of Clinical Gastroenterology.* 2005;39:757–773.
Clark B, McKendrick M. A review of viral gastroenteritis. *Current Opinion in Infectious Diseases.* 2004;17:461–469.
Diagnosis and Management of Foodborne Illnesses: A Primer for Physicians *MMWR.* 2001; 50(RR02):1-69. Accessed from http://www.cdc.gov/mmwr/preview/mmwrhtml/rr5002a1.htm on 8/16/2006.
Guerrant RL, Van Gilder T, Steiner TS, et al. Practice guidelines for the management of infectious diarrhea. *Clinical Infectious Diseases* 2001;32:331–351.
Ilnyckyj A. Clinical evaluation and management of acute infectious diarrhea in adults. *Gastroenterology Clinics of North America.* 2001;30:599–609.
Musher D, Musher B. Contagious acute gastrointestinal infections. *The New England Journal of Medicine.* 2004;351:2417–2327.
Lodfield E, Wallace M. The role of antibiotics in the treatments of infectious diarrhea. *Gastroenterology Clinics of North America.* 2001;30:817–835.
Roe A, Gally D. Enteropathogenic and enterohaemorrhagic Escherichia coli and diarrhoea. *Current Opinion in Infectious Diseases.* 2000;13:511–517.
Su C, Brandt L. Escherichia coli 0157:H7 infection in humans. *Annals of Internal Medicine.* 1995;123:698–707.
Turgeon D, Fritsche T. Laboratory approaches to infectious diarrhea. *Gastroenterology Clinics of North America.* 2001;30:693–707.

Chapter 8
Hepatitis

Michele Lamoreux

Introduction

Most cases of infectious hepatitis are caused by the viral hepatitis viruses A, B, C, D, and E. Although other infections may cause hepatitis as part of the overall illness, they are not considered primarily hepatotrophic. This chapter focuses on the diagnosis and management of hepatitis A through E.

Hepatitis A

Introduction

Hepatitis A virus (HAV) infection occurs worldwide and is the most common cause of hepatitis reported in the United States.[1,2] The Centers for Disease Control and Prevention (CDC) estimates that in 2003 there were 33,000 clinical cases of hepatitis A and 61,000 new infections.

Pathophysiology

HAV is an RNA virus in the *Picornaviridae* family.[1] It is transmitted primarily by the fecal–oral route through person-to-person contact or ingestion of contaminated food (e.g., especially raw shellfish) or water.[3] The incubation period is 2 to 6 weeks.[4] After ingestion and absorption, the virus replicates in the liver and is transported through the bile to the stool.[5] Viral titers peak in the stool 2 weeks before the onset of symptoms, the highest period of infectivity, and remain detectable for approximately 2 weeks after jaundice begins.[1,3] Although parenteral spread is not a significant route of transmission, infection has been reported occasionally through blood transfusion, receipt of clotting factors, injection drug use, sexual contact, and tattooing.[3]

N.S. Skolnik (ed.), *Essential Infectious Disease Topics for Primary Care.*
© Humana Press, Totowa, NJ

Clinical Presentation (History and Physical Exam)

HAV infection is often symptomatic in adults (75%) and often asymptomatic in children younger than 6 years of age (70%).[5] When symptoms do occur, they appear suddenly, and include fever, malaise, fatigue, nausea, and loss of appetite followed by abdominal pain, dark urine, light stool, jaundice, and pruritus.[6] Clinical illness lasts an average of 2 months.[2] The physical exam may reveal fever, jaundice, lymphadenopathy, hepatomegaly, abdominal tenderness, and splenomegaly. However, the results of the physical exam may also be normal.

Laboratory Investigations

Diagnosis of acute hepatitis A infection (Fig. 8.1) depends on the presence of IgM antibody to HAV (anti-HAV IgM) and the absence of other viral markers in serum. Anti-HAV IgM is usually present in serum 5 to 10 days after infection and remains detectable for up to 6 months.[1] Anti-HAV IgG rises to high titer as anti-HAV IgM falls, and anti-HAV IgG persists for life.[1]

Additional tests should be ordered to look for liver injury (alanine aminotransferase [ALT] and aspartate aminotransferase [AST]) and signs of abnormal liver

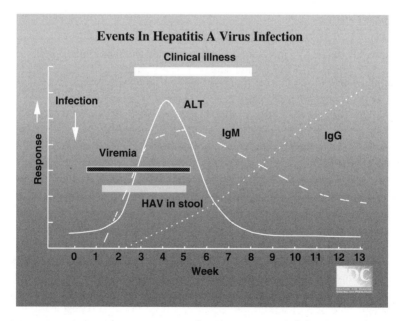

Fig. 8.1 HAV serology (http://www.cdc.gov/ncidod/diseases/hepatitis/slideset/hep_a/hep_a.ppt #753,6,Slide 6; accessed 7/16/07).

function (prothrombin time and albumin) as well as to exclude other possible diagnoses. Serum transaminases, ALT and AST, are markers of hepatocellular injury or necrosis. ALT is more specific for hepatic injury because it is present mainly in the liver.[7] AST can be found in tissues of the liver, heart, skeletal muscle, kidney, brain, pancreas, lungs, and in white and red blood cells.[7]

In acute hepatitis infection, ALT and AST are usually >500 U/L and often >1,000 U/L, with ALT higher than AST.[4] The height of the ALT elevation generally correlates with the level of destruction of hepatocytes but not with clinical outcome.[1] The serum alkaline phosphatase level, a marker of biliary epithelial cell damage, may be normal or only slightly elevated.[4] The conjugated and unconjugated serum bilirubin fractions are variably elevated.[4] In fulminant cases, prothrombin time prolongs, serum albumin falls, and higher bilirubin levels are seen, indicating impending hepatic failure.[1]

Differential Diagnosis and Differentiating Features

The differential diagnosis of acute viral hepatitis is summarized in Table 8.1. Hepatitis A, B, C, D, and E all may cause acute hepatitis. Several other infections may involve the liver and cause an acute hepatitis as well: cytomegalovirus (CMV), Epstein-Barr virus (EBV), herpes simplex virus (HSV), varicella zoster virus (VZV), adenovirus, rubella, mumps, influenza, echovirus, reovirus, Coxsackie B virus, HIV, yellow fever, malaria, and Q fever. In patients with alcoholic liver disease, serum transaminase levels rarely rise above 500 U/L, and, typically, serum AST levels are >serum ALT levels. Clinical clues to the diagnosis of drug-induced liver disease are the presence of serum eosinophilia and jaundice that tends to lag behind the rise of aminotransferases.[1] In viral hepatitis, in contrast, the serum aminotransferase levels tend to peak with the onset of jaundice.[1] Autoimmune hepatitis and Wilson's disease may be differentiated by the presence of smooth muscle antibodies or serum ceruloplasmin, respectively.

Hypotension from cardiovascular failure or sepsis can result in ischemic injury to the liver. In this setting, serum aminotransferase levels may be >20-fold the

Table 8.1 Differential diagnosis of acute viral hepatitis[1,4]

Alcohol abuse
Autoimmune hepatitis
Biliary tract disease (acute cholecystitis, common duct stone, ascending cholangitis)
Drug toxicity (e.g., isoniazid, acetaminophen, halothane, phenytoin, valproic acid)
Graft/versus host disease in bone marrow transplant patients
Hemolysis, elevated liver enzymes, and low platelet count (HELLP) syndrome in pregnancy
Infections: hepatitis A through E, CMV, EBV, HSV, VZV, adenovirus, rubella, mumps, influenza, echovirus, reovirus, Coxsackie B virus, HIV, yellow fever, malaria, Q fever
"Shock liver" secondary to hypotension
Wilson's disease
Toxic injury: mushrooms, carbon tetrachloride

upper limit of normal, mimicking acute viral hepatitis; however, bilirubin levels usually are only mildly elevated.[1] Mushroom poisoning from ingestion of Amanita phalloides and exposure to carbon tetrachloride are two examples of toxic injury leading to markedly elevated aminotransferase levels.[1] When abdominal pain is prominent, acute viral hepatitis may be confused with biliary tract disease.[4] However, an elevated serum alkaline phosphatase level and appropriate radiologic evaluation will aid in the correct diagnosis.

Treatment

Treatment is supportive for the majority of patients with acute hepatitis A infection. Patients should be monitored for signs of hepatic failure and, if present, considered for liver transplantation.

Expected Outcomes and Complications

Most individuals recover without sequelae. Approximately 15% of individuals have prolonged or relapsing symptoms during a 6- to 9-month period of time.[3] Relapses are generally benign, with eventual complete resolution.[4] In < 1% of cases, fulminant hepatic failure results from acute infection.[3,4] Systemic manifestations are uncommon and include cryoglobulinemia, nephritis, and leucytoclastic vasculitis.[4] Cholestatic hepatitis with protracted cholestatic jaundice and pruritus can occur as a variant of acute hepatitis A.[4] There is no chronic state.[2]

Prevention and Screening

General measures to prevent hepatitis A involve careful hand washing, effective public water sanitation, and food hygiene.[2] The Advisory Committee of Immunization Practices (ACIP) of the CDC recommends hepatitis A vaccination for all children beginning at 1 year of age and for persons with specific risk factors: travelers or those working in countries with high or intermediate rates of HAV infection, men who have sex with men (MSM), users of illicit drugs, those who work with HAV in laboratories or with nonhuman primates, those with clotting factor disorders, and those with chronic liver disease.[6]

There are two hepatitis A vaccines: Havrix (GlaxoSmithKline) and VAQTA (Merck and Co.). In 2005, the FDA approved the use of the pediatric/adolescent form of both vaccines for persons 1 to 18 years of age.[8,9] Previously, pediatric use was approved for use in persons aged 2 to 18 years. In children and adults, more than 97% develop antibodies after one dose, and approximately 100% respond after two doses.[2] A two-dose schedule is recommended for both vaccines.[5] If the second dose

Table 8.2 Table of doses for vaccination against Hepatitis A

	Age group	Dose	Volume	No. of doses	Schedule
Havrix	1–18 years	720 ELU	0.5 mL	2	0, 6–12 months
	>19 years	1440 ELU	1.0 mL	2	0, 6–12 months
VAQTA	1–18 years	25 U	0.5 mL	2	0, 6–18 months
	>19 years	50 U	1.0 mL	2	0, 6–12 months

is delayed, it can still be given without the need to repeat the primary dose, and the two brands of vaccines are considered to be interchangeable.[5]

Preexposure and postexposure prophylaxis with hepatitis A immunoglobulin (HAIG; concentrated solution of antibodies prepared from pooled plasma) can be given in certain situations. For those traveling to high-risk areas, preexposure prophylaxis HAIG at a dose of 0.02 mL/kg intramuscularly provides up to 3 months of protection; a dose of 0.06 mL/kg intramuscularly provides protection for up to 5 months.[6]

The dose for postexposure IG prophylaxis is 0.02 mL/kg; and, if given within 2 weeks of exposure, it is 85% effective in preventing disease.[2,6] Immunoglobulin is recommended within 2 weeks of the last exposure for all unvaccinated household/sexual contacts of those with laboratory-confirmed hepatitis A and for those who have shared illicit drugs with an infected person.[2,6] HAIG may also be given to children and employees at day-care centers where hepatitis A has been identified, and coworkers of food handlers with hepatitis A.[2]

Hepatitis B

Introduction

Hepatitis B occurs worldwide.[1] It is estimated that 5% of the US population carries antibody evidence of past hepatitis B virus (HBV) infection, with 0.1 to 0.5% being chronic carriers (1.25 million people).[11, 12]

Pathophysiology

Hepatitis B is a DNA virus in the *Hepadnaviridae* family.[13] HBV is transmitted primarily by percutaneous or mucous membrane exposure to infectious body fluids.[12] Highest titers of virus are seen in serum and blood with intermediate titers in semen, vaginal fluid, and saliva.[1] The incubation period is 30 to 180 days.[3] HBV replicates in hepatocytes but is not directly cytotoxic.[13] The host immune response to viral antigens on infected hepatocytes causes hepatocellular injury.[13]

Transfusion of blood products was the major route of transmission before the introduction of blood screening in 1985.[1] Today, sexual transmission among adults accounts for most HBV infection in the USA.[11] Injection drug use is next most common.[1] In endemic areas, perinatal (vertical) transmission is a common mode of spread.[1] Fetal exposure to blood during passage through the birth canal is thought to be the cause of infection, rather transplacental spread.[1] Other potential routes include blood transfusion, needle stick, and dialysis.[1,11]

Clinical Presentation (History and Physical Exam)

Primary HBV infection can be either symptomatic or asymptomatic. Asymptomatic infection is more common, especially in children.[13] Symptomatic acute HBV infection begins with a prodrome of malaise, fatigue, nausea, and low-grade fever followed by jaundice, dark urine, light stool, and pruritus.[3] In 5 to 10% of patients with acute HBV infection, a serum sickness-like syndrome occurs.[4]

Laboratory Investigations

In acute infection (Fig. 8.2), hepatitis B surface (HBs) antigen (HBsAg) becomes detectable in the blood after 4 to 10 weeks, followed shortly by IgM antibody against the HBV core antigen (anti-HBc IgM).[13] The presence of anti-HBc IgM is diagnostic of acute HBV infection.[11] HBV DNA titers are very high in acute infection, and circulating hepatitis B e (HBe) antigen (HBeAg) becomes detectable in most cases.[13] With clearance of the infection, the viral antigens HBsAg and HBeAg disappear from the circulation, and free anti-HBs antibodies become detectable.[13] Antibody to HBsAg (anti-HBs) is the only HBV antibody marker present after immunization.[11]

In persistent HBV infection (Fig. 8.3), virus production continues and HBsAg remains detectable, often for life.[13] Individuals who also remain HBeAg positive often have high titer of HBV in the blood and are highly infectious.[13]

Differential Diagnosis

The differential diagnosis for acute HBV is listed in Table 8.1. The differential diagnosis of chronic HBV includes alcohol abuse, medication or supplement use, chronic hepatitis C, autoimmune hepatitis, fatty liver, hemochromatosis Wilson's disease, primary biliary cirrhosis, and α-1-antitrypsin deficiency.[4] Laboratory studies and liver histopathology help to determine the diagnosis.

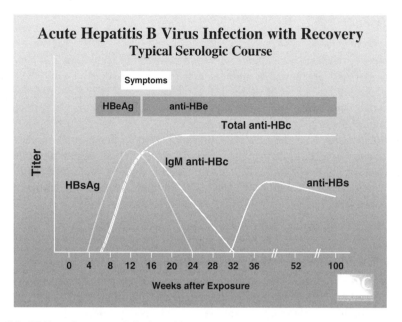

Fig. 8.2 HBV serology, acute infection with recovery (http://www.cdc.gov/ncidod/diseases/hepatitis/slideset/101/101_hbv.ppt#442,9,Slide 9; accessed 7/16/07).

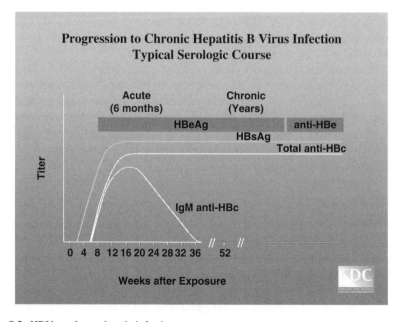

Fig. 8.3 HBV serology, chronic infection.

Treatment

Treatment is indicated for patients who have chronic to severe hepatitis: >twofold elevation of ALT or significant findings on liver biopsy associated with HBV DNA > 10^5 copies/ml.[14] Markers of successful therapy are loss of HBeAg, seroconversion to anti-HBe antibodies, and reduction of the circulating viral load.[13] True cure of infection occurs in only 1 to 5% of patients.[13]

Currently approved drugs for treatment of chronic hepatitis B in the USA include interferon α-2a, lamivudine, adefovir, entecavir, and peginterferon α-2a.[14] For patients with liver failure, liver transplantation may be performed, with post-transplantation administration of hepatitis B immune globulin and lamivudine to prevent reinfection.[13]

Expected Outcomes and Complications

HBV results in chronic infection in approximately 90% of infected infants, 30% of infected children aged younger than 5 years, and <5% of infected persons aged at least 5 years.[12] People with subclinical persistent infection, normal ALT and AST levels, and normal or nearly normal findings on liver biopsy are called asymptomatic chronic HBV carriers; those with abnormal liver function and histologic features are classified as having chronic hepatitis B.[13] Cirrhosis develops in approximately 20% of people with chronic hepatitis B.[3]

Individuals with chronic hepatitis B have a risk of hepatocellular carcinoma (HCC) that is 100 times as high as that for noncarriers.[13] HBeAg-positive carriers have the highest risk of HCC.[4] Given these facts, twice-a-year screening of chronically infected patients with measurements of serum α-fetoprotein (AFP) or hepatic ultrasonography (USN), or both is often recommended.[13]

Polyarteritis nodosa (PAN) is well described in association with HBV infection.[1] Additional possible extrahepatic manifestations include essential mixed cryoglobulinemia, renal disease (most commonly membranous and membranoproliferative glomerulonephritis), myocarditis, pericarditis, bradycardia, pericardial and pleural effusion, encephalitis, meningoencephalitis, mononeuritis multiplex, transverse myelitis, Guillain-Barré syndrome, pure red cell aplasia, pancytopenia, aplastic anemia, and hemolytic anemia.[1]

Prevention

There are two available monovalent hepatitis B vaccines for use in children and adults: Recombivax HB (Merck and Co., Inc.) and Engerix-B (SmithKline Beecham Biologicals). If a dose of the vaccination series is missed, it should be given as soon as possible; however, the series does not need to be restarted.[11]

Table 8.3 Table of doses for vaccination against Hepatitis B[12]

	Age group	Dose	Volume	No. of doses	Schedule (months)
Recombivax	<20 years	5 µg	0.5 ml	3	0, 1, 6 or 0, 2, 4 or 0, 1, 4 or 0, 12, 24
	≥20 years	10 µg	1.0 ml	3	as above
Engerix-B	<20 years	10 µg	0.5 ml	3	as above
	≥20 years	20 µg	1.0 ml	3	as above

Hepatitis B immunoglobulin (HBIG) is prepared from plasma known to contain high titer of anti-HBs and is used for postexposure prophylaxis. The recommended dose of HBIG for children and adults is 0.06 mL/kg.[11] To prevent perinatal HBV infection among infants born to HBsAg-positive mothers, a dose of 0.5 ml is given.[11]

CDC's national immunization strategy to eliminate transmission of HBV infection includes 1) prevention of perinatal infection through maternal HBsAg screening and postexposure prophylaxis of at-risk infants, 2) universal infant immunization, 3) universal immunization of previously unvaccinated adolescents aged 11 to 12 years, and 4) vaccination of adolescents and adults at increased risk for infection.[11]

The following persons are considered at high risk and should be vaccinated: 1) persons with a history of sexually transmitted disease (STD), persons who have had multiple sex partners, those who have had sex with an infected-drug user, and sexually active MSM; 2) persons engaging in illegal drug use; 3) household members, sex partners, and drug-sharing partners of a person with chronic HBV infection; and 4) persons on hemodialysis, persons receiving clotting factor concentrates, or persons who have occupational exposure to blood.[11] In addition, hepatitis B vaccine should be offered to all persons who have not been previously vaccinated who receive services in drug treatment programs and long-term correctional facilities.[11]

Hepatitis C

Introduction

Approximately 3% of the world's population is thought to be infected with hepatitis C virus (HCV) based on blood donor studies.[1] In the US, the CDC estimates that HCV has infected 3.9 million (1.8% of Americans), of whom, 2.7 million are chronically infected.[15]

Pathophysiology

Hepatitis C is an RNA virus in the family *Flaviviridae*.[1] It has six different genotypes and more than 50 serotypes.[16] In the USA, approximately 74% of those infected have genotype 1; genotypes 2 and 3 account for most of the remaining cases.[3] HCV transmission occurs primarily through exposure to infected blood.[16] The incubation period ranges from 2 to 26 weeks.[3] HCV replicates preferentially in hepatocytes but is not directly cytopathic.[16] Highest viral titers are seen in blood and serum.[1]

Transfusion of blood or blood products was a major source of infection before the introduction of blood-screening procedures.[1] The current risk of acquiring hepatitis C through blood transfusion in the USA is < 1 per 2 million transfused units.[15] Today, injection drug use accounts for more than two thirds of all new infections in the USA.[16] Transmission may also occur through occupational exposure to infected blood, sex with multiple partners, body piercing, tattoos, long-term hemodialysis, perinatal transmission and intranasal cocaine use (due to sharing drug paraphernalia contaminated with blood).[16,17] The risk of HCV infection from a needle stick injury is estimated to be 2%.[16] The rate of sexual transmission from an infected case to a partner is low in a monogamous relationship, estimated to be only 0 to 0.6% annually.[16] Perinatal transmission occurs in approximately 4% of infants born to mothers not infected with HIV-1 and in 19% of infants of HIV-1-positive women.[15] Transmission of HCV through breast feeding has not been reported.[1]

Clinical Presentation (History and Physical Exam)

Acute HCV is asymptomatic in 70 to 80% of infected adults.[3] For those with symptoms, the manifestations are similar to acute hepatitis A or B infection (listed previously) and may last for 2 to 12 weeks.[18] Fulminant hepatic failure is rare in acute HCV infection.[3] For patients with chronic disease, the physical examination may reveal signs of liver disease, such as spider angiomata, jaundice, splenomegaly, ascites, and hepatic encephalopathy.[18]

Laboratory Investigations

A third-generation HCV antibody (enzyme immunoassay [EIA]) is recommended for use as the initial test in patients suspected of having HCV, and is at least 99% sensitive and 99% specific (see Figs. 8.4 and 8.5).[19] Anti-HCV EIA determines whether a person has been exposed to HCV but not the presence of active infection.[19] False positive results may occur when EIA is used as a screening test in a population with a low risk of disease. False negative results may occur in immunosuppressed persons, including those with HIV, renal failure, and HCV-associated essential mixed cryoglobulinemia.[19,20]

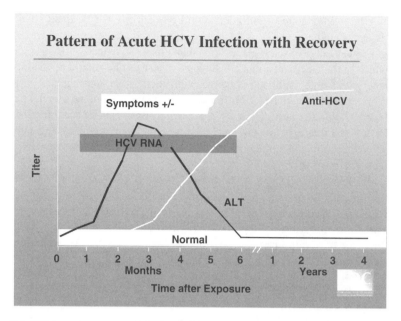

Fig. 8.4 HCV serology, acute infection with recovery (http://www.cdc.gov/ncidod/diseases/hepatitis/slideset/101/101_hcv.ppt#448,10,Slide10; accessed 7/16/07).

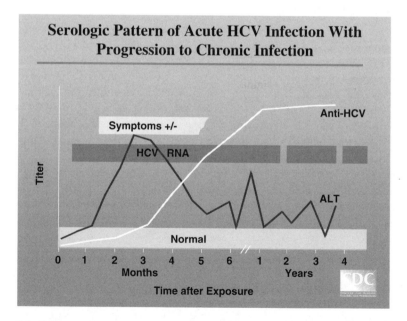

Fig. 8.5 HCV serology, chronic infection (http://www.cdc.gov/ncidod/diseases/hepatitis/slideset/101/101_hcv.ppt#449,9,Slide 9; accessed 7/16/07).

Active infection, acute or chronic, should be confirmed by a qualitative HCV RNA assay.[16] Qualitative HCV RNA tests detect (but do not count) the presence of HCV at a lower range (5 to 50 copies/mL) than quantitative tests (50 to 500 copies/mL), which both detect and count.[19] All negative test results should be reconfirmed in patients with a high likelihood of disease with another test approximately 1 month later to be certain that active HCV infection is not present.[19] Patients with a positive anti-HCV EIA but a negative HCV RNA assay may have cleared the infection, may have HCV RNA that is below the level of detection, or may be have false positive results.[17] A recombinant immunoblot assay will confirm that the anti-HCV EIA result is a true positive.[17]

Elevated levels of AST and ALT have only a weak correlation with the degree of liver injury.[19] Liver biopsy is recommended to assess the severity of liver disease and the need for antiviral therapy; however, it is optional in patients with genotypes 2 and 3 because of the high likelihood of viral response to treatment.[17] Liver biopsies have two serious limitations: sampling variability and the number of adverse events.[20] The coefficient of variation of the staging of a standard 15-mm biopsy sample is 55%.[20] The incidence of severe adverse events in 98,445 liver biopsy samples from nine studies was 3.1 per 1,000 with a mortality rate of 0.3 per 1,000.[20]

Differential Diagnosis and Differentiating Features—See Hepatitis A and B

Treatment

Treatment should be considered for all patients with hepatitis C.[16] Combination therapy using pegylated interferon and ribavirin is currently the treatment of choice and cures in up to 50% persons for genotype 1 and in up to 80% persons for genotypes 2 and 3.[15] The goal of therapy is the absence of hepatitis C RNA 6 months after the completion of treatment.[17] If hepatitis C RNA does not drop by at least 2 logs at month 3 of therapy, treatment should be discontinued because the likelihood of a sustained response is only 0 to 3%.[17] Absolute contraindications to treatment with pegylated interferon and ribavirin are allergy to either medication, decompensated cirrhosis, active intravenous drug use or heavy alcohol use, and pregnancy.[19] Liver transplantation is reserved for patients with decompensated liver disease.[16]

Expected Outcomes and Complication

Only 15 to 45% of newly infected patients clear the infection; most (55 to 85%) will develop chronic HCV.[3,18] Factors associated with spontaneous clearance of HCV are younger age at infection, female sex, development of jaundice during acute infection, and non-African American ethnicity.[3] Chronic liver disease occurs in 70% of chronically infected persons.[15] Cirrhosis and HCC usually occur two to three decades after initial exposure.[3] An increased rate of fibrosis progression is seen in patients with the following cofactors: age older than 40 years at time of infection, daily consumption of >50 g/day of alcohol, and male sex.[3] HCV accounts for an estimated one third of HCC cases in the USA.[16] Screening for HCC with AFP testing and hepatic USN at 6 month internals is a common practice in the USA; however, there is a lack of evidence for this practice.[16]

Patients with chronic hepatitis C can present with extrahepatic manifestations such as rheumatoid symptoms, keratoconjunctivitis sicca, lichen planus, glomerulonephritis, lymphoma, and essential mixed cryoglobulinemia.[16] Cryoglobulins have been detected in the serum of approximately 40% of patients with chronic hepatitis C, but symptomatic mixed cryoglobulinemia is rare.[19] In 20 to 30% of individuals with HCV infection, psychological disorders including depression have been associated.[16]

Prevention

There is no vaccine to prevent hepatitis C. The CDC recommends screening in persons who have any of the following risk factors: history of intravenous drug use, blood transfusion or organ transplant before 1992, receipt of clotting factors before 1987, long-term hemodialysis and people with undiagnosed liver problems, infants born to infected mothers, and healthcare/public safety workers after known exposure.[15]

Sexual partners of male and female patients with hepatitis C should be considered for testing.[16] Household items such as razors or toothbrushes that may be contaminated with blood should not be shared.[18] There is no evidence that food, water, or contact such as kissing, hugging, sneezing, coughing, sharing eating utensils or drinking glasses without exposure to blood is associated with transmission.[16]

Currently, immune globulin or antiviral prophylaxis is not recommended after needle-stick exposure.[16] The exposed individual should be tested for HCV antibody, HCV RNA, and ALT at exposure and again between 2 and 8 weeks after injury.[16] If seroconversion occurs, the person should be considered for treatment.

Hepatitis D

Introduction

Hepatitis D virus (HDV) depends on the presence of HBV for its life cycle.[1] Worldwide, HDV is present in <5% of chronic HBV carriers.[21]

Pathophysiology

HDV is an RNA virus in an unclassified family.[4] Exposure to blood products was the major route of transmission before screening procedures for HBV were instituted.[1] In developed countries, injection drug use and sexual transmission are the major routes of spread.[1] The incubation period is 30 to 180 days.[1] HDV cannot make its own envelope protein; instead, its envelope consists of HBsAg.[4] Therefore, HDV infection and replication can occur only in an individual with HBV infection.[4] Unlike HBV, HDV virus is thought to be directly cytopathic.[4]

Clinical Presentation (History, Physical Exam, and Laboratory Investigations)

Acute co-infection of HBV and HDV (Fig. 8.6) and acute superinfection of HDV on a chronic HBV patient (Fig. 8.7) both cause a severe hepatitis.[4] Anti-HDV IgM and IgG detect acute and chronic infection, respectively.[1]

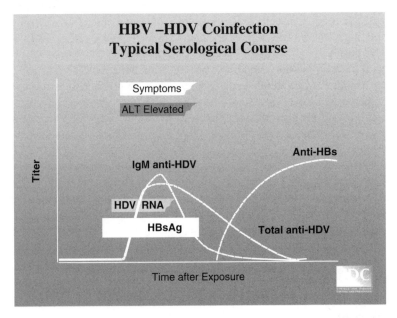

Fig. 8.6 HDV serology, acute co-infection with HBV (http://www.cdc.gov/ncidod/diseases/hepatitis/slideset/101/101_hdv.ppt#355,5,Slide 5; accessed 7/16/07).

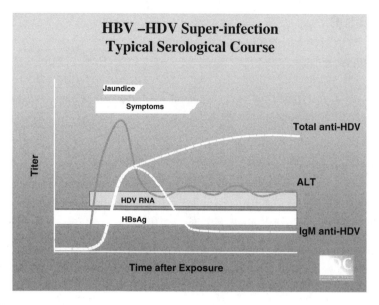

Fig. 8.7 HDV serology, super infection in patient with HBV (http://www.cdc.gov/ncidod/
diseases/hepatitis/slideset/101/101_hdv.ppt#357,6,Slide 6; accessed 7/16/07).

Treatment

Treatment for chronic HDV is currently limited to α-interferon, although a sustained response is unusual and incomplete.[21,22] Other therapies, including acyclovir, ribavirin, and lamivudine, have been tried but have not been successful.[22] Liver transplantation is a treatment option for patients with end-stage liver disease.

Expected Outcomes and Complications

Acute co-infection of HBV and HDV resolves in 80 to 95% of cases.[4] However, HDV superinfection results in chronic HDV–HBV in more than 70 to 80% of cases.[4] In both co-infection and superinfection, fulminant hepatitis develops in 2 to 20% of cases.[4] Chronic HDV progresses to cirrhosis frequently and is more rapid than for chronic HBV or chronic HCV.[4]

Prevention

Vaccination against HBV will protect against HDV.[21] There is no effective vaccine, however, for preventing delta superinfection in HBsAg carriers.[4]

Hepatitis E

Introduction

Hepatitis E virus (HEV) infection is endemic in India and Southeast and Central Asia.[1,4] HEV infection is rare in the USA.[4]

Pathophysiology

HEV is a small RNA virus that is currently classified in the genus *Hepatitis E-like viruses*.[23] There are two main strains, Burmese (or Asian) and Mexican.[4] Transmission is through the fecal–oral route.[1,4] The incubation period ranges from 2 to 10 weeks.[4] Person-to-person spread is rare, occurring in 0.7 to 2.2% of household contacts of hepatitis E, compared with rates of 50 to 75% in susceptible household contacts of hepatitis A.[1]

Clinical Presentation (History, Physical Exam, and Laboratory Investigations)

The clinical course is similar to hepatitis A, but usually is more severe.[4] Acute HEV infection is diagnosed by the presence of anti-HEV IgM (Fig. 8.8).[4] Anti-HEV IgM is detectable for approximately 2 to 3 months after the onset of illness. Anti-HEV IgG persists for several years.[4] Polymerase chain reaction (PCR) for the detection of HEV RNA in the stool or serum is also available.

Treatment

Treatment is supportive.

Expected Outcomes and Complications

Acute hepatitis E is self-limiting; the illness usually lasts 1 to 4 weeks, although some patients have a prolonged cholestatic hepatitis lasting 2 to 6 months.[4] There is no chronic infection. The case fatality rate is 1 to 2%, although there is a much higher mortality (10–30%) in pregnant women, particularly if they are in the third trimester.[4]

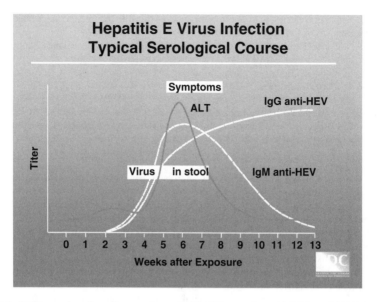

Fig. 8.8 HEV serology(http://www.cdc.gov/ncidod/diseases/hepatitis/slideset/101/101_hev.ppt #361,6,Slide 6; accessed 7/16/07).

Prevention

Prevention involves improved sanitation and sanitary handling of food and water.[4] The efficacy of passive immunization with immunoglobulin for prevention of HEV infection is under evaluation.[4] Currently, vaccines are under development.[23]

References

1. Ghany MG, Kiang TJ. Acute viral hepatitis. In: Textbook of Gastroenterology. 4th ed. Philadelphia: Lippincott Williams and Wilkins, 2003:2276–2301.
2. Leach CT. Hepatitis A in the United States. Pediatr Infect Dis J 2004;23:551–552.
3. Rawls RA, Vega KJ. Viral hepatitis in minority America. J Clin Gastroenterol 2005;39:144–151.
4. Fox RF, Wright TL. Viral hepatitis. In: Current Diagnosis and Treatment in Gastroenterology. 2nd ed. New York: McGraw-Hill, 2003:545–562.
5. Craig AS, Schaffner W. Prevention of hepatitis A with the hepatitis A vaccine. N Engl J Med 2004;350:476–481.
6. Campos-Outcalt D. Hepatitis A: matching preventive resources to needs. J Fam Prac 2004;53:292–295.
7. Giboney PT. Mildly elevated liver transaminase levels in the asymptomatic patient. Am Fam Phy 2005;71:1105–1110.

8. CDC. Notice to Readers: FDA approval of Havrix (Hepatitis A vaccine, inactivated) for persons aged 1–18 years. MMWR Weekly 12/9/2005;54:1235–1236.

9. CDC. Notice to Readers: FDA approval of VAQTA (Hepatitis A vaccine, inactivated) for children aged ≥ 1 year. MMWR Weekly 10/14/2005;54:1026.

10. CDC. Prevention of Hepatitis A through Active and Passive Immunization. Recommendations of the ACIP. MMWR 2006;55(RR07):1–23.

11. CDC. Sexually transmitted diseases treatment guidelines. MMWR 2002:51:59–66.

12. CDC. Recommendation of the Immunization Practices Advisory Committee (ACIP). A comprehensive immunization strategy to eliminate transmission of hepatitis B virus infection in the United States. MMWR 2005;54(RR16):1–23.

13. Ganem D, Prince AM. Hepatitis B virus infection—natural history and clinical consequences. N Engl J Med 2004;350:1118–1129.

14. Crockett SD, Keeffe EB. Natural history and treatment of hepatitis B virus and hepatitis C virus coinfection. Ann Clin Micro Antimicrobials 2005;4:13.

15. CDC. Hepatitis C fact sheet. 2005. Available at http://www.cdc.gov/hepatitis.

16. Management of hepatitis C:2002. NIH Consens State Sci Statement 2002;19:1–46.

17. Kim AI, Saab S. Treatment of hepatitis C. Am J Med 2005;118:080–815.

18. Wong T, Lee SS. Hepatitis C: a review for primary care physicians. CMAJ 2006;174:649–659.

19. Ward RP, Kugelmas M, Libsch KD. Management of hepatitis C: evaluating suitability for drug therapy. Am Fam Physician 2004;69:1429–1438.

20. Poynard T, Yuen MF, Ratziu V, Lai CL. Viral hepatitis C. Lancet 2003;362:2095–2100.

21. Taylor JM. Hepatitis delta virus. Virology 2006;344:71–76.

22. Niro GA, Rosina F, Rizzetto M. Treatment of hepatitis D. J Vir Hep 2005;12:2–9.

23. Wang L, Zhuang H. Hepatitis E: an overview and recent advances in vaccine research. World J Gastroenterol 2004;10:2157–2162.

Part III
Sexually Transmitted Diseases

Chapter 9
Sexually Transmitted Diseases

Neil S. Skolnik

In August, 2006 the Centers for Disease Control and Prevention (CDC) issued the Sexually Transmitted Diseases Treatment Guidelines, 2006, which were updated in April of 2007 with revised treatment regimens to account for increasing resistance of gonorrhea to the fluoroquinolone class of antibiotics. The guidelines contain and establish the standard of care for the treatment of sexually transmitted diseases (STDs) nationwide. This chapter summarizes the most important points and the updated treatment regimens recommended in the guidelines. All treatment regimens, as well as selected text below, are taken essentially verbatim from the guidelines. In addition to treatment, it is essential to understand that counseling patients routinely about prevention of STD acquisition is an important aspect of routine clinical care of adolescents and adults.

Partner Management

Treatment of the partners of patients who are treated is important, because when partners are treated, the index patient has less chance of reinfection, and there is a decreased chance of the partners spreading the STD to another individual. Clinicians should encourage patients treated for STDs to inform their sexual partners of the presence of an STD and encourage their partners to seek treatment. Another option for partner treatment is expedited partner therapy (EPT). In EPT, partners of infected patients are treated without medical evaluation or prevention counseling by giving the treated patient an extra prescription to be used for treatment of their partner. In the treatment of chlamydia and gonorrhea, EPT has been shown to prevent reinfection of the index case and is associated with a higher likelihood of partner notification, compared with recommending that a treated patient refer their partners. It should always be given with appropriate precautions and the recommendation that it would be best for the partner to seek medical care. A potential problem with EPT is the unclear legal status of this approach in many states. The legal status of EPT is reviewed in detail, and the CDC has delineated state-specific legal status of EPT, which is available at: http://www.cdc.gov/std/ept/legal/default.htm.

N.S. Skolnik (ed.), *Essential Infectious Disease Topics for Primary Care.*
© Humana Press, Totowa, NJ

Special Populations

Adolescents

Adolescents have one of the highest rates of STDs, therefore, emphasis on both preventing and treating STDs among adolescents is important. Adolescents are at higher risk for STDs because they often have unprotected intercourse, are biologically more susceptible to infection than older individuals, often have multiple partners over time, and often face real obstacles to getting appropriate healthcare. With rare exceptions, adolescents in the United States can legally consent to the confidential diagnosis and treatment of STDs. The guidelines state explicitly that, "in all 50 states and the District of Columbia, medical care for STDs can be provided to adolescents without parental consent or knowledge."

Men Who Have Sex with Men

Men who have sex with men (MSM) are at high risk for STDs. Routine screening is indicated for all sexually active MSM, and the following tests are recommended on an annual basis:

- HIV serology, if HIV-negative or not tested within the previous year
- Syphilis serology
- A test for urethral infection with *Neisseria gonorrhoeae* and *Chlamydia trachomatis* in men who have had insertive intercourse during the preceding year
- A test for rectal infection with *N. gonorrhoeae* and *C. trachomatis* in men who have had receptive anal intercourse during the preceding year
- A test for pharyngeal infection with *N. gonorrhoeae* in men who have acknowledged participation in receptive oral intercourse during the preceding year; testing for *C. trachomatis* pharyngeal infection is not recommended

In addition, clinicians can consider serologic tests for herpes simplex virus (HSV)-2. Routine testing for anal cytologic abnormalities or anal HPV infection is not recommended.

More frequent screening, at 3 to 6 month intervals, is indicated for MSM who have multiple or anonymous partners, have sex while using illicit drugs or methamphetamine, or whose sex partners participate in these activities.

Vaccination against hepatitis A (HAV) and B (HBV) is recommended for all MSM.

Detection of HIV Infection: Screening and Diagnostic Testing

All persons who seek evaluation and treatment for STDs should be screened for HIV infection. Screening should be routine, regardless of whether the patient is known or suspected to have specific behavioral risks for HIV infection.

HIV antibody is positive in >95% of patients within 3 months after infection, therefore, a negative test indicates that a person has very likely not had HIV for more than 3 months. The majority of HIV infections in the United States are caused by HIV-1; however, HIV-2 infection may be suspected in persons who have epidemiologic risk factors linking infection that possibly originated in West Africa.

Clinicians should be aware of acute retroviral syndrome, which is characterized by fever, malaise, lymphadenopathy, and skin rash. Acute retroviral syndrome occurs in the first few weeks after HIV infection, before antibody test results become positive, and can be detected by checking a HIV nucleic acid (RNA) test. Patients with acute retroviral syndrome may benefit from antiretroviral therapy.

Diseases Characterized by Genital Ulcers

Management of Patients Who Have Genital Ulcers

The majority of young, sexually active patients who have genital ulcers in the United States have genital herpes, syphilis, or chancroid. Herpes is the most common of the three infections. Because clinical assessment is often inaccurate, all patients with genital ulcers should have 1) syphilis serology and either darkfield examination or direct immunofluorescence test for *Treponema pallidum*; 2) culture or antigen test for HSV; and 3) in areas where chancroid is present, a culture for *Haemophilus ducreyi*. After complete testing, 25% of patients with genital ulcers still do not have a laboratory-confirmed diagnosis.

Chancroid

Diagnosis

Chancroid typically has a combination of a painful genital ulcer and tender suppurative inguinal adenopathy. Culture testing results are only positive in <80% of cases. A case can be considered probable if 1) the patient has one or more painful genital ulcers; 2) the patient has no evidence of *T. pallidum* infection by darkfield examination or by a serologic testing at least 7 days after onset of ulcers; 3) the clinical presentation is typical for chancroid; and 4) HSV testing is negative. There is a high rate of co-infection in patients with chancroid. Patients should be retested for syphilis and HIV 3 months after the diagnosis, if the initial test results were negative.

Treatment

Recommended Regimens

- 1 g azithromycin orally in a single dose **OR**
- 250 mg ceftriaxone intramuscularly in a single dose **OR**

- 500 mg ciprofloxacin orally twice a day for 3 days **OR**
- 500 mg erythromycin base orally three times a day for 7 days

Ciprofloxacin is contraindicated for pregnant and lactating women. Azithromycin and ceftriaxone offer the advantage of single-dose therapy. Worldwide, several isolates with intermediate resistance to either ciprofloxacin or erythromycin have been reported.

Genital ulcers should improve within 3 to 7 days of treatment. Improvement of adenopathy often takes longer and sometimes requires incision and drainage.

Genital HSV Infections

More than 50 million Americans have genital HSV infections. The majority of cases of recurrent genital herpes are caused by HSV-2, although HSV-1 can cause genital herpes. The majority of persons infected with HSV-2 have mild or rarely recurrent infection and are undiagnosed; therefore, the majority of transmission occurs from individuals who shed virus intermittently and are often not aware that they are infected.

Diagnosis

The clinical diagnosis of HSV infection is imprecise. More than 50% of first episodes of genital herpes are HSV-1, although recurrence is less frequent for HSV-1 than HSV-2. Clinical diagnosis of genital herpes should be confirmed by laboratory testing. HSV culture is the preferred virologic test, although it is not as sensitive as polymerase chain reaction (PCR) assays for HSV.

Accurate type-specific HSV serologic assays are available that can distinguish HSV-1 from HSV-2. Because nearly all HSV-2 infections are sexually acquired, the presence of HSV-2 antibody is strong evidence of anogenital infection, and counseling regarding genital herpes and risk of asymptomatic shedding should be provided.

Treatment

First Clinical Episode of Genital Herpes

Patients with an initial episode should be treated with oral antiviral medication.

Recommended Regimens

- 400 mg acyclovir orally three times a day for 7 to 10 days **OR**
- 200 mg acyclovir orally five times a day for 7 to 10 days **OR**

- 250 mg famciclovir orally three times a day for 7 to 10 days **OR**
- 1 g valacyclovir orally twice a day for 7 to 10 days

Treatment might be extended if healing is incomplete after 10 days of therapy.

Established HSV-2 Infection

Intermittent asymptomatic shedding occurs with genital HSV-2 infection, even with long-standing or clinically silent infection. Antiviral therapy for established genital herpes can be given either episodically to diminish or shorten the duration of and outbreak or continuously as suppressive therapy to decrease the frequency of recurrences. Continuous suppressive therapy has the additional advantage of decreasing the risk of asymptomatic genital HSV-2 shedding and transmission to susceptible partners.

Suppressive Therapy for Recurrent Genital Herpes

Suppressive therapy reduces the frequency of genital herpes recurrences by 70 to 80% in patients with frequent recurrences, and often eliminates recurrences. The frequency of recurrent genital herpes outbreaks diminishes over time, so that once a year it may be reasonable to consider a trial off suppressive therapy.

Recommended Regimens

- 400 mg acyclovir orally twice a day **OR**
- 250 mg famciclovir orally twice a day **OR**
- 500 mg valacyclovir orally once a day **OR**
- 1.0 g valacyclovir orally once a day

Five hundred milligrams valacyclovir once a day might be less effective than other valacyclovir or acyclovir dosing regimens in patients who have very frequent recurrences (i.e., > 10 episodes per year).

Episodic Therapy for Recurrent Genital Herpes

When episodic treatment is chosen, it should be started within 1 day of lesion onset or during the prodrome before lesions are apparent.

Recommended Regimens

- 400 mg acyclovir orally three times a day for 5 days **OR**
- 800 mg acyclovir orally twice a day for 5 days **OR**
- 800 mg acyclovir orally three times a day for 2 days **OR**

- 125 mg famciclovir orally twice daily for 5 days **OR**
- 1000 mg famciclovir orally twice daily for 1 day **OR**
- 500 mg valacyclovir orally twice a day for 3 days **OR**
- 1.0 g valacyclovir orally once a day for 5 days

Severe Disease

Intravenous acyclovir therapy is recommended for severe HSV disease or complications that necessitate hospitalization (e.g., disseminated infection, pneumonitis, or hepatitis) or central nervous system (CNS) complications (e.g., meningitis or encephalitis). The recommended dose is 5 to 10 mg/kg body weight acyclovir intravenously every 8 hours for 2 to 7 days, followed by oral antiviral therapy to complete at least 10 days of total therapy.

Special Situations

Co-infection with HIV

Immunocompromised patients may have outbreaks that are more severe.

*Recommended Regimens for Daily Suppressive Therapy in
Persons Infected with HIV*

- 400 to 800 mg acyclovir orally twice to three times a day **OR**
- 500 mg famciclovir orally twice a day **OR**
- 500 mg valacyclovir orally twice a day

Recommended Regimens for Episodic Infection in Persons Infected with HIV

- 400 mg acyclovir orally three times a day for 5 to 10 days **OR**
- 500 mg famciclovir orally twice a day for 5 to 10 days **OR**
- 1.0 g valacyclovir orally twice a day for 5 to 10 days

Genital Herpes in Pregnancy

Most neonatal herpes infections occur in infants whose mothers lack a history of clinical herpes. The risk for transmission from an infected mother is 30 to 50% among women who acquire herpes near the time of delivery and is low, <1%, among women with histories of recurrent herpes at term or who acquire herpes earlier in pregnancy. Prevention of neonatal herpes relies both on preventing late acquisition of herpes infection in women near the end of their pregnancy and in avoiding vaginal delivery for infants in mothers who have active herpes lesions.

Women without herpes should avoid intercourse or oral sex during the third trimester with partners who may have genital or oral herpes. It may be helpful to offer type-specific serologic testing to women at risk for acquiring HSV during pregnancy, particularly if their partner may have herpes, to better be able to provide accurate counseling.

At the onset of labor, women should be questioned about symptoms of genital herpes and prodromal symptoms, as well as examined carefully for lesions. Women without symptoms or signs can deliver vaginally. If a woman has genital herpetic lesions at the onset of labor delivery, she should be delivered by cesarean section to decrease the probability of neonatal herpes.

The safety of antiviral therapy in pregnant women has not been established, although available data for acyclovir does not indicate an increased risk for major birth defects. Acyclovir may be administered orally to pregnant women with first-episode genital herpes or severe recurrent herpes and should be administered intravenously to pregnant women with severe HSV infection. Some specialists recommend acyclovir in pregnancy to women with frequently recurrent genital herpes to decrease the chances of having active lesions when in labor. For women who acquire genital HSV during late pregnancy, expert consultation should be sought, and some experts recommend acyclovir therapy, some recommend routine cesarean section to reduce the risk for neonatal herpes, and some recommend both.

Granuloma Inguinale (Donovanosis)

Granuloma inguinale is caused by the intracellular gram-negative bacterium *Klebsiella granulomatis*. It is rare in the United States, and endemic in some tropical areas, including India; Papua, New Guinea; central Australia; and southern Africa. It causes painless, progressive ulcerative lesions without regional lymphadenopathy. The lesions have a beefy red appearance and bleed easily. Diagnosis is made by visualization of dark-staining Donovan bodies on tissue preparation or biopsy. PCR tests have not been FDA approved, but are available.

Recommended Regimen

- 100 mg doxycycline orally twice a day for at least 3 weeks and until all lesions have completely healed. Relapse can occur 6 to 18 months after therapy

Alternative Regimens

- 1 g azithromycin orally once per week for at least 3 weeks and until all lesions have completely healed **OR**
- 750 mg ciprofloxacin orally twice a day for at least 3 weeks and until all lesions have completely healed **OR**

- 500 mg erythromycin base orally four times a day for at least 3 weeks and until all lesions have completely healed **OR**
- One double-strength (160 mg/800 mg) trimethoprim–sulfamethoxazole tablet orally twice a day for at least 3 weeks and until all lesions have completely healed

Some specialists recommend the addition of an aminoglycoside (e.g., 1 mg/kg gentamicin intravenously every 8 hours) to these regimens if improvement is not evident within the first few days of therapy.

Special Considerations

Pregnancy

Pregnant and lactating women should be treated with the erythromycin regimen, and consideration should be given to the addition of a parenteral aminoglycoside (e.g., gentamicin). Azithromycin might prove useful for treating granuloma inguinale during pregnancy, but published data are lacking.

HIV Infection

Persons with both granuloma inguinale and HIV infection should receive the same regimens as those who are HIV negative. Consideration should be given to the addition of a parenteral aminoglycoside (e.g., gentamicin).

Lymphogranuloma Venereum

Lymphogranuloma venereum (LGV) is caused by *C. trachomatis*. LGV manifests with tender inguinal and/or femoral lymphadenopathy that is typically unilateral. A self-limited genital ulcer or papule can occur at the site of inoculation, although this has often resolved by the time patients seek care. Rectal exposure in women or MSM can cause proctocolitis. If proctocolitis is not treated, it can lead to chronic colorectal fistulas and strictures.

   Genital and lymph node specimens (i.e., lesion swab or bubo aspirate) may be tested for *C. trachomatis* by culture, direct immunofluorescence, or nucleic acid detection.

   Chlamydia serology (complement fixation titers >1:64) can support the diagnosis in the appropriate clinical context.

   In the absence of specific LGV diagnostic testing, patients with a clinical syndrome consistent with LGV, including proctocolitis or genital ulcer disease with lymphadenopathy, should be treated for LGV.

Treatment

Treatment cures infection and prevents ongoing tissue damage, although tissue reaction to the injection can result in scarring. Buboes can require aspiration through intact skin or incision and drainage.

Recommended Regimen

- 100 mg doxycycline orally twice a day for 21 days

Alternative Regimen

- 500 mg erythromycin base orally four times a day for 21 days

Some STD specialists think that 1.0 g azithromycin orally once weekly for 3 weeks is probably effective, although trial data is lacking.

Special Considerations

Pregnancy

Pregnant and lactating women should be treated with erythromycin. Azithromycin might prove useful for treatment of LGV in pregnancy, but no published data are available regarding its safety and efficacy.

HIV Infection

Persons with both LGV and HIV infection should receive the same regimens as those who are HIV negative. Prolonged therapy might be required, and delay in resolution of symptoms might occur.

Syphilis

General Principles

Background

The clinical diagnosis of syphilis is divided into stages. Primary infection is characterized by an ulcer or chancre at the infection site. Secondary infection manifests with skin rash, mucocutaneous lesions, and lymphadenopathy. Tertiary infection can have cardiac and ophthalmic manifestations, auditory abnormalities, or gummatous lesions. Latent infection lacks clinical manifestations and is detected by serologic testing. Latent syphilis acquired within the preceding year is referred to as early latent syphilis; all other cases of latent syphilis are either late latent syphilis or latent syphilis of unknown duration.

Serologic Testing

Darkfield examinations and direct fluorescent antibody (DFA) tests of lesion exudate or tissue are used for diagnosing early syphilis. A presumptive diagnosis is possible with the use of two types of serologic tests: 1) nontreponemal tests (e.g., Venereal Disease Research Laboratory [VDRL] and rapid plasma reagin [RPR]) and 2) treponemal tests (e.g., fluorescent treponemal antibody absorbed [FTA-ABS] and *T. pallidum* particle agglutination [TP-PA]). The use of only one type of serologic test is insufficient for diagnosis because false-positive nontreponemal test results are sometimes associated with various medical conditions unrelated to syphilis.

Nontreponemal test antibody titers usually correlate with disease activity. Nontreponemal tests usually become nonreactive with time after treatment; however, they may persist at a low titer in some patients. Treponemal tests usually remain positive long term, regardless of treatment or disease activity.

Treatment

The Jarisch–Herxheimer reaction is an acute febrile reaction frequently accompanied by headache, myalgia, and other symptoms that usually occurs within the first 24 hours after any therapy for syphilis. It occurs most frequently among patients who have early syphilis.

Management of Sex Partners

Sexual transmission of *T. pallidum* occurs only when mucocutaneous syphilitic lesions are present. However, persons exposed sexually to a patient who has syphilis in any stage should be evaluated according to the following recommendations:

- Persons who were exposed within the 90 days preceding the diagnosis of primary, secondary, or early latent syphilis in a sex partner might be infected even if seronegative; therefore, such persons should be treated presumptively
- Persons who were exposed more than 90 days before the diagnosis of primary, secondary, or early latent syphilis in a sex partner should be treated presumptively if serologic test results are not available immediately and the opportunity for follow-up is uncertain
- For purposes of partner notification and presumptive treatment of exposed sex partners, patients with syphilis of unknown duration who have high nontreponemal

serologic test titers (i.e., >1:32) can be assumed to have early syphilis. However, serologic titers should not be used to differentiate early from late latent syphilis for the purpose of determining treatment (see the "Treatment" section in "Latent Syphilis")

- Long-term sex partners of patients who have latent syphilis should be evaluated clinically and serologically for syphilis and treated on the basis of the evaluation findings

For identification of at-risk sexual partners, the periods before treatment are 1) 3 months plus duration of symptoms for primary syphilis, 2) 6 months plus duration of symptoms for secondary syphilis, and 3) 1 year for early latent syphilis.

Primary and Secondary Syphilis

Recommended Regimen for Adults

- 2.4 million U benzathine penicillin G intramuscularly in a single dose

Other Management Considerations

All patients who have syphilis should be tested for HIV infection. If the person is a high risk for HIV, then they should be retested for HIV after 3 months.

Follow-Up

Serologic follow-up is recommended at 6 months and 12 months after treatment.

Patients who have persistent or recurrent signs or symptoms or who have a sustained fourfold increase in nontreponemal test titer are likely to have failed treatment or have been reinfected. These patients should be retreated as well as evaluated for HIV infection and have a cerebrospinal fluid (CSF) analysis. 15% of patients with early syphilis treated with the recommended therapy will not achieve a two-dilution decline in nontreponemal titer used to define response at 1 year after treatment.

For retreatment, administer weekly injections of 2.4 million U benzathine penicillin G intramuscularly for 3 weeks, unless CSF examination indicates that neurosyphilis is present.

Special Considerations

Penicillin Allergy

If the patient is allergic to penicillin, alternatives are 100 mg doxycycline orally twice daily for 14 days or 500 mg tetracycline four times daily for 14 days.

Although limited clinical studies, along with biologic and pharmacologic evidence, suggest that ceftriaxone is effective for treating early syphilis, the optimal dose and duration of ceftriaxone therapy have not been defined. Some specialists recommend 1 g daily either intramuscularly or intravenously for 8 to 10 days. Preliminary data suggest that azithromycin might be effective as a single oral dose of 2 g. However, several cases of azithromycin treatment failure have been reported, and resistance to azithromycin has been documented in several geographic areas.

Patients with penicillin allergy whose compliance with therapy or follow-up cannot be ensured should be desensitized and treated with benzathine penicillin.

Pregnancy

Pregnant patients who are allergic to penicillin should be desensitized and treated with penicillin.

HIV Infection

See "Syphilis in HIV-Infected Persons."

Latent Syphilis

Latent syphilis is defined as syphilis characterized by seroreactivity without other evidence of disease. Patients who have latent syphilis and who acquired syphilis within the preceding year are classified as having early latent syphilis.

Treatment

Treatment of latent syphilis usually does not affect transmission and is intended to prevent late complications.

Recommended Regimens for Adults

Early Latent Syphilis

- 2.4 million U benzathine penicillin G intramuscularly in a single dose

Late Latent Syphilis or Latent Syphilis of Unknown Duration

- 7.2 million U total benzathine penicillin G, administered as three doses of 2.4 million U intramuscularly each at 1-week intervals

Other Management Considerations

All persons who have latent syphilis should be evaluated clinically for evidence of tertiary disease (e.g., aortitis and gumma) and syphilitic ocular disease (e.g., iritis and uveitis). Patients who have syphilis and who demonstrate any of the following criteria should have a CSF examination:

- Neurologic or ophthalmic signs or symptoms
- Evidence of active tertiary syphilis (e.g., aortitis and gumma)
- Treatment failure
- HIV infection with late latent syphilis or syphilis of unknown duration

A CSF examination may be performed for patients who do not meet these criteria. Some specialists recommend performing a CSF examination on all patients who have latent syphilis and a nontreponemal serologic test of >1:32 or if the patient is HIV-infected with a serum CD4 count <350 cells. However, the likelihood of neurosyphilis in this circumstance is unknown.

If a patient misses a dose of penicillin in a course of weekly therapy for late syphilis, the appropriate course of action is unclear. Pharmacologic considerations suggest that an interval of 10 to 14 days between doses of benzathine penicillin for late syphilis or latent syphilis of unknown duration might be acceptable before restarting the sequence of injections. Missed doses are not acceptable for pregnant patients receiving therapy for late latent syphilis; pregnant women who miss any dose of therapy must repeat the full course of therapy.

Follow-Up

Quantitative nontreponemal serologic tests should be repeated at 6, 12, and 24 months. Patients with a normal CSF examination should be retreated for latent syphilis if 1) titers increase fourfold, 2) an initially high titer (>1:32) fails to decline at least fourfold (i.e., two dilutions) within 12 to 24 months of therapy, or 3) signs or symptoms attributable to syphilis develop.

Special Considerations

Penicillin Allergy

Nonpregnant patients allergic to penicillin who have clearly defined early latent syphilis should respond to therapies recommended as alternatives to penicillin for the treatment of primary and secondary syphilis. The only acceptable alternatives for the treatment of late latent syphilis or latent syphilis of unknown duration are 100 mg doxycycline orally twice daily or 500 mg tetracycline orally four times daily, both for 28 days. These therapies should be used only in conjunction with close serologic and clinical follow-up. Limited clinical studies, along with biologic and pharmacologic evidence, suggest that ceftriaxone might be effective for treating late latent syphilis or syphilis of unknown duration. However, the optimal dose and duration of ceftriaxone therapy have not been defined, and treatment decisions should be discussed in consultation with a specialist.

Pregnancy

Pregnant patients who are allergic to penicillin should be desensitized and treated with penicillin (see the full guidelines for "Management of Patients Who Have a History of Penicillin Allergy and Syphilis During Pregnancy").

HIV Infection

See "Syphilis in HIV-Infected Persons."

Tertiary Syphilis

Tertiary syphilis refers to gumma and cardiovascular syphilis but not to all neurosyphilis. Patients who are not allergic to penicillin and have no evidence of neurosyphilis should be treated with the following regimen.

Recommended Regimen

- 7.2 million U total benzathine penicillin G, administered as three doses of 2.4 million U intramuscularly each at 1-week intervals

Other Management Considerations

Patients who have symptomatic late syphilis should be treated in consultation with a specialist.

Special Considerations

Penicillin Allergy

Patients allergic to penicillin should be treated according to treatment regimens recommended for late latent syphilis.

Pregnancy

Pregnant patients who are allergic to penicillin should be desensitized, if necessary, and treated with penicillin.

HIV Infection

See "Syphilis in HIV-Infected Persons."

Neurosyphilis

Treatment

CNS involvement can occur during any stage of syphilis. A patient who has clinical evidence of neurologic involvement with syphilis should have a CSF examination.

Patients who have neurosyphilis or syphilitic eye disease (e.g., uveitis, neuroretinitis, and optic neuritis) should be treated with the following regimen.

Recommended Regimen

- 18 to 24 million U/day aqueous crystalline penicillin G, administered as 3 to 4 million U intravenously every 4 hours or continuous infusion, for 10 to 14 days

If compliance with therapy can be ensured, patients may be treated with the following alternative regimen.

Alternative Regimen

- 2.4 million U procaine penicillin intramuscularly once daily **PLUS**
- 500 mg probenecid orally four times a day, both for 10 to 14 days.

The durations of the recommended and alternative regimens for neurosyphilis are shorter than that of the regimen used for late syphilis in the absence of neurosyphilis. Therefore, some specialists administer 2.4 million U benzathine penicillin intramuscularly once per week for up to 3 weeks after completion of these neurosyphilis treatment regimens to provide a comparable total duration of therapy.

Follow-Up

If CSF pleocytosis was present initially, a CSF examination should be repeated every 6 months until the cell count is normal. Follow-up CSF examinations also can be used to evaluate changes in the VDRL-CSF or CSF protein after therapy; however, changes in these two parameters occur more slowly than cell counts, and persistent abnormalities might be less important. If the cell count has not decreased after 6 months or if the CSF is not normal after 2 years, retreatment should be considered. Recent data on HIV-infected persons with neurosyphilis suggest that CSF abnormalities might persist for extended periods in these persons, and close clinical follow-up is warranted.

Special Considerations

Penicillin Allergy

Ceftriaxone can be used as an alternative treatment for patients with neurosyphilis. Some specialists recommend ceftriaxone 2 g daily either intramuscularly or intravenously for 10 to 14 days. Other regimens have not been adequately evaluated for treatment of neurosyphilis.

Pregnancy

Pregnant patients who are allergic to penicillin should be desensitized, if necessary, and treated with penicillin (see "Syphilis During Pregnancy").

HIV Infection

See "Syphilis in HIV-Infected Patients."

Syphilis in HIV-Infected Persons

Diagnostic Considerations

Unusual serologic responses have been observed among HIV-infected persons who have syphilis. Unusual serologic responses are uncommon, and the majority of specialists think that both treponemal and nontreponemal serologic tests for syphilis can be interpreted in the usual manner for the majority of patients who are co-infected with *T. pallidum* and HIV.

Treatment

Compared with HIV-negative patients, HIV-positive patients who have early syphilis might be at increased risk for neurologic complications and might have higher rates of treatment failure with currently recommended regimens. The magnitude of these risks is not defined precisely but is likely minimal.

Primary and Secondary Syphilis in HIV-Infected Persons

Treatment

Treatment with 2.4 million U benzathine penicillin G intramuscularly in a single dose is recommended. Some specialists recommend additional treatments (e.g., benzathine penicillin G administered at 1-week intervals for 3 weeks, as recommended for late syphilis) in addition to 2.4 million U benzathine penicillin G intramuscularly.

Other Management Considerations

Because CSF abnormalities (e.g., mononuclear pleocytosis and elevated protein levels) are common in patients with early syphilis and in persons with HIV infection, the clinical and prognostic significance of such CSF abnormalities in HIV-infected persons with primary or secondary syphilis is unknown. Although the majority of HIV-infected persons respond appropriately to standard benzathine penicillin therapy, some specialists recommend intensified therapy when CNS syphilis is suspected in these persons. Therefore, some specialists recommend CSF examination before treatment of HIV-infected persons with early syphilis, with follow-up CSF examination conducted after treatment in persons with initial abnormalities.

Follow-Up

HIV-infected persons should be evaluated clinically and serologically for treatment failure at 3, 6, 9, 12, and 24 months after therapy. Although of unproven benefit, some specialists recommend a CSF examination 6 months after therapy.

HIV-infected persons who meet the criteria for treatment failure (i.e., signs or symptoms that persist or recur or persons who have fourfold increase in nontreponemal test titer) should be managed in the same manner as HIV-negative patients (i.e., a CSF examination and retreatment). CSF examination and retreatment also should be strongly considered for persons whose nontreponemal test titers do not decrease fourfold within 6 to 12 months of therapy. The majority of specialists would retreat patients with benzathine penicillin G administered as three doses of 2.4 million U intramuscularly each at weekly intervals, if CSF examination results are normal.

Special Considerations

Penicillin Allergy

Penicillin-allergic patients who have primary or secondary syphilis and HIV infection should be managed according to the recommendations for penicillin-allergic, HIV-negative patients. The use of alternatives to penicillin has not been well studied in HIV-infected patients.

Latent Syphilis in HIV-Infected Persons

Diagnostic Considerations

HIV-infected patients who have early latent syphilis should be managed and treated according to the recommendations for HIV-negative patients who have primary and secondary syphilis. HIV-infected patients who have either late latent syphilis or syphilis of unknown duration should have a CSF examination before treatment.

Treatment

Patients with late latent syphilis or syphilis of unknown duration and normal CSF examination results can be treated with benzathine penicillin G, at weekly doses of 2.4 million U for 3 weeks. Patients who have CSF results consistent with neurosyphilis should be treated and managed as patients who have neurosyphilis.

Follow-Up

Patients should be evaluated clinically and serologically at 6, 12, 18, and 24 months after therapy. If, at any time, clinical symptoms develop or nontreponemal titers rise fourfold, a repeat CSF examination should be performed and treatment administered accordingly. If during 12 to 24 months, the nontreponemal titer does not decline fourfold, the CSF examination should be repeated and treatment administered accordingly.

Special Considerations

Penicillin Allergy

The efficacy of alternative nonpenicillin regimens in HIV-infected persons has not been well studied.

Syphilis During Pregnancy

All women should be screened serologically for syphilis during the early stages of pregnancy. For communities and populations in which the prevalence of syphilis is high or for patients at high risk, serologic testing should be performed twice during the third trimester, at 28 to 32 weeks' gestation, and at delivery.

Diagnostic Considerations

Seropositive pregnant women should be considered infected unless an adequate treatment history is documented clearly in the medical records and sequential serologic antibody titers have declined.

Treatment

Penicillin is effective for preventing maternal transmission to the fetus and for treating fetal infection. Evidence is insufficient to determine specific, recommended penicillin regimens that are optimal.

Recommended Regimen

Treatment during pregnancy should be the penicillin regimen appropriate for the stage of syphilis.

Other Management Considerations

Some specialists recommend additional therapy for pregnant women in some settings (e.g., a second dose of 2.4 million U benzathine penicillin intramuscularly administered 1 week after the initial dose for women who have primary, secondary, or early latent syphilis). During the second half of pregnancy, syphilis management may be facilitated by a sonographic fetal evaluation for congenital syphilis, but this evaluation should not delay therapy. Sonographic signs of fetal or placental syphilis (i.e., hepatomegaly, ascites, hydrops, or a thickened placenta) indicate a greater risk for fetal treatment failure; such cases should be managed in consultation with obstetric specialists. Evidence is insufficient to recommend specific regimens for these situations.

Women treated for syphilis during the second half of pregnancy are at risk for premature labor and/or fetal distress if the treatment precipitates the Jarisch-Herxheimer reaction. These women should be advised to seek obstetric attention after treatment, if they notice any contractions or decrease in fetal movements. Stillbirth is a rare complication of treatment, but concern for this complication should not delay necessary treatment. All patients who have syphilis should be offered testing for HIV infection.

Follow-Up

Serologic titers should be repeated at 28 to 32 weeks' gestation, at delivery, and following the recommendations for the stage of disease. Serologic titers can be checked monthly in women at high risk for reinfection. The clinical and antibody response should be appropriate for the stage of disease.

Special Considerations

Penicillin Allergy

For treatment of syphilis during pregnancy, no proven alternatives to penicillin exist. Pregnant women who have a history of penicillin allergy should be desensitized and treated with penicillin.

HIV Infection

Placental inflammation from congenital infection might increase the risk for perinatal transmission of HIV. All HIV-infected women should be evaluated for infectious syphilis and treated. Data are insufficient to recommend a specific regimen.

Management of Patients Who Have a History of Penicillin Allergy

See the full STD Guidelines for further information regarding skin testing and desensitization.

Diseases Characterized by Urethritis and Cervicitis

Management of Male Patients Who Have Urethritis

Urethritis can result from infectious and noninfectious conditions. Patients can be symptomatic or asymptomatic. *N. gonorrhoeae* and *C. trachomatis* are clinically important infectious causes of urethritis. If Gram stain is not available, patients should be treated for both gonorrhea and chlamydia. Further testing to determine the specific etiology is recommended. Culture, nucleic acid hybridization tests, and nucleic acid amplification tests (NAAT) are available for the detection of both *N. gonorrhoeae* and *C. trachomatis*. Culture and hybridization tests require urethral swab specimens, whereas amplification tests can be performed on urine specimens. Because of their higher sensitivity, amplification tests are preferred for the detection of *C. trachomatis*.

Etiology

Several organisms can cause infectious urethritis. The presence of Gram-negative intracellular diplococci (GNID) on urethral smear is indicative of gonorrhea infection. Nongonoccocal urethritis (NGU) is diagnosed when microscopy indicates inflammation without GNID. *C. trachomatis* is a frequent cause of NGU (i.e., 15–55% of cases); however, the prevalence varies by age group, with lower prevalence among older men. The proportion of NGU cases caused by chlamydia has been declining gradually.

The etiology of the majority of cases of nonchlamydial NGU is unknown. *Ureaplasma urealyticum* and *Mycoplasma genitalium* have been implicated as etiologic agents of NGU in some studies. *Trichomonas vaginalis*, HSV, and adenovirus might also cause NGU. Diagnostic and treatment procedures for these organisms are reserved for situations in which these infections are suspected or when NGU is not responsive to therapy. Enteric bacteria have been identified as an uncommon cause of NGU and might be associated with insertive anal sex.

Confirmed Urethritis

Clinicians should document that urethritis is present. Urethritis can be documented on the basis of any of the following signs or laboratory tests:

- Mucopurulent or purulent discharge
- Gram stain of urethral secretions demonstrating more than five white blood cells (WBC) per oil immersion field. The Gram stain is the preferred rapid diagnostic test for evaluating urethritis. It is highly sensitive and specific for documenting both urethritis and the presence or absence of gonococcal infection. Gonococcal infection is established by documenting the presence of WBC containing GNID
- Positive leukocyte esterase test on first-void urine or microscopic examination of first-void urine sediment demonstrating more than 10 WBC per high power field.

If none of these criteria are present, treatment should be deferred, and the patient should be tested for *N. gonorrhoeae* and *C. trachomatis*.

Management of Patients Who Have Nongonococcal Urethritis Diagnosis

All patients who have confirmed or suspected urethritis should be tested for gonorrhea and chlamydia.

Treatment

Treatment should be initiated as soon as possible after diagnosis. Azithromycin and doxycycline are highly effective for chlamydial urethritis; however, infections with *M. genitalium* may respond better to azithromycin.

Recommended Regimens

- 1 g azithromycin orally in a single dose **OR**
- 100 mg doxycycline orally twice a day for 7 days

Alternative Regimens

- 500 mg erythromycin base orally four times a day for 7 days **OR**
- 800 mg erythromycin ethylsuccinate orally four times a day for 7 days **OR**
- 300 mg ofloxacin orally twice a day for 7 days **OR**
- 500 mg levofloxacin orally once daily for 7 days

Follow-Up for Patients Who Have Urethritis

Patients should be instructed to abstain from sexual intercourse until 7 days after therapy is initiated. Persistence of pain, discomfort, and irritative voiding symptoms beyond 3 months leads to the possibility of chronic prostatitis/chronic pelvic pain syndrome in men. Persons whose conditions have been diagnosed as a new STD should receive testing for other STDs, including syphilis and HIV.

Recurrent and Persistent Urethritis

Consider retreatment if a patient did not finish the initial treatment or may have been reexposed to infection. *T. vaginalis* culture should be performed using an intraurethral swab or a first-void urine specimen. Some cases of recurrent urethritis after doxycycline treatment might be caused by tetracycline-resistant *U. urealyticum*. If the patient was compliant with the initial regimen and reexposure can be excluded, the following regimen is recommended.

Recommended Regimens

- 2 g metronidazole orally in a single dose **OR**
- 2 g tinidazole orally in a single dose **PLUS**
- 1 g azithromycin orally in a single dose (if not used for initial episode)

Management of Patients Who Have Cervicitis

Cervicitis frequently is asymptomatic, or can cause abnormal vaginal discharge and intermenstrual vaginal bleeding (e.g., after sexual intercourse). A finding of leukorrhea (>10 WBC per high power field on microscopic examination of vaginal fluid) has been associated with chlamydial and gonococcal infection of the cervix. In the absence of inflammatory vaginitis, leukorrhea might be a sensitive indicator of cervical inflammation with a high negative predictive value.

Etiology

When an etiologic organism is isolated in the setting of cervicitis, it is typically *C. trachomatis* or *N. gonorrhoeae*. Cervicitis also can accompany trichomoniasis and genital herpes (especially primary HSV-2 infection). However, in the majority of cases of cervicitis, no organism is isolated, especially in women at relatively low risk for recent acquisition of these STDs (for example, women aged >30 years). Limited data indicate that infection with *M. genitalium* and bacterial vaginosis (BV) as well as frequent douching might cause cervicitis. For reasons that are unclear, cervicitis can persist despite repeated courses of antimicrobial therapy. Because the majority of persistent cases of cervicitis are not caused by relapse or reinfection with *C. trachomatis* or *N. gonorrhoeae*, other determinants (e.g., persistent abnormality of vaginal flora, douching or exposure to chemical irritants, or idiopathic inflammation in the zone of ectopy) might be involved.

Diagnosis

Because cervicitis might be a sign of upper genital tract infection (endometritis), women who seek medical treatment for a new episode of cervicitis should be assessed for signs of pelvic inflammatory disease (PID) and should be tested for *C. trachomatis* and for *N. gonorrhoeae*. Women with cervicitis also should be evaluated for the presence of BV and trichomoniasis, and these conditions should be treated, if present. Because the sensitivity of microscopy to detect *T. vaginalis* is relatively low (approximately 50%), symptomatic women with cervicitis and negative microscopy for trichomonads should receive further testing (i.e., culture or antigen-based detection). Although HSV-2 infection has been associated with cervicitis, the usefulness of specific testing (i.e., culture or serologic testing) for HSV-2 in this setting is unclear. Standardized diagnostic tests for *M. genitalium* are not commercially available.

Treatment

Recommended Regimens for Presumptive Treatment

- 1 g azithromycin orally in a single dose **OR**
- 100 mg doxycycline orally twice a day for 7 days

Consider concurrent treatment for gonococcal infection if prevalence of gonorrhea is high in the patient population under assessment.

Management of Sex Partners

Sex partners of women treated for cervicitis should be treated. Patients and their sex partners should abstain from sexual intercourse until therapy is completed (i.e., 7 days after a single-dose regimen or after completion of a 7-day regimen).

Special Considerations

HIV Infection

Patients who have cervicitis and also are infected with HIV should receive the same treatment regimen as those who are HIV negative.

Chlamydial Infections

Chlamydial Infections in Adolescents and Adults

In the United States, chlamydial genital infection is the most frequently reported infectious disease, and the prevalence is highest in persons aged younger than 25 years. Asymptomatic infection is common among both men and women, and to detect chlamydial infections, healthcare providers frequently rely on screening tests. Annual screening of all sexually active women aged younger than 25 years is recommended, as is screening of older women with risk factors (e.g., those who have a new sex partner or multiple sex partners). Evidence is insufficient to recommend routine screening for *C. trachomatis* in sexually active young men, based on feasibility, efficacy, and cost-effectiveness. However, screening of sexually active young men should be considered in clinical settings with a high prevalence of chlamydia (e.g., adolescent clinics, correctional facilities, and STD clinics).

Diagnostic Considerations

C. trachomatis urogenital infection in women can be diagnosed by testing urine or swab specimens collected from the endocervix or vagina. Diagnosis of *C. trachomatis* urethral infection in men can be made by testing a urethral swab or urine specimen. Rectal *C. trachomatis* infections in persons that engage in receptive anal intercourse can be diagnosed by testing a rectal swab specimen. Culture, direct immunofluorescence, enzyme immunoassay (EIA), nucleic acid hybridization tests, and NAATs are available for the detection of *C. trachomatis* on endocervical and male urethral swab specimens.

Treatment

Treating infected patients prevents transmission to sex partners. In addition, treating pregnant women usually prevents transmission of *C. trachomatis* to infants during birth. Treatment of sex partners helps to prevent reinfection of the index patient and infection of other partners.

Coinfection with *C. trachomatis* frequently occurs among patients who have gonococcal infection; therefore, presumptive treatment of such patients for chlamydia is appropriate. The following recommended treatment regimens and alternative regimens:

Recommended Regimens

- 1 g azithromycin orally in a single dose **OR**
- 100 mg doxycycline orally twice a day for 7 days

Alternative Regimens

- 500 mg erythromycin base orally four times a day for 7 days **OR**
- 800 mg erythromycin ethylsuccinate orally four times a day for 7 days **OR**
- 300 mg ofloxacin orally twice a day for 7 days **OR**
- 500 mg levofloxacin orally once daily for 7 days

Follow-Up

Except in pregnant women, test-of-cure (repeat testing 3–4 weeks after completing therapy) is *not* recommended. Repeat infections confer an elevated risk for PID and other complications when compared with the initial infection. Therefore, recently infected women are a major priority for repeat testing for *C. trachomatis*. Clinicians and healthcare agencies should consider advising all women with chlamydial infection to be retested approximately 3 months after treatment. Providers also are strongly encouraged to retest all women treated for chlamydial infection whenever they next seek medical care within the following 3 to 12 months, regardless of whether the patient thinks that her sex partners were treated. Recognizing that retesting is distinct from a test-of-cure is vital. Limited evidence is available regarding the benefit of retesting for chlamydia in men previously infected; however, some specialists suggest retesting men approximately 3 months after treatment.

Management of Sex Partners

Patients should be instructed to refer their sex partners for evaluation, testing, and treatment. Sex partners should be evaluated, tested, and treated if they had sexual contact with the patient during the 60 days preceding onset of symptoms in the patient or diagnosis of chlamydia. The most recent sex partner should be evaluated and treated, even if the time of the last sexual contact was more than 60 days before symptom onset or diagnosis.

If concerns exist that sex partners will not seek evaluation and treatment, then delivery of antibiotic therapy (either a prescription or medication) by heterosexual male or female patients to their partners might be an option (see "Partner Management"). Patient-delivered partner therapy is not routinely recommended for MSM because of a high risk for coexisting infections, especially undiagnosed HIV infection, in their partners.

Patients should be instructed to abstain from sexual intercourse until they and their sex partners have completed treatment. Abstinence should be continued until 7 days after a single-dose regimen or after completion of a 7-day regimen. Timely treatment of sex partners is essential for decreasing the risk for reinfecting the index patient.

Special Considerations

Pregnancy

Azithromycin is likely to be safe and effective. Repeat testing 3 weeks after completion of therapy with the following regimens is recommended for all pregnant women to ensure therapeutic cure, considering the sequelae that might occur in the mother and neonate if the infection persists. The frequent gastrointestinal side effects associated with erythromycin might discourage patient compliance with the alternative regimens.

Recommended Regimens

- 1 g azithromycin orally in a single dose **OR**
- 500 mg amoxicillin orally three times a day for 7 days

Alternative Regimens

- 500 mg erythromycin base orally four times a day for 7 days **OR**
- 250 mg erythromycin base orally four times a day for 14 days **OR**
- 800 mg erythromycin ethylsuccinate orally four times a day for 7 days **OR**
- 400 mg erythromycin ethylsuccinate orally four times a day for 14 days

Erythromycin estolate is contraindicated during pregnancy because of drug-related hepatotoxicity. The lower-dose 14-day erythromycin regimens may be considered if gastrointestinal tolerance is a concern.

HIV Infection

Patients who have chlamydial infection and also are infected with HIV should receive the same treatment regimen as those who are HIV negative.

Gonococcal Infections

Gonococcal Infections in Adolescents and Adults

Gonorrhea is the second most commonly reported bacterial STD. Because gono-coccal infections among women frequently are asymptomatic, an essential compo-nent of gonorrhea control in the United States continues to be the screening of women at high risk for STDs. The US Preventive Services Task Force (USPSTF) recommends that clinicians screen all sexually active women, including those who are pregnant, for gonorrhea infection if they are at increased risk. Women aged younger than 25 years are at highest risk for gonorrhea infection. Other risk factors for gonorrhea include a previous gonorrhea infection, other sexually transmitted infections, new or multiple sex partners, inconsistent condom use, commercial sex work, and drug use. The prevalence of gonorrhea infection varies widely among communities and patient populations. The USPSTF does not recommend screening for gonorrhea in men and women who are at low risk for infection.

Diagnostic Considerations

A Gram stain of a male urethral specimen that demonstrates polymorphonuclear leukocytes with intracellular gram-negative diplococci can be considered diagnostic for infection with *N. gonorrhoeae* in symptomatic men. A negative Gram stain should not be considered sufficient for excluding infection in asymptomatic men. Specific diagnosis of infection with *N. gonorrhoeae* may be performed by testing endocervical, vaginal, male urethral, or urine specimens. Culture, nucleic acid hybridization tests, and NAAT are available for the detection of genitourinary infec-tion with *N. gonorrhoeae*. In making the diagnosis of gonorrhoeae, it is important to know the indications and the limitations of the available tests at your clinical site.

All patients tested for gonorrhea should be tested for other STDs, including chlamydia, syphilis, and HIV.

Dual Therapy for Gonococcal and Chlamydial Infections

Patients treated for gonococcal infection should also be treated routinely with a regimen that is effective against uncomplicated genital *C. trachomatis* infection.

Quinolone-Resistant **N. gonorrhoeae**

In April 2007, the CDC published updated guidelines for the treatment of gonorrhea. Due to the increasing prevalence of quinolone-resistant *N. gonorrhoeae* (QRNG), **fluoroquinolones are no longer recommended for the treatment of gonococcal**

infections and associated conditions, such as PID. Only one class of antibiotics, the cephalosporins, is still recommended for the treatment of gonorrhea. Beginning in 2000, fluoroquinolones were no longer recommended for gonorrhea treatment in persons who acquired their infections in Asia or the Pacific Islands (including Hawaii); in 2002, this recommendation was extended to California. In 2004, CDC recommended that fluoroquinolones not be used in the United States to treat gonorrhea in MSM.

QRNG prevalence was < 1% from 1990 to 2001, increased to 2.2% in 2002, to 4.1% in 2003, and to 6.8% in 2004. In 2005, 9.4% of isolates were resistant to ciprofloxacin, and during January to June 2006, 13.3% of 3,005 isolates collected were resistant.

In addition, since 2001, the Gonococcal Isolate Surveillance Project (GISP) has observed QRNG increases among isolates from MSM, and more recently, from heterosexual males. In 2001, QRNG prevalence was 1.6% and 0.6% among MSM and heterosexual males, respectively. The QRNG prevalence among isolates from MSM increased to:

- 1.6% in 2001
- 7.2% in 2002
- 15% in 2003
- 23.8% in 2004
- 29% in 2005
- 38.3% in January to June 2006

Among heterosexual males, the prevalence increased more slowly, but still in an important manner, to:

- 0.6% in 2001
- 0.9% in 2002
- 1.5% in 2003
- 2.9% in 2004
- 3.8% in 2005
- 6.7% in January to June 2006

As a result of the increasing prevalence of QRNG, and consistent with a long-term plan of changing the recommendations for treatment when the prevalence of QRNG increased to be above 5%, the CDC no longer recommends fluoroquinolones for treatment of gonorrhea in the United States; similarly, the CDC no longer recommends fluoroquinolones for treatment of other conditions that might be caused by *N. gonorrhoeae.*

Uncomplicated Gonococcal Infections of the Cervix, Urethra, and Rectum

Recommended Regimens

- 125 mg ceftriaxone intramuscularly in a single dose **OR**

- 400 mg cefixime orally (the tablet formulation of cefixime is currently not available in the United States) in a single dose, or 400 mg cefixime by suspension (200 mg/5 ml) **PLUS**
- Treatment for chlamydia if chlamydial infection is not excluded

These regimens are recommended for all adult and adolescent patients, regardless of travel history or sexual behavior.

Alternative Regimens

- 2 g spectinomycin (spectinomycin is currently not available in the United States) in a single intramuscular dose **OR**
- Single-dose cephalosporin regimens

Other single-dose cephalosporin therapies that are considered alternative treatment regimens for uncomplicated urogenital and anorectal gonococcal infections include 500 mg ceftizoxime intramuscularly; or 2 g cefoxitin intramuscularly administered with 1 g probenecid orally; or 500 mg cefotaxime intramuscularly. Some evidence indicates that 400 mg cefpodoxime and 1 g cefuroxime axetil might be oral alternatives.

Uncomplicated Gonococcal Infections of the Pharynx

Recommended Regimens

- 125 mg ceftriaxone intramuscularly in a single dose **PLUS**
- Treatment for chlamydia if chlamydial infection is not excluded

This regimen is recommended for all adult and adolescent patients, regardless of travel history or sexual behavior.

Follow-Up

There is no need to perform a test of cure if symptoms resolve. Patients who have symptoms that persist after treatment should be evaluated by culture for *N. gonorrhoeae*, and any gonococci isolated should be tested for antimicrobial susceptibility. Clinicians should consider advising all patients with gonorrhea to be retested 3 months after treatment. If patients do not seek medical care for retesting in 3 months, providers are encouraged to test these patients whenever they next seek medical care within the following 12 months.

Management of Sex Partners

Sex partners within 60 days of treatment or the index patient's last sexual partner, should be referred for evaluation and treatment. If it is thought to be unlikely that a partner will be referred or come in for treatment, delivery of antibiotic therapy (i.e., either a prescription or medication) by heterosexual male or female patients to their partners is an option. Undertreatment of PID in female partners and missed opportunities to diagnose other STDs are concerns with patient-delivered therapy. Patient-delivered therapy for patients with gonorrhea should routinely include treatment for chlamydia. This approach should not be considered a routine partner management strategy in MSM because of the high risk of coexisting undiagnosed STDs or HIV infection.

Special Considerations

Allergy, Intolerance, and Adverse Reactions

Persons who cannot tolerate cephalosporins or quinolones should be treated with spectinomycin. Because spectinomycin is unreliable (52% effective) against pharyngeal infections, patients who have suspected or known pharyngeal infection should have a pharyngeal culture 3 to 5 days after treatment to verify eradication of infection.

Pregnancy

Pregnant women infected with *N. gonorrhoeae* should be treated with a recommended or alternate cephalosporin. Women who cannot tolerate a cephalosporin should be administered a single 2-g dose of spectinomycin intramuscularly. Either azithromycin or amoxicillin is recommended for treatment of presumptive or diagnosed *C. trachomatis* infection during pregnancy (see "Chlamydial Infections").

Administration of Quinolones to Adolescents

There has been caution around the use of fluoroquinolones in persons aged younger than 18 years based on studies showing damage to articular cartilage in young animals. No joint damage attributable to quinolone therapy has been observed in children treated with prolonged ciprofloxacin regimens. Therefore, children who weigh more than 45 kg can be treated with any regimen recommended for adults.

HIV Infection

Patients who have gonococcal infection and also are infected with HIV should receive the same treatment regimen as those who are HIV negative.

Gonococcal Conjunctivitis

Recommended Regimen

- 1 g ceftriaxone intramuscularly in a single dose

  Consider lavage of the infected eye with saline solution once.

Disseminated Gonococcal Infection

Disseminated gonococcal infection (DGI) is the result of gonococcal bacteremia.

Treatment

Hospitalization is recommended for initial therapy, especially for patients who might not comply with treatment, for those in whom diagnosis is uncertain, and for those who have purulent synovial effusions or other complications. Patients should be examined for clinical evidence of endocarditis and meningitis. Patients treated for DGI should be treated presumptively for concurrent *C. trachomatis* infection, unless appropriate testing excludes this infection.

Recommended Regimen

- 1 g ceftriaxone intramuscularly or intravenously every 24 hours

Alternative Regimens

- 1 g cefotaxime intravenously every 8 hours **OR**
- 1 g ceftizoxime intravenously every 8 hours **OR**
- 2 g spectinomycin (spectinomycin is currently not available in the United States) intramuscularly every 12 hours

A cephalosporin-based intravenous regimen is recommended for the initial treatment of DGI. This is particularly important when gonorrhea is detected at mucosal sites by nonculture tests. Spectinomycin is not currently available in the United States; updated information regarding its availability can be found at: http://www.cdc.gov/std/gonorrhea/arg. Treatment should be continued for 24 to 48 hours after clinical improvement, at which time, therapy may be switched to one of the following regimens to complete at least 1 week of antimicrobial therapy.

- 400 mg cefixime (the tablet formulation of cefixime is currently not available in the United States) orally twice daily **OR**
- 400 mg cefixime suspension (200 mg/5 ml) twice daily **OR**
- 400 mg cefpodoxime orally twice daily

Fluoroquinolones may be an alternative treatment option if antimicrobial susceptibility can be documented by culture. With use of nonculture tests to diagnose *N. gonorrhoeae* increasing and with local data on antimicrobial susceptibility less available, laboratories should maintain the capacity to conduct such testing or form partnerships with laboratories that can.

Gonococcal Meningitis and Endocarditis

Recommended Regimen

- 1 to 2 g ceftriaxone intravenously every 12 hours

Therapy for meningitis should be continued for 10 to 14 days; therapy for endocarditis should be continued for at least 4 weeks. Treatment of complicated DGI should be undertaken in consultation with a specialist.

Diseases Characterized by Vaginal Discharge

Management of Patients Who Have Vaginal Infections

Vaginitis is usually characterized by a vaginal discharge and/ or vulvar itching and irritation, and a vaginal odor might be present. The three diseases most frequently associated with vaginal discharge are BV (replacement of the normal vaginal flora by an overgrowth of anaerobic microorganisms, mycoplasmas, and *Gardnerella vaginalis*), trichomoniasis (*T. vaginalis*), and candidiasis (usually caused by *Candida albicans*). Cervicitis can sometimes cause a vaginal discharge. Although vulvovaginal candidiasis (VVC) usually is not transmitted sexually, it is included in this section because it is frequently diagnosed in women being evaluated for STDs.

Laboratory testing fails to identify the cause of vaginitis in a minority of women. The pH of the vaginal secretions can be determined by narrow-range pH paper; an elevated pH (i.e., >4.5) is common with BV or trichomoniasis but might not be highly specific. Discharge can be further examined by diluting one sample in one to two drops of 0.9% normal saline solution on one slide and a second sample in 10% potassium hydroxide (KOH) solution. An amine odor detected immediately after applying KOH suggests BV.

Bacterial Vaginosis

BV is a polymicrobial clinical syndrome resulting from replacement of the normal H_2O_2-producing *Lactobacillus* sp. in the vagina with high concentrations of anaerobic bacteria (e.g., *Prevotella* sp. and *Mobiluncus* sp.), *G. vaginalis*, and *Mycoplasma hominis*. BV is the most prevalent cause of vaginal discharge or malodor; however, more than 50% of women with BV are asymptomatic. It is not clear whether BV results from sexual transmission. Treatment of male sex partners has not been beneficial in preventing the recurrence of BV.

Diagnostic Considerations

BV can be diagnosed by the use of clinical criteria or Gram stain. Clinical criteria require three of the following symptoms or signs:

- Homogeneous, thin, white discharge that smoothly coats the vaginal walls
- Presence of clue cells on microscopic examination
- pH of vaginal fluid >4.5
- A fishy odor of vaginal discharge before or after addition of 10% KOH (i.e., the whiff test)

When a Gram stain is used, determining the relative concentration of lactobacilli (long gram-positive rods), gram-negative and gram-variable rods and cocci (i.e., *G. vaginalis, Prevotella, Porphyromonas*, and peptostreptococci), and curved gram-negative rods (*Mobiluncus*) characteristic of BV is considered the gold standard laboratory method for diagnosing BV. Culture of *G. vaginalis* is not recommended as a diagnostic tool because it is not specific. A DNA probe-based test for high concentrations of *G. vaginalis* (Affirm™ VP III, Becton Dickinson, Sparks, MD) might have clinical use. Cervical Papanicolaou tests have no clinical use for the diagnosis of BV because of low sensitivity. Other commercially available tests that might be useful for the diagnosis of BV include a card test for the detection of elevated pH and trimethylamine (QuickVue Advance Quidel, San Diego, CA) and prolineaminopeptidase (Pip Activity TestCard™, Quidel).

Treatment

The established benefits of therapy for BV in nonpregnant women are to 1) relieve vaginal symptoms and signs of infection and 2) reduce the risk for infectious complications after abortion or hysterectomy.

BV during pregnancy is associated with adverse pregnancy outcomes, including premature rupture of the membranes, preterm labor, preterm birth, intraamniotic infection, and postpartum endometritis. The established benefit of therapy for BV in pregnant women is to relieve vaginal symptoms and signs of infection. Additional potential benefits of therapy include 1) reducing the risk for infectious complications associated with BV during pregnancy and 2) reducing the risk for other infections (e.g., other STDs or HIV). The results of several investigations indicate that treatment of pregnant women with BV who are at high risk for preterm delivery (i.e., those who previously delivered a premature infant) might reduce the risk for prematurity. Therefore, clinicians should consider evaluation and treatment of high-risk pregnant women with asymptomatic BV.

The results of two randomized controlled trials have indicated that treatment of BV with metronidazole substantially reduced postabortion PID. Three trials that evaluated the use of anaerobic antimicrobial coverage (i.e., metronidazole) for routine operative prophylaxis before abortion and seven trials that evaluated this additional coverage for women undergoing hysterectomy demonstrated a substantial reduction in postoperative infectious complications. Because of the increased risk for postoperative infectious complications associated with BV, some specialists recommend that, before performing surgical abortion or hysterectomy, providers should screen and treat women with BV in addition to providing routine prophylaxis. However, more information is needed before recommending treatment of asymptomatic BV before other invasive procedures.

Recommended Regimens

- 500 mg metronidazole orally twice a day for 7 days **OR**
- 0.75% metronidazole gel, one full applicator (5 g) intravaginally, once a day for 5 days **OR**
- 2% clindamycin cream, one full applicator (5 g) intravaginally at bedtime for 7 days

Patients should be advised to avoid consuming alcohol during treatment with metronidazole and for 24 hours thereafter. Clindamycin cream is oil-based and might weaken latex condoms and diaphragms for 5 days after use. Topical clindamycin preparations should not be used in the second half of pregnancy.

The recommended metronidazole regimens are equally efficacious. The recommended intravaginal clindamycin regimen might be less efficacious than the metronidazole regimens.

Alternative Regimens

- 300 mg clindamycin orally twice a day for 7 days **OR**
- 100 g clindamycin ovules intravaginally once at bedtime for 3 days

The 2 g metronidazole single-dose therapy has the lowest efficacy for BV and is no longer a recommended or alternative regimen. FDA has cleared 750 mg metronidazole extended-release tablets once daily for 7 days and a single dose of clindamycin intravaginal cream.

Management of Sex Partners

The results of clinical trials indicate that a woman's response to therapy and the likelihood of relapse or recurrence are not affected by treatment of her sex partner(s). Therefore, routine treatment of sex partners is not recommended.

Special Considerations

Allergy or Intolerance to the Recommended Therapy

Intravaginal clindamycin cream is preferred in case of allergy or intolerance to metronidazole. Intravaginal metronidazole gel can be considered for patients who do not tolerate systemic metronidazole, but patients allergic to oral metronidazole should not be administered intravaginal metronidazole.

Pregnancy

All pregnant women who have symptomatic disease require treatment. BV has been associated with adverse pregnancy outcomes (e.g., premature rupture of the membranes, chorioamnionitis, preterm labor, preterm birth, intraamniotic infection, postpartum endometritis, and postcesarean wound infection). Some specialists prefer using systemic therapy to treat possible subclinical upper genital tract infections.

Treatment of BV in asymptomatic pregnant women at high risk for preterm delivery (i.e., those who have previously delivered a premature infant) with a recommended oral regimen has reduced preterm delivery in three of four randomized controlled trials; some specialists recommend screening and oral treatment of these women. Screening (if conducted) and treatment should be performed during the first prenatal visit.

Multiple studies and meta-analyses have not demonstrated an association between metronidazole use during pregnancy and teratogenic or mutagenic effects in newborns.

Recommended Regimens for Pregnant Women

- 500 mg metronidazole orally twice a day for 7 days **OR**
- 250 mg metronidazole orally three times a day for 7 days **OR**
- 300 mg clindamycin orally twice a day for 7 days

Whether treatment of asymptomatic pregnant women with BV who are at low risk for preterm delivery reduces adverse outcomes of pregnancy is unclear. One trial in which oral clindamycin was used demonstrated a reduction in spontaneous preterm birth. Several trials have evaluated the use of intravaginal clindamycin during pregnancy to reduce preterm birth and treat asymptomatic BV. One trial in which women were treated before 20 weeks' gestation demonstrated a reduction in preterm birth. In three other trials, intravaginal clindamycin cream was administered at 16 to 32 weeks' gestation, and an increase in adverse events (e.g., low birthweight and neonatal infections) was observed in newborns. Therefore, intravaginal clindamycin cream should only be used during the first half of pregnancy.

Follow-Up of Pregnant Women

Treatment of BV in asymptomatic pregnant women who are at high risk for preterm delivery might prevent adverse pregnancy outcomes. Therefore, a follow-up evaluation 1 month after completion of treatment should be considered to evaluate whether the therapy was effective.

HIV Infection

Patients who have BV and also are infected with HIV should receive the same treatment regimen as those who are HIV negative. BV seems to be more persistent in HIV-positive women.

Trichomoniasis

Trichomoniasis is caused by the protozoan *T. vaginalis*. Men may be asymptomatic or have symptoms of urethritis. Women can be asymptomatic or can have a diffuse, malodorous, yellow-green vaginal discharge with vulvar irritation. Microscopy of vaginal secretions has a sensitivity of 60 to 70%. Other FDA-cleared tests for trichomoniasis in women include OSOM Trichomonas Rapid Test (Genzyme Diagnostics, Cambridge, MA), an immunochromatographic capillary flow dipstick technology, and the Affirm™ VP III (Becton Dickenson, San Jose, CA), a nucleic acid probe test that evaluates for *T. vaginalis, G. vaginalis,* and *C. albicans.* These tests are both performed on vaginal secretions and have a sensitivity >83% and a specificity >97%. Culture is the most sensitive and specific commercially available method of diagnosis. In women in whom trichomoniasis is suspected but not confirmed by microscopy, vaginal secretions should be cultured for *T. vaginalis*.

Recommended Regimens

- 2 g metronidazole orally in a single dose **OR**
- 2 g tinidazole orally in a single dose

Alternative Regimen

- 500 mg metronidazole orally twice a day for 7 days

Metronidazole gel is considerably less efficacious for the treatment of trichomoniasis (<50%) than oral preparations of metronidazole.

Follow-Up

If treatment failure occurs with a 2-g metronidazole single dose and reinfection is excluded, the patient can be treated with 500 mg metronidazole orally twice daily for 7 days or a 2-g tinidazole single dose. For patients failing either of these regimens, clinicians should consider treatment with 2 g tinidazole or 2 g metronidazole orally for 5 days.

Management of Sex Partners

Sex partners of patients with *T. vaginalis* should be treated.

Special Considerations

Allergy, Intolerance, and Adverse Reactions

Metronidazole and tinidazole are both nitroimidazoles. Patients with an immediate-type allergy to a nitroimidazole can be managed by metronidazole desensitization in consultation with a specialist. Topical therapy with drugs other than nitroimidazoles can be attempted, but cure rates are low (<50%).

Pregnancy

Vaginal trichomoniasis has been associated with adverse pregnancy outcomes, particularly premature rupture of membranes, preterm delivery, and low birthweight. However, data do not suggest that metronidazole treatment results in a reduction in perinatal morbidity. Although some trials suggest the possibility of increased prematurity or low birthweight after metronidazole treatment, limitations of the studies prevent definitive conclusions regarding risks of treatment. Treatment of *T. vaginalis* might relieve symptoms of vaginal discharge in pregnant women and might prevent respiratory or genital infection of the newborn and further sexual transmission. Clinicians should counsel patients regarding the potential risks and benefits of treatment. Some specialists would defer therapy in asymptomatic pregnant women until after 37 weeks' gestation.

Women may be treated with 2 g of metronidazole in a single dose. Metronidazole is pregnancy category B (animal studies have revealed no evidence of harm to the fetus, but no adequate, well-controlled studies among pregnant women have been conducted). Multiple studies and meta-analyses have not demonstrated a consistent association between metronidazole use during pregnancy and teratogenic or mutagenic effects in infants. Tinidazole is pregnancy category C (animal studies have demonstrated an adverse event, and no adequate, well-controlled studies in pregnant women have been conducted), and its safety in pregnant women has not been well evaluated.

In lactating women who are administered metronidazole, withholding breast-feeding during treatment and for 12 to 24 hours after the last dose will reduce the exposure of metronidazole to the infant. While using tinidazole, interruption of breastfeeding is recommended during treatment and for 3 days after the last dose.

HIV Infection

Patients who have trichomoniasis and also are infected with HIV should receive the same treatment regimen as those who are HIV negative.

Vulvovaginal Candidiasis

VVC usually is caused by *C. albicans* but occasionally is caused by other *Candida* sp. or yeasts. Typical symptoms of VVC include pruritus, vaginal soreness, dyspareunia, external dysuria, and abnormal vaginal discharge. VVC can be classified as either uncomplicated or complicated. Uncomplicated VVC is characterized by sporadic or infrequent VVC that is mild-to-moderate in severity, is likely to be *C. albicans*, and occurs in a nonimmunocompromised woman. Complicated VVC is recurrent, severe, and is often nonalbicans candidiasis, occurring in women with uncontrolled diabetes, debilitation, or immunosuppression or pregnancy.

Uncomplicated VVC

Diagnostic Considerations in Uncomplicated VVC

A diagnosis of *Candida* vaginitis is suggested clinically by the presence of external dysuria and vulvar pruritus, pain, swelling, and redness. Signs include vulvar edema, fissures, excoriations, or thick curdy vaginal discharge. The diagnosis can be made in a woman who has signs and symptoms of vaginitis when either 1) a wet preparation (saline, 10% KOH) or Gram stain of vaginal discharge demonstrates yeasts or pseudohyphae or 2) a culture or other test yields a positive result for a yeast species. *Candida* vaginitis is associated with a normal vaginal pH (<4.5). Use of 10% KOH in wet preparations improves the visualization of yeast and mycelia by disrupting cellular material that might obscure the yeast or pseudohyphae. If KOH is negative, a culture should be done. If *Candida* cultures cannot be done, empiric treatment can be considered for symptomatic women with any sign of VVC on examination when the wet mount is negative.

Treatment

Short-course topical formulations (i.e., single dose and regimens of 1–3 days) effectively treat uncomplicated VVC. The topically applied azole drugs are more effective than nystatin. Treatment with azoles results in relief of symptoms and negative cultures in 80 to 90% of patients who complete therapy.

Recommended Regimens

Intravaginal Agents

- 5 g of 2% butoconazole cream intravaginally for 3 days* **OR**
- 5 g of 2% butoconazole cream (Butaconazole1-sustained release), single intravaginal application **OR**
- 5 g of 1% clotrimazole cream intravaginally for 7 to 14 days* **OR**
- 100 mg clotrimazole vaginal tablet for 7 days **OR**
- 100 mg clotrimazole vaginal tablet, two tablets for 3 days **OR**
- 5 g of 2% miconazole cream intravaginally for 7 days* **OR**
- 100 mg miconazole vaginal suppository, one suppository for 7 days* **OR**
- 200 mg miconazole vaginal suppository, one suppository for 3 days* **OR**
- 1,200 mg miconazole vaginal suppository, one suppository for 1 day* **OR**
- 100,000-U nystatin vaginal tablet, one tablet for 14 days **OR**
- 5 g of 6.5% tioconazole ointment intravaginally in a single application* **OR**
- 5 g of 0.4% terconazole cream intravaginally for 7 days **OR**
- 5 g of 0.8% terconazole cream intravaginally for 3 days **OR**
- 80 mg terconazole vaginal suppository, one suppository for 3 days

*Over-the-counter preparations. The creams and suppositories in this regimen are oil-based and might weaken latex condoms and diaphragms. Intravaginal preparations of butoconazole, clotrimazole, miconazole, and tioconazole are available over-the-counter.

Oral Agent

- 150 mg fluconazole oral tablet, one tablet in single dose

Management of Sex Partners

VVC is not usually acquired through sexual intercourse; treatment of sex partners is not recommended but may be considered in women who have recurrent infection. A minority of male sex partners might have balanitis, which is characterized by erythematous areas on the glans of the penis in conjunction with pruritus or irritation. These men benefit from treatment with topical antifungal agents to relieve symptoms.

Complicated VVC

Recurrent VVC

Recurrent VVC (RVVC), usually defined as four or more episodes of symptomatic VVC in 1 year, affects a small percentage of women (<5%). The pathogenesis of RVVC is poorly understood, and the majority of women with RVVC have no apparent predisposing or underlying conditions. Vaginal cultures should be obtained from patients with RVVC to confirm the clinical diagnosis and to identify unusual species, including nonalbicans species, particularly *Candida glabrata* (*C. glabrata* does not form pseudohyphae or hyphae and is not easily recognized on microscopy). *C. glabrata* and other nonalbicans *Candida* species are observed in 10 to 20% of patients with RVVC. Conventional antimycotic therapies are not as effective against these species as against *C. albicans.*

Treatment

Each individual episode of RVVC caused by *C. albicans* responds well to short duration oral or topical azole therapy. However, to maintain clinical and mycologic control, some specialists recommend a longer duration of initial therapy (e.g., 7–14 days of topical therapy or a 100-mg, 150-mg, or 200-mg oral dose of fluconazole every third day for a total of three doses (days 1, 4, and 7) to attempt mycologic remission before initiating a maintenance antifungal regimen.

Maintenance Regimens

Oral fluconazole (i.e., 100-mg, 150-mg, or 200-mg dose) weekly for 6 months is the first line of treatment. If this regimen is not feasible, some specialists recommend topical 200 mg clotrimazole twice a week, clotrimazole (500-mg dose vaginal suppositories once weekly), or other topical treatments used intermittently.

Suppressive maintenance antifungal therapies are effective in reducing RVVC. However, 30 to 50% of women will have recurrent disease after maintenance therapy is discontinued. Routine treatment of sex partners is controversial. *C. albicans* azole resistance is rare in vaginal isolates, and susceptibility testing is usually not warranted for individual treatment guidance.

Severe VVC

Severe vulvovaginitis (i.e., extensive vulvar erythema, edema, excoriation, and fissure formation) is associated with lower clinical response rates in patients treated with short courses of topical or oral therapy. Either 7 to 14 days of topical azole or 150 mg of fluconazole in two sequential doses (second dose 72 hours after initial dose) is recommended.

Nonalbicans VVC

The optimal treatment of nonalbicans VVC remains unknown. Options include longer duration of therapy (7–14 days) with a nonfluconazole azole drug (oral or topical) as first-line therapy. If recurrence occurs, 600 mg of boric acid in a gelatin capsule is recommended, administered vaginally once daily for 2 weeks. This regimen has clinical and mycologic eradication rates of approximately 70%. If symptoms recur, referral to a specialist is advised.

Compromised Host

Women with underlying debilitating medical conditions (e.g., those with uncontrolled diabetes or those receiving corticosteroid treatment) do not respond as well to short-term therapies. Efforts to correct modifiable conditions should be made, and more prolonged (i.e., 7–14 days) conventional antimycotic treatment is necessary.

Pregnancy

VVC frequently occurs during pregnancy. Only topical azole therapies, applied for 7 days, are recommended for use among pregnant women.

HIV Infection

The incidence of VVC in HIV-infected women is unknown. Vaginal *Candida* colonization rates among HIV-infected women are higher than among those for seronegative women with similar demographic characteristics and high-risk behaviors, and the colonization rates correlate with increasing severity of immunosuppression. Based on available data, therapy for VVC in HIV-infected women should not differ from that for seronegative women.

Pelvic Inflammatory Disease

PID comprises a spectrum of inflammatory disorders of the upper female genital tract, including any combination of endometritis, salpingitis, tubo-ovarian abscess, and pelvic peritonitis. Sexually transmitted organisms, especially *N. gonorrhoeae* and *C. trachomatis*, are implicated in many cases; however, microorganisms that comprise the vaginal flora (e.g., anaerobes, *G. vaginalis, Haemophilus influenzae*, enteric gram-negative rods, and *Streptococcus agalactiae*) also have been associated with PID. In addition, cytomegalovirus (CMV), *M. hominis, U. urealyticum*, and *M. genitalium* might be associated with some cases of PID. All women who are diagnosed with acute PID should be tested for *N. gonorrhoeae* and *C. trachomatis* and should be screened for HIV infection.

Diagnostic Considerations

Acute PID is difficult to diagnose, yet delay in diagnosis and treatment probably contributes to inflammatory sequelae in the upper reproductive tract. The diagnosis of PID usually is based on clinical findings.

The clinical diagnosis of acute PID is imprecise. Data indicate that a clinical diagnosis of symptomatic PID has a positive predictive value (PPV) for salpingitis of 65 to 90% compared with laparoscopy.

Empiric treatment of PID should be initiated in sexually active young women and other women at risk for STDs if they are experiencing pelvic or lower abdominal pain, if no cause for the illness other than PID can be identified, and if one or more of the following minimum criteria are present on pelvic examination:

- Cervical motion tenderness **OR**
- Uterine tenderness **OR**
- Adnexal tenderness

Diagnostic evaluation that is more elaborate is frequently needed because incorrect diagnosis and management might cause unnecessary morbidity. These additional criteria may be used to enhance the specificity of the minimum criteria. The following additional criteria can be used to enhance the specificity of the minimum criteria and support a diagnosis of PID:

- Oral temperature > 101 °F (>38.3 °C)
- Abnormal cervical or vaginal mucopurulent discharge
- Presence of abundant numbers of WBC on saline microscopy of vaginal secretions
- Elevated erythrocyte sedimentation rate
- Elevated C-reactive protein
- Laboratory documentation of cervical infection with *N. gonorrhoeae* or *C. trachomatis*

The majority of women with PID have either mucopurulent cervical discharge or evidence of WBC on a microscopic evaluation of a saline preparation of vaginal fluid. If the cervical discharge appears normal and no WBCs are observed on the wet preparation of vaginal fluid, the diagnosis of PID is unlikely, and alternative causes of pain should be investigated.

Treatment

Treatment should be initiated as soon as the presumptive diagnosis has been made because prevention of long-term sequelae is dependent on immediate administration of appropriate antibiotics.

Some specialists have recommended that all patients with PID be hospitalized so that bed rest and supervised treatment with parenteral antibiotics can be initiated. However, in women with PID of mild or moderate clinical severity, outpatient therapy can provide short- and long-term clinical outcomes similar to inpatient therapy. Limited data support the use of outpatient therapy in women with clinical presentations that are more severe.

The following criteria for hospitalization are suggested:

- Surgical emergencies (e.g., appendicitis) cannot be excluded
- The patient is pregnant
- The patient does not respond clinically to oral antimicrobial therapy
- The patient is unable to follow or tolerate an outpatient oral regimen
- The patient has severe illness, nausea and vomiting, or high fever
- The patient has a tubo-ovarian abscess

Many practitioners have preferred to hospitalize adolescent women whose condition is diagnosed as acute PID. No evidence is available suggesting that adolescents benefit from hospitalization for treatment of PID. Younger women with mild-to-moderate acute PID have similar outcomes with either outpatient therapy or inpatient therapy. The decision to hospitalize adolescents with acute PID should be based on the same criteria used for older women.

Parenteral Treatment

For women with PID of mild or moderate severity, parenteral and oral therapy seems to have similar clinical efficacy. Clinical experience should guide decisions regarding transition to oral therapy, which usually can be initiated within 24 hours of clinical improvement. The majority of clinicians recommend at least 24 hours of direct inpatient observation for patients who have tuboovarian abscesses.

Recommended Parenteral Regimen A

- 2 g cefotetan intravenously every 12 hours **OR**
- 2 g cefoxitin intravenously every 6 hours **PLUS**
- 100 mg doxycycline orally or intravenously every 12 hours

Because of the pain associated with infusion, doxycycline should be administered orally when possible, even when the patient is hospitalized. Oral and intravenous administration of doxycycline provide similar bioavailability.

Parenteral therapy may be discontinued 24 hours after a patient improves clinically, and oral therapy with 100 mg doxycycline twice a day should continue to completion of 14 days of therapy. When tubo-ovarian abscess is present, many healthcare providers use clindamycin or metronidazole with doxycycline for continued therapy, rather than doxycycline alone, because it provides anaerobic coverage that is more effective.

Clinical data are limited regarding the use of other second- or third-generation cephalosporins (e.g., ceftizoxime, cefotaxime, and ceftriaxone), which also might be effective therapy for PID and may replace cefotetan or cefoxitin. However, these cephalosporins are less active than cefotetan or cefoxitin against anaerobic bacteria.

Recommended Parenteral Regimen B

- 900 mg clindamycin intravenously every 8 hours **PLUS**
- 2 mg/kg of body weight gentamicin loading dose intravenously or intramuscularly, followed by a maintenance dose (1.5 mg/kg) every 8 hours. Single daily dosing may be substituted

Although the use of a single daily dose of gentamicin has not been evaluated for the treatment of PID, it is efficacious in analogous situations. Parenteral therapy can be discontinued 24 hours after a patient improves clinically; continuing oral therapy should consist of 100 mg doxycycline orally twice a day or 450 mg clindamycin orally four times a day to complete a total of 14 days of therapy. When tubo-ovarian abscess is present, many healthcare providers use clindamycin for continued therapy, rather than doxycycline, because clindamycin provides anaerobic coverage that is more effective.

Alternative Parenteral Regimens

- 3 g ampicillin/sulbactam intravenously every 6 hours **PLUS**
- 100 mg doxycycline orally or intravenously every 12 hours

One trial demonstrated high short-term clinical cure rates with azithromycin, either alone for 1 week (at least one intravenous dose followed by oral therapy) or with a 12-day course of metronidazole (*184*). Ampicillin/sulbactam plus doxycycline is effective coverage against *C. trachomatis, N. gonorrhoeae*, and anaerobes, and for patients who have a tubo-ovarian abscess.

Oral Treatment

Oral therapy can be considered for women with mild-to-moderately severe acute PID, because the clinical outcomes among women treated with oral therapy are similar to those treated with parenteral therapy. The following regimens provide coverage against the frequent etiologic agents of PID. Patients who do not respond to oral therapy within 72 hours should be reevaluated to confirm the diagnosis and should be administered parenteral therapy on either an outpatient or an inpatient basis.

Recommended Oral Regimen

- 250 mg ceftriaxone intramuscularly in a single dose **PLUS**
- 100 mg doxycycline orally twice a day for 14 days **WITH OR WITHOUT**
- 500 mg metronidazole orally twice a day for 14 days **OR**
- 2 g cefoxitin intramuscularly in a single dose and 1 g probenecid orally administered concurrently in a single dose **PLUS**
- 100 mg doxycycline orally twice a day for 14 days **WITH OR WITHOUT**
- 500 mg metronidazole orally twice a day for 14 days **OR**
- Other parenteral third-generation cephalosporin (e.g., ceftizoxime or cefotaxime)
  PLUS
- 100 mg doxycycline orally twice a day for 14 days **WITH OR WITHOUT**
- 500 mg metronidazole orally twice a day for 14 days

Alternative Oral Regimens

If parenteral cephalosporin therapy is not feasible, use of fluoroquinolones (500 mg
levofloxacin orally once daily or 400 mg ofloxacin twice daily for 14 days) with or
without 500 mg metronidazole orally twice daily for 14 days may be considered if
the community prevalence and individual risk (see "Gonococcal Infections in
Adolescents and Adults" in Sexually Transmitted Disease Treatment Guidelines,
2006) of gonorrhea is low. Tests for gonorrhea must be performed before instituting
therapy, and the patient managed as follows if the test results are positive:

- If NAAT test results are positive, parenteral cephalosporin is recommended
- If culture for gonorrhea is positive, treatment should be based on the results of
  antimicrobial susceptibility. If the isolate is QRNG, or antimicrobial susceptibility
  cannot be assessed, parenteral cephalosporin is recommended

Although information regarding other outpatient regimens is limited, amoxicillin–
clavulanic acid and doxycycline or azithromycin with metronidazole has demonstrated short-term clinical cure. No data has been published regarding the use of
oral cephalosporins for the treatment of PID.

Follow-Up

Patients should demonstrate substantial clinical improvement (e.g., defervescence;
reduction in direct or rebound abdominal tenderness; and reduction in uterine, adnexal,
and cervical motion tenderness) within 3 days after initiation of therapy. Patients
who do not improve within this period usually require hospitalization, additional
diagnostic tests, and surgical intervention.

If no clinical improvement has occurred within 72 hours after outpatient oral
or parenteral therapy, an examination should be performed. Subsequent hospitalization,
parenteral therapy, and diagnostic evaluation, including the consideration of diagnostic
laparoscopy for alternative diagnoses, are recommended in women without clinical
improvement. All women diagnosed with acute PID should be offered HIV testing.

Management of Sex Partners

Male sex partners of women with PID should be examined and treated if they had sexual contact with the patient during the 60 days preceding the patient's onset of symptoms.

Prevention

Prevention of chlamydial infection by screening and treating high-risk women reduces the incidence of PID. Theoretically, the majority of cases of PID can be prevented by screening all women or those determined to be at high risk (based on age or other factors) by using DNA amplification on cervical specimens (in women receiving pelvic examinations) and on urine specimens (in women not undergoing examinations).

Special Considerations

Pregnancy

Because of the high risk for maternal morbidity and preterm delivery, pregnant women who have suspected PID should be hospitalized and treated with parenteral antibiotics.

HIV Infection

Differences in the clinical manifestations of PID between HIV-infected women and HIV-negative women have not been well delineated. HIV-infected women with PID have similar symptoms when compared with uninfected controls.

Intrauterine Device

The risk of PID associated with intrauterine device (IUD) use is primarily confined to the first 3 weeks after insertion and is uncommon thereafter. No evidence suggests that IUDs should be removed in women diagnosed with acute PID. The rate of treatment failure and recurrent PID in women continuing to use an IUD is unknown.

Epididymitis

Acute epididymitis is a clinical syndrome consisting of pain, swelling, and inflammation of the epididymis of <6 weeks. Chronic epididymitis is characterized by a 3-month or longer history of symptoms of discomfort and/or pain in the scrotum, testicle, or epididymis that is localized on clinical examination. Among sexually active men aged younger than 35 years, acute epididymitis is most frequently caused by *C. trachomatis* or *N. gonorrhoeae*. Acute epididymitis caused by sexually transmitted enteric organisms (e.g., *Escherichia coli*) also occurs among men who are the insertive partner during anal intercourse.

Diagnostic Considerations

Men with epididymitis usually have unilateral testicular pain and tenderness. Emergency testing for torsion might be indicated when the onset of pain is sudden, pain is severe, or the test results available during the initial examination do not support a diagnosis of urethritis or urinary tract infection. If the diagnosis is questionable, a specialist should be consulted immediately because testicular viability might be compromised. Radionuclide scanning of the scrotum is the most accurate radiologic method of diagnosis, although it is not routinely available. Color duplex Doppler ultrasonography has a sensitivity of 70% and a specificity of 88% in diagnosing acute epididymitis.

The evaluation of men for epididymitis should include one of the following:

- Gram stain of urethral secretions demonstrating >five WBC per oil immersion field
- Positive leukocyte esterase test on first-void urine or microscopic examination of first-void urine sediment demonstrating >10 WBC per high power field

Treatment

As an adjunct to therapy, bed rest, scrotal elevation, and analgesics are recommended until fever and local inflammation have subsided. Because empiric therapy is often initiated before laboratory tests are available, it is recommended that all patients receive ceftriaxone plus doxycycline for the initial therapy of epididymitis. Additional therapy may include a quinolone if acute epididymitis is not caused by gonorrhea (i.e., results from culture or NAAT are negative for *N. gonorrhoeae*) or if the infection is most likely caused by enteric organisms.

Recommended Regimens

- 250 mg ceftriaxone intramuscularly in a single dose **PLUS**
- 100 mg doxycycline orally twice a day for 10 days

For acute epididymitis most likely caused by enteric organisms or with negative gonococcal culture or NAAT:

- 300 mg ofloxacin orally twice a day for 10 days **OR**
- 500 mg levofloxacin orally once daily for 10 days

Management of Sex Partners

Patients who have acute epididymitis, confirmed or suspected to be caused by
N. gonorrhoeae or *C. trachomatis*, should be instructed to refer sex partners for
evaluation and treatment if their contact with the index patient was within the 60
days preceding onset of the patient's symptoms.

Special Considerations

HIV Infection

Patients who have uncomplicated acute epididymitis and also are infected with HIV
should receive the same treatment regimen as those who are HIV negative.

HPV Infection

Genital HPV infection can cause genital warts, usually associated with HPV types
6 or 11. Other HPV types that infect the anogenital region (e.g., high-risk HPV
types 16, 18, 31, 33, and 35) are strongly associated with cervical neoplasia.
Persistent infection with high-risk types of HPV is the most important risk factor
for cervical neoplasia.

HPV Tests

A definitive diagnosis of HPV infection is based on detection of viral nucleic acid
(i.e., DNA or RNA) or capsid protein. Tests that detect several types of HPV
DNA in cells scraped from the cervix are available and might be useful in the
triage of women with atypical squamous cells of undetermined significance
(ASC-US) or in screening women aged older than 30 years in conjunction with
the Papanicolaou test. Screening women or men with the HPV test, outside of recommendations for use of the test with cervical cancer screening, is not recommended.

Treatment

In the absence of genital warts or cervical squamous intraepithelial lesion (SIL),
treatment is not recommended for subclinical genital HPV infection, whether it is
diagnosed by colposcopy, biopsy, acetic acid application, or through the detection
of HPV by laboratory tests. Genital HPV infection frequently goes away on its own,
and no therapy has been identified that can eradicate infection.

Genital Warts

Genital warts are usually flat, papular, or pedunculated growths on the genital mucosa. HPV types 6 or 11 are commonly found in genital warts

Treatment

If left untreated, visible genital warts might resolve on their own, remain unchanged, or increase in size or number. Treatment possibly reduces, but does not eliminate, HPV infection. Whether the reduction in HPV viral DNA, resulting from treatment, impacts future transmission remains unclear.

Regimens

Treatment of genital warts should be guided by the preference of the patient, the available resources, and the experience of the healthcare provider. The treatment modality should be changed if a patient has not improved substantially. Treatment regimens are classified into patient-applied and provider-applied modalities.

Recommended Regimens for External Genital Warts

Patient Applied

- 0.5% podofilox solution or gel. Patients should apply podofilox solution with a cotton swab, or podofilox gel with a finger, to visible genital warts twice a day for 3 days, followed by 4 days of no therapy. This cycle may be repeated, as necessary, for up to four cycles. The total wart area treated should not exceed $10\,cm^2$, and the total volume of podofilox should be limited to 0.5 ml per day. If possible, the healthcare provider should apply the initial treatment to demonstrate the proper application technique and identify which warts should be treated. The safety of podofilox during pregnancy has not been established **OR**
- 5% imiquimod cream. Patients should apply imiquimod cream once daily at bedtime, three times a week for up to 16 weeks. The treatment area should be washed with soap and water 6 to 10 hours after the application. The safety of imiquimod during pregnancy has not been established

Provider Administered

- Cryotherapy with liquid nitrogen or cryoprobe. Repeat applications every 1 to 2 weeks **OR**
- 10 to 25% podophyllin resin in a compound tincture of benzoin. A small amount should be applied to each wart and allowed to air dry. The treatment can be repeated weekly, if necessary. To avoid the possibility of complications associated

with systemic absorption and toxicity, two important guidelines should be followed: 1) application should be limited to <0.5 ml of podophyllin or an area of <10 cm² of warts per session, and 2) no open lesions or wounds should exist in the area to which treatment is administered. Some specialists suggest that the preparation should be thoroughly washed off 1 to 4 hours after application to reduce local irritation. The safety of podophyllin during pregnancy has not been established **OR**

- 80 to 90% trichloroacetic acid (TCA) or bichloracetic acid (BCA). A small amount should be applied only to the warts and allowed to dry, at which time, a white "frosting" develops. If an excess amount of acid is applied, the treated area should be powdered with talc, sodium bicarbonate (i.e., baking soda), or liquid soap preparations to remove unreacted acid. This treatment can be repeated weekly, if necessary **OR**
- Surgical removal either by tangential scissor excision, tangential shave excision, curettage, or electrosurgery

Alternative Regimens

- Intralesional interferon **OR**
- Laser surgery

Interferons, both natural or recombinant, have been used for the treatment of genital warts. The efficacy and recurrence rates of intralesional interferon are comparable to other treatment modalities. Administration of intralesional interferon is associated with stinging, burning, and pain at the injection site. Interferon therapy is not recommended as a primary modality because of inconvenient routes of administration, frequent office visits, and the association between its use and a high frequency of systemic adverse effects.

Because of the shortcomings associated with all available treatments, some clinics use combination therapy (i.e., the simultaneous use of two or more modalities on the same wart at the same time).

Recommended Regimens for Cervical Warts

For women who have exophytic cervical warts, high-grade SIL must be excluded before treatment is initiated. Management of exophytic cervical warts should include consultation with a specialist.

Recommended Regimens for Vaginal Warts

- Cryotherapy with liquid nitrogen. The use of a cryoprobe in the vagina is not recommended because of the risk for vaginal perforation and fistula formation. **OR**
- 80 to 90% TCA or BCA applied to warts. A small amount should be applied only to warts and allowed to dry, at which time a white "frosting" develops. If

an excess amount of acid is applied, the treated area should be powdered with talc, sodium bicarbonate, or liquid soap preparations to remove unreacted acid. This treatment can be repeated weekly, if necessary

Recommended Regimens for Urethral Meatus Warts

- Cryotherapy with liquid nitrogen **OR**
- 10 to 25% podophyllin in compound tincture of benzoin. The treatment area must be dry before contact with normal mucosa. This treatment can be repeated weekly, if necessary. The safety of podophyllin during pregnancy has not been established

Although data evaluating the use of podofilox and imiquimod for the treatment of distal meatal warts are limited, some specialists recommend their use in some patients.

Recommended Regimens for Anal Warts

- Cryotherapy with liquid nitrogen **OR**
- 80 to 90% TCA or BCA applied to warts. A small amount should be applied only to warts and allowed to dry, at which time a white "frosting" develops. If an excess amount of acid is applied, the treated area should be powdered with talc, sodium bicarbonate, or liquid soap preparations to remove unreacted acid. This treatment can be repeated weekly, if necessary **OR**
- Surgical removal

Warts on the rectal mucosa should be managed in consultation with a specialist. Many persons with warts on the anal mucosa also have warts on the rectal mucosa, so persons with anal warts can benefit from an inspection of the rectal mucosa by digital examination or anoscopy.

Counseling Genital HPV Infection

Attempts should be made to convey the following key messages:

- Genital HPV infection is common among sexually active adults. The majority of sexually active adults will have it at some point in their lives
- Genital HPV infection is usually sexually transmitted. The incubation period (i.e., the interval between initial exposure and established infection or disease) is variable, and determining the timing and source of infection is frequently difficult
- No recommended uses of the HPV test to diagnose HPV infection in sex partners have been established. HPV infection is commonly transmitted to partners but usually goes away on its own

Management of Sex Partners

Examination of sex partners is not necessary for the management of genital warts.

Special Considerations

Pregnancy

Imiquimod, podophyllin, and podofilox should not be used during pregnancy. However, because genital warts can proliferate and become friable during pregnancy, many specialists advocate their removal during pregnancy. HPV types 6 and 11 can cause respiratory papillomatosis in infants and children. The route of transmission (i.e., transplacental, perinatal, or postnatal) is not completely understood. Whether cesarean section prevents respiratory papillomatosis in infants and children is unclear; therefore, cesarean delivery should not be performed solely to prevent transmission of HPV infection to the newborn.

HIV Infection

No data suggest that treatment modalities for external genital warts should be different in the setting of HIV-infection. Squamous cell carcinomas arising in or resembling genital warts might occur more frequently among immunosuppressed persons, therefore, requiring biopsy for confirmation of diagnosis.

Cervical Cancer Screening for Women Who Attend STD Clinics or Have a History of STDs

Women with a history of STDs might be at increased risk for cervical cancer, and should receive cervical cancer screening according to current guidelines. The American Cancer Society and American College of Obstetricians and Gynecologists guidelines recommend annual screening for women aged 21 to 30 years and then every 2 to 3 years for women aged older than 30 years if three consecutive annual Papanicolaou tests are negative.

Vaccine Preventable STDs

Some STDs can be effectively prevented through preexposure vaccination. Every person being evaluated or treated for an STD, who is not already vaccinated, should receive HBV vaccination. In addition, some persons (e.g., MSM and illegal drug users) should receive HAV vaccination.

Hepatitis A

HAV has an incubation period of approximately 28 days (range, 15–50 days). HAV is shed in high concentrations in feces from 2 weeks before to 1 week after the onset of clinical illness. It does cause chronic infection or chronic liver disease, although 10 to 15% of patients might experience a relapse of symptoms during the 6 months after acute illness. Acute liver failure from HAV is rare (overall case fatality rate, 0.5%). The risk for symptomatic infection is directly related to age, with >80% of adults having symptoms compatible with acute viral hepatitis and the majority of children having either asymptomatic or unrecognized infection. Antibody produced in response to HAV infection persists for life and confers protection against reinfection.

Diagnosis

The presence of IgM antibody to HAV is diagnostic of acute HAV infection.

Treatment

Patients with acute hepatitis A usually require only supportive care, with no restrictions in diet or activity.

Prevention

Two products are available for the prevention of HAV infection: HAV vaccine and immune globulin (Ig) for intramuscular administration. When administered intramuscularly before, or within 2 weeks after, exposure to HAV, Ig is >85% effective in preventing HAV infections.

Preexposure Immunization

Persons in the following groups should be offered HAV vaccine: 1) all MSM; 2) illegal drug users (both injecting and noninjecting drugs); and 3) persons with chronic liver disease.

Prevaccination Serologic Testing for Susceptibility

Approximately one third of the US population has serologic evidence of previous HAV infection, which increases directly with age and reaches 75% among persons aged older than 70 years. Screening for HAV infection might be cost-effective in populations in which the prevalence of infection is likely to be high (e.g., persons aged >40 years and persons born in areas of high HAV endemicity).

Postvaccination Serologic Testing

Postvaccination serologic testing is not indicated.

Postexposure Prophylaxis

Previously unvaccinated persons exposed to HAV (e.g., through household or sexual contact or by sharing illegal drugs with a person who has hepatitis A) should be administered a single intramuscular dose of Ig (0.02 ml/kg) as soon as possible but not longer than 2 weeks after exposure. Persons who have had one dose of HAV vaccine at least 1 month before exposure to HAV do not need Ig. If HAV vaccine is recommended for a person receiving Ig, it can be administered simultaneously at a separate anatomic injection site.

Hepatitis B

The incubation period from the time of exposure to onset of symptoms is 6 weeks to 6 months. HBV is efficiently transmitted by percutaneous or mucous membrane exposure to infectious blood or body fluids that contain blood.

All unvaccinated adults seeking services for STDs should be assumed to be at risk for HBV and should receive HBV vaccination.

Diagnosis

The presence of IgM antibody to HBV core antigen (HBc; IgM anti-HBc) is diagnostic of acute or recently acquired HBV infection. Antibody to HBV surface antigen (HBsAg; anti-HBs) is produced after a resolved infection and is the only HBV antibody marker present after immunization. The presence of HBsAg and total anti-HBc, with a negative test for IgM anti-HBc, indicates chronic HBV infection. The presence of anti-HBc alone might indicate a false-positive result or acute, resolved, or chronic infection.

Treatment

No specific therapy is available for persons with acute hepatitis B; treatment is supportive. For evaluation, persons with chronic HBV infection should be referred to a physician experienced in the management of chronic liver disease. Therapeutic agents approved by FDA for treatment of chronic hepatitis B can achieve sustained suppression of HBV replication and remission of liver disease in some persons. In addition, patients with chronic hepatitis B might benefit from screening to detect hepatocellular carcinoma (HCC) at an early stage.

Prevention

Two products have been approved for HBV prevention: HBV Ig (HBIG) and HBV vaccine. HBIG provides temporary (i.e., 3–6 months) protection from HBV infection and is typically used as postexposure prophylaxis (PEP) either as an adjunct to HBV vaccination in previously unvaccinated persons or alone in persons who have not responded to vaccination. The recommended dose of HBIG is 0.06 ml/kg.(see Table 9.1).

For details of vaccination, see approved adolescent and adult schedules.

In adolescents and healthy adults aged younger than 40 years, approximately 30 to 55% acquire a protective antibody response (anti-HBs >10 mIU/ml) after the first vaccine dose, 75% after the second, and >90% after the third.

Postexposure Prophylaxis

Both passive-active PEP with HBIG and HBV vaccination and active PEP with HBV vaccination alone have been demonstrated to be highly effective in preventing transmission after exposure to HBV. HBIG alone also has been demonstrated to be effective in preventing HBV transmission, but, with the availability of HBV vaccine, HBIG typically is used as an adjunct to vaccination.

Table 9.1 Interpretation of serologic test results for HBV infection

Serologic marker				
HBsAg	Total anti-HBc	IgM anti-HBc	Anti-HBs	Interpretation
−	−	−	−	Never infected
+[a]	−	−	−	Early acute infection; transient (up to 18 days) after vaccination
+	+	+	−	Acute infection
−	+	+	−	Acute resolving infection
−	+	−	+	Recovered from previous infection and immune
+	+	−	−	Chronic infection
−	+	−	−	False-positive (i.e., susceptible); previous infection; low-level chronic infection,[b] passive transfer to infant born to HBsAg-positive mother
−	−	−	+	Immune if concentration is >10 mIU/ml; passive transfer after HBIG administration

[a] To ensure that an HBsAg-positive test result is not a false positive, samples with repeatedly reactive HBsAg results should be tested with a licensed (and, if appropriate, neutralizing confirmatory) test.

[b] Persons positive for only anti-HBc are unlikely to be infectious except under unusual circumstances involving direct percutaneous exposure to large quantities of blood (e.g., blood transfusion and organ transplantation).

Exposure to HBsAg-Positive Source

Unvaccinated persons or persons known not to have responded to a complete HBV vaccine series should receive both HBIG and hepatitis vaccine as soon as possible (preferably <24 hours) after a discrete, identifiable exposure to blood or body fluids that contain blood from an HBsAg-positive source. See current recommendations for HBV for details.

Hepatitis C

Hepatitis C virus (HCV) infection is the most common chronic bloodborne infection in the United States. Although HCV is not efficiently transmitted sexually, persons at risk for infection through injection drug use might seek care in STD treatment facilities, HIV counseling and testing facilities, correctional facilities, drug treatment facilities, and other public health settings where STD and HIV prevention and control services are available. See Hepatitis C guidelines for details.

Proctitis, Proctocolitis, and Enteritis

Sexually transmitted gastrointestinal syndromes include proctitis, proctocolitis, and enteritis. Evaluation for these syndromes should include appropriate diagnostic procedures (e.g., anoscopy or sigmoidoscopy, stool examination, and culture).

Proctitis is inflammation of the rectum (i.e., the distal 10–12 cm) that might be associated with anorectal pain, tenesmus, or rectal discharge. *N. gonorrhoeae, C. trachomatis* (including LGV serovars), *T. pallidum*, and HSV are the most common sexually transmitted pathogens involved. In patients co-infected with HIV, herpes proctitis might be especially severe. Proctitis occurs predominantly among persons who participate in receptive anal intercourse.

When outbreaks of gastrointestinal illness occur among social or sexual networks of MSM, clinicians should consider sexual transmission as a mode of spread and provide counseling accordingly. Diagnostic and treatment recommendations for all enteric infections are beyond the scope of these guidelines.

Treatment

Acute proctitis of recent onset among persons who have recently practiced receptive anal intercourse is usually sexually acquired. Such patients should be examined by anoscopy and should be evaluated for infection with HSV, *N. gonorrhoeae, C. trachomatis*, and *T. pallidum*. If an anorectal exudate is detected on examination or if polymorphonuclear leukocytes are detected on a Gram-stained smear of anorectal secretions, the following therapy may be prescribed while awaiting additional laboratory tests.

Recommended Regimen

- 125 mg ceftriaxone intramuscularly (or another agent effective against rectal and genital gonorrhea) **PLUS**
- 100 mg doxycycline orally twice a day for 7 days

Patients with suspected or documented herpes proctitis should be managed in the same manner as those with genital herpes (see "Genital HSV Infections").

Ectoparasitic Infections

Pediculosis Pubis

Recommended Regimens

- 1% permethrin cream rinse applied to affected areas and washed off after 10 minutes **OR**
- Pyrethrins with piperonyl butoxide applied to the affected area and washed off after 10 minutes

Alternative Regimens

- 0.5% Malathion lotion applied for 8 to 12 hours and washed off **OR**
- 250 μg/kg ivermectin, repeated in 2 weeks

Reported resistance to pediculicides has been increasing and is widespread. Malathion may be used when treatment failure is thought to have occurred because of resistance. The odor and long duration of application for Malathion make it a less attractive alternative than the recommended pediculicides. Ivermectin has been successfully used to treat lice but has only been evaluated in small studies.

Lindane is not recommended as first-line therapy because of toxicity.

Other Management Considerations

The recommended regimens should not be applied to the eyes. Pediculosis of the eyelashes should be treated by applying occlusive ophthalmic ointment to the eyelid margins twice a day for 10 days. Bedding and clothing should be decontaminated (i.e., machine-washed, machine-dried using the heat cycle, or dry cleaned) or removed from body contact for at least 72 hours. Fumigation of living areas is not necessary.

Follow-Up

Patients should be evaluated after 1 week if symptoms persist. Retreatment might be necessary if lice are found or if eggs are observed at the hair–skin junction. Patients who do not respond to one of the recommended regimens should be retreated with an alternative regimen.

Special Considerations

Pregnancy

Pregnant and lactating women should be treated with either permethrin or pyrethrins with piperonyl butoxide; lindane is contraindicated in pregnancy.

Scabies

Recommended Regimen

- 5% permethrin cream applied to all areas of the body from the neck down and washed off after 8 to 14 hours **OR**
- 200 µg/kg ivermectin orally, repeated in 2 weeks

Alternative Regimens

- 1 oz lindane (1%) lotion or 30 g of cream applied in a thin layer to all areas of the body from the neck down and thoroughly washed off after 8 hours

  Permethrin is effective and safe and less expensive than ivermectin.

Other Management Considerations

Bedding and clothing should be decontaminated (i.e., either machine-washed, machine-dried using the hot cycle, or dry cleaned) or removed from body contact for at least 72 hours. Fumigation of living areas is unnecessary.

Crusted Scabies

Crusted scabies (i.e., Norwegian scabies) is an aggressive infestation that usually occurs in immunodeficient, debilitated, or malnourished persons. Crusted scabies is associated with greater transmissibility than scabies. Substantial treatment failure might occur with a single topical scabicide or with oral ivermectin treatment.

Some specialists recommend combined treatment with a topical scabicide and oral ivermectin or repeated treatments with 200 µg/kg ivermectin on days 1, 15, and 29.

Follow-Up

Patients should be informed that the rash and pruritus of scabies might persist for up to 2 weeks after treatment.

Management of Sex Partners and Household Contacts

Both sexual and close personal or household contacts within the preceding month should be examined and treated.

Management of Outbreaks in Communities, Nursing Homes, and Other Institutional Settings

Scabies epidemics frequently occur in nursing homes, hospitals, residential facilities, and other communities. Control of an epidemic can only be achieved by treatment of the entire population at risk. Ivermectin can be considered in this setting, especially if treatment with topical scabicides fails.

Special Considerations

Infants, Young Children, and Pregnant or Lactating Women

Infants, young children, and pregnant or lactating women can be treated with permethrin.

Ivermectin is not recommended for pregnant or lactating patients. The safety of ivermectin in children who weigh < 15 kg has not been determined.

Sexual Assault and STDs

Adults and Adolescents

The recommendations in this report are limited to the identification, prophylaxis, and treatment of sexually transmitted infections and conditions commonly identified in the management of such infections. The documentation of findings, collection of specimens for forensic purposes, and the management of potential pregnancy or physical and psychological trauma are beyond the scope of this report.

Trichomoniasis, BV, gonorrhea, and chlamydial infection are the most frequently diagnosed infections among women who have been sexually assaulted. Because the prevalence of these infections is high among sexually active women, their presence after an assault does not necessarily signify acquisition during the assault.

See the full guidelines for further information on Sexual Assault or Abuse of Children.

Evaluation for Sexually Transmitted Infections
Initial Examination

An initial examination should include the following procedures:

- Testing for *N. gonorrhoeae* and *C. trachomatis* from specimens collected from any sites of penetration or attempted penetration
- Culture or FDA-cleared NAAT for either *N. gonorrhoeae* or *C. trachomatis*. NAATs offer the advantage of increased sensitivity in detection of *C. trachomatis*
- Wet mount and culture of a vaginal swab specimen for *T. vaginalis* infection. If vaginal discharge, malodor, or itching is evident, the wet mount also should be examined for evidence of BV and candidiasis
- Collection of a serum sample for immediate evaluation for HIV, HBV, and syphilis

Follow-Up Examinations

After the initial postassault examination, follow-up examinations provide an opportunity to 1) detect new infections acquired during or after the assault; 2) complete HBV immunization, if indicated; 3) complete counseling and treatment for other STDs; and 4) monitor side effects and adherence to postexposure prophylactic medication, if prescribed.

Examination for STDs should be repeated within 1 to 2 weeks of the assault. Because infectious agents acquired through assault might not have produced sufficient concentrations of organisms to result in positive test results at the initial examination, testing should be repeated during the follow-up visit, unless prophylactic treatment was provided. Serologic tests for syphilis and HIV infection should be repeated 6 weeks, 3 months, and 6 months after the assault, if the initial test results were negative.

Prophylaxis

Many specialists recommend routine preventive therapy after a sexual assault because follow-up of survivors of sexual assault can be difficult. The following prophylactic regimen is suggested as preventive therapy:

- Postexposure HBV vaccination, without HBIG. HBV vaccination should be administered to sexual assault victims at the time of the initial examination if they have not been previously vaccinated. Follow-up doses of vaccine should be administered 1 to 2, and 4 to 6 months after the first dose
- An empiric antimicrobial regimen for chlamydia, gonorrhea, trichomonas, and BV
- Emergency contraception should be offered if the assault could result in pregnancy in the survivor

Recommended Regimens

- 125 mg ceftriaxone intramuscularly in a single dose **PLUS**
- 2 g metronidazole orally in a single dose **PLUS**
- 1 g azithromycin orally in a single dose **OR** 100 mg doxycycline orally twice a day for 7 days

For patients requiring alternative treatments, refer to the sections in this report relevant to the specific agent. Providers might also consider antiemetic medications, particularly if emergency contraception also is provided.

Risk for Acquiring HIV Infection

HIV seroconversion has occurred in persons whose only known risk factor was sexual assault or sexual abuse, but the frequency of this occurrence is probably low. In consensual sex, the risk for HIV transmission from vaginal intercourse is 0.1 to 0.2% and for receptive rectal intercourse is 0.5 to 3%. The risk for HIV transmission from oral sex is substantially lower. Specific circumstances of an assault might increase risk for HIV transmission (e.g., trauma, including bleeding) with vaginal, anal, or oral penetration; site of exposure to ejaculate; viral load in ejaculate; and the presence of an STD or genital lesions in the assailant or survivor.

Although a definitive statement of benefit cannot be made regarding PEP after sexual assault, the possibility of HIV exposure from the assault should be assessed at the time of the postassault examination. The possible benefit of PEP in preventing HIV infection also should be discussed with the assault survivor if risk exists for HIV exposure from the assault. If PEP is offered, the following information should be discussed with the patient: 1) the unproven benefit and known toxicities of antiretrovirals; 2) the close follow-up that will be necessary; 3) the benefit of adherence to recommended dosing; and 4) the necessity of early initiation of PEP to optimize potential benefits (as soon as possible after rand up to 72 hours after the assault). Specialist consultation on PEP regimens is recommended if HIV exposure during the assault was possible and if PEP is being considered (for more details see CDC. Antiretroviral postexposure prophylaxis after sexual, injection-drug use, or other nonoccupational exposure to HIV in the United States. Recommendations from the U.S. Department of Health and Human Services. MMWR 2005; 54:[No. RR-2]).

Bibliography

Workowski KA, Berman SM. Sexually transmitted diseases treatment guidelines, 2006; MMWR
    Recommendations and Reports August 4, 2006;55:RR-11.
CDC. Update to CDC's *STD Treatment Guidelines, 2006*: Fluoroquinolones no longer recom-
    mended for treatment of gonococcal infections. MMWR April 13, 2007;56(14):332–336.
CDC. Antiretroviral postexposure prophylaxis after sexual, injection-drug use, or other nonoccu-
    pational exposure to HIV in the United States. Recommendations from the U.S. Department
    of Health and Human Services. MMWR 2005;54:(No. RR-2).

Chapter 10
Human Immunodeficiency Virus

Rosemary Harris

Introduction

In 1981 a cluster of *Pneumocystis carinii* (now *jiroveci*) pneumonia (PCP) and Kaposi's sarcoma seen in gay male Californians was recognized as a syndrome related to profound immunosuppression, ultimately named acquired immune deficiency syndrome (AIDS). Twenty-five years later, the human immunodeficiency virus (HIV) is responsible for a devastating global pandemic, already killing 25 million people and infecting 40 million. Heterosexual transmission is now the most common mode of infection worldwide. The AIDS epidemic ushered in a new era of medical response to an unfolding disease, forcing society to confront sexuality issues and highlighting the vast disparity in resources.

HIV infection began as a primate retrovirus that crossed over to human hosts. Direct exposure to infected bodily fluids is the only means of transmission. The largest amounts of infective virus are in blood, followed by semen, vaginal secretions, and breast milk. Saliva, tears, sweat, and urine have minimal virus and are not considered infectious unless contaminated by blood. Practices with the highest risk for infection are anal, vaginal, and receptive oral intercourse and needle sharing through intravenous (IV) drug abuse (IVDA) or tattooing. Transmission from mother to child (vertical transmission) can occur at birth or during breast-feeding. Infection can occur from transfusion with infected blood or transplantation of infected body parts. Risk per act is shown in Table 10.1.

More than a million Americans are infected with HIV, and one third of them are undiagnosed. AIDS is now more prevalent among ethnic minorities. Black men who have sex with men (MSM) have a prevalence of 46% with 67% undiagnosed (see Fig. 10.2). Effective treatment has markedly reduced the number of deaths, and HIV infection is now regarded as a chronic disease. The rate of new infections has remained constant, at 20,000 to 40,000 new cases annually, contributing to the increase in patients living with infection. Complacency about the virus and increased drug usage among young gay men is contributing to an increase in new infection.

N.S. Skolnik (ed.), *Essential Infectious Disease Topics for Primary Care.*
© Humana Press, Totowa, NJ

Table 10.1 Risk of infection for a single exposure

Exposure route	Risk per 10,000 exposures to an HIV-infected source
Blood transfusion	9,000
Needle-sharing injection drug use	67
Receptive anal intercourse	50
Percutaneous needle stick	30
Receptive penile–vaginal intercourse	10
Insertive anal intercourse	6.5
Insertive penile–vaginal intercourse	5
Receptive oral intercourse	1
Insertive oral intercourse	0.5

Antiretroviral post-exposure prophylaxis after sexual, injection drug use, or other non-occupational exposures to HIV in the US. MMWR Jan 21, 2005; 54(RR02):1–20.

Pathophysiology

HIV attaches, enters, and then replicates in CD4 "helper" T cells, killing the cells and producing up to a billion virus particles daily during acute infection. Viral numbers are highest during initial infection, kept in check for varying lengths of time, and increase as the immune system fails. "Viral load" is the burden of virus within the bloodstream and is used as a practical marker for infection and to monitor efficacy of treatment. CD4 cells decline from a normal range of 400 to 1,000 in adults as infection progresses, with a concomitant decline in cell-mediated immunity.

Clinical Presentation

Acute retroviral syndrome occurs days to weeks after exposure to the virus and is usually overlooked as a source of illness. Fever, fatigue, maculopapular rash, headache, pharyngitis, and lymphadenopathy are the most common symptoms, last usually for 2 weeks and resolve. Careful history taking, with an eye to high-risk practices for HIV infection, will raise the index of suspicion for HIV. Antibody testing will most often be negative and CD4 counts normal, but viral loads reach detectable amounts within a week or two. Once this phase of the illness resolves, viral replication enters a steady state of infection. Viral loads remain stable, and CD4 cells decline steadily. Most patients remain asymptomatic for an average of 10 years, depending on the virulence of the particular strain. HIV infection is a reportable illness, along with the presence of the opportunistic infections (OIs) that arise with waning immunity. AIDS is diagnosed by the criteria listed in Table 10.3.

OIs and Treatment

As CD4 cells and immunity decline, patients develop OIs. When the CD4 count drops below 500, bacterial pneumonias, recurrent vulvovaginal candidiasis and oral thrush, herpes zoster, Kaposi's sarcoma, cryptosporidiosis, pulmonary tuberculosis

Table 10.2 HIV infections in the USA; total, female, and transmission mode, by race. Tot, total; MSM, male sex with male; IDU, IV drug use; Het, heterosexual; Fem, female

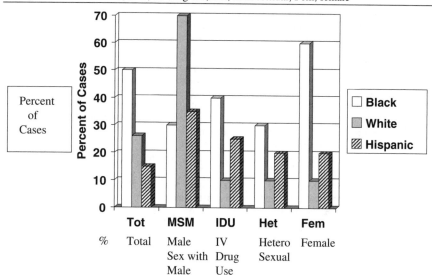

Cases of HIV: infection and AIDS in the United States and dependent areas 2005. Available at http://www.cdc.gov/hiv/topics/surveillance/basic.htm. (Tables 1, 3, and 5b)

(TB), and oral hairy leukoplakia may develop. When the CD4 count is 200 or less, a patient meets the definition of full-blown AIDS. More severe OIs may occur, such as PCP, Candida esophagitis, toxoplasmosis, and extrapulmonary and miliary TB, along with anemia, weight loss, and chronic diarrhea. As the CD4 count drops below 50, the profoundly immunocompromised develop cytomegalovirus (CMV), mycobacterium avium complex/intracellulare (MAC/MAI), significant wasting, and neurological deterioration, and die.

PCP, remains the prototypic OI. It is the primary presenting infection in men, followed by Candida esophagitis and toxoplasmosis. Classic features are a prodrome of weight loss, progressive exertional dyspnea, and fatigue, with a dry cough lasting for weeks. Physical exam is notable for a cachexia, lymphadenopathy, and dry, inspiratory crackles. Chest x-ray (CXR) shows bilateral hilar and interstitial infiltrates. Results from a complete blood cell count (CBC) are normal or even low, and laboratory examinations show increased lactate dehydrogenase (LDH). Treatment is with IV trimethoprim/sulfamethoxisole (TMP)/sulfamethoxazole TMP/(SMX) at 5 mg/kg (as the TMP component) every 8 hours, or orally as 2 TMP/SMX 160/800 (DS) three times daily for 3 weeks, followed by one tablet daily until the CD4 count rebounds to 200 or more with therapy for at least 3 months. Alternate regimens are IV pentamidine or dapsone with trimethhoprim for severe cases while clindamycin plus primaquine or atavaquone can be used in milder cases. Corticosteroids are indicated if the PaO_2 is <70 and should be administered early, at 80 mg of prednisone, tapering by ½ every 5 days.

Table 10.3 Case-defining illness for AIDS

A diagnosis of AIDS is made whenever a person is HIV positive and:
- Has a CD4+ cell count below 200 cells/ml OR
- CD4+ cells account for < 14% of all lymphocytes OR
- Has been diagnosed with one or more of the AIDS-defining illnesses listed below:
  - Candidiasis of bronchi, trachea, lungs, esophagus
  - Cervical cancer, invasive
  - Coccidioidomycosis, disseminated
  - Cryptococcosis, extrapulmonary
  - Cytomegalovirus retinitis or disease (other than liver, spleen, or lymph nodes)
  - Encephalopathy, HIV-related or progressive multifocal leukoencephalopathy
  - Herpes simplex: ulcers for longer than 1 month or bronchitis, pneumonitis, or esophagitis
  - Histoplasmosis, disseminated
  - Isosporiasis or cryptosporidiosis, chronic intestinal (>1 month duration)
  - Kaposi's sarcoma
  - Lymphoma; Burkitt's, immunoblastic, or primary brain/CNS
  - MAC or disease caused by *M. Kansasii*, disseminated
  - Disease caused by *Mycobacterium tuberculosis*, any site (pulmonary or extrapulmonary) or other nontype *Mycobacterium*
  - PCP
  - Pneumonia, recurrent
  - *Salmonella* septicemia, recurrent
  - Toxoplasmosis of brain (encephalitis)
  - Wasting syndrome caused by HIV infection
- Additional illnesses that are AIDS-defining in children, but not adults:
  - Multiple, recurrent bacterial infections
  - Lymphoid interstitial pneumonia/pulmonary lymphoid hyperplasia

CDC. 1993 Revised Classification System for HIV Infection and Expanded Surveillance Case Definition for AIDS Among Adolescents and Adults. MMWR Dec 18, 1992; 41(RR 17).

Candida esophagitis is the presenting OI in 19% of women versus only 9% of men. Although 77% of patients with thrush will have some degree of esophagitis, only 40% of those with esophagitis will have symptomatic thrush. Candida esophagitis is characterized by odynophagia, dysphagia, and retrosternal pain, with a sticking sensation while eating. Diagnosis is by endoscopic confirmation and biopsy, or the less specific and lower yield barium swallow showing cobblestoning and irregularity. Treatment is with fluconazole in dosages up to 400 mg or itraconazole. Oral treatments, such as miconazole suspension or pastilles for thrush are not effective for esophagitis. Oral thrush can manifest as the classic patchy white exudates or a hyperemic form with significant glossitis. HIV testing is indicated for all patients with Candida esophagitis and extensive or recurrent oral thrush in the absence of risk factors for thrush, such as diabetes and antibiotic treatment.

Cryptococcal meningitis and central nervous system (CNS) toxoplasmosis develop as CD4 counts drop below 100. Cryptococcal meningitis presents as an indolent change in mental status, headache, and vague neurological complaints without focality. Cerebrospinal fluid (CSF) examination shows budding yeast forms and will be positive for cryptococcal antigen. India ink staining is no longer indicated. Treatment is with IV amphotericin combined with flucytosine for 2 weeks followed by flluconazole 400 mg daily for 8 weeks; patients require prophylactic fluconazole at 200 mg daily pending helper cell rebound >200 with ART. Mortality for cryptococcal meningitis is at least 10% even with treatment, relapse rates are high and neurologic outcomes are unpredictable and these patients should be transferred to a tertiary care center. Toxoplasmosis can have a similar presentation, but with focal neurological findings and seizures. CT scanning will show the classic "ring-enhancing lesion," often multiple, considered pathognomonic for CNS toxoplasmosis but seen also in neoplasms and inflammation. Treatment is pyrimethamine with leucovorin plus either sulfadiazine or clindamycin, for 6 weeks, progress is monitored radiographically; secondary prophylaxis with trimethoprim/sulfamethoxisole is given until CD4 rebounds above 200 with ART. Steroids can be used short term for vasogenic edema if needed; anticonvulsants can be discontinued if lesions resolve.

With profound immunosuppression (CD4 count below 50), CMV, MAC/MAI, and cryptosporidium may develop. CMV is usually gastrointestinal or ocular and is treated with IV ganciclovir, valgangcyclovir or foscarnet. MAC/MAI is an atypical mycobacterium that causes gastrointestinal (GI) and constitutional symptoms. Diagnosis is through blood culture or even bone marrow or tissue aspirate; treatment is with azithromycin or clairthromycin with ethambutol. Cryptosporidium causes a chronic diarrhea with weight loss, steatorrhea, and crampy abdominal pain; treatment is effective antiretroviral therapy (ART).

HIV infection can alter the presentation of other infectious processes, causing a more aggressive and harder to treat condition. Herpes zoster in HIV patients can involve several dermatomes and be disseminated. Herpes antivirals are administered in much higher doses, with acyclovir at 800 mg four times daily for outbreaks and 800 twice daily for prophylaxis.

Testing for syphilis by Rapid Plasma Reagin (RPR) with VDRL confirmation of positives should be done on all patients newly diagnosed with HIV, with any intercurrent sexually transmitted disease (STD), and in sex workers and those who trade sex for drugs. Syphilis in HIV patients progresses more rapidly; neurosyphilis is more common. CDC recommendations for treatment are 2.4 million U of benzathine penicillin G intramuscularly (IM) once for early syphilis. CSF examination for neurosyphilis with Venereal Disease Research Laboratory test (VDRL) on CSF should be done for all patients with late latent or disease of unknown latency. If the results of the CSF VDRL are negative, IM benzathine penicillin G 2.4 million units is given weekly for 3 weeks. If the patient has neurosyphilis with a positive CSF VDRL result, then procaine penicillin G 2.4 million units is administered IM daily for 14 days with oral probenecid 500 four times daily or intravenous aqueous penicillin G at 3–4 million U is administered every 4 hours for 10–14 days. Follow-up RPR testing should be done at 3, 6, 9, 12, and 24 months to document at least a fourfold drop in titer. HIV patients often never return to baseline; re-infection is diagnosed by a fourfold increase in baseline titer. Neurosyphilis patients undergo repeat CSF exam at 3 and 6 months or biannually until CSF VDRL normalizes. ID consultation is advised for all patients with neurosyphilis or tertiary disease.

Chancroid, genital herpes, and HPV are more frequent and aggressive in HIV patients. Genital warts can be massive and multiple, involving the entire perineal and anal area. Pelvic inflammatory disease in HIV-positive women may take longer to resolve, and tuboovarian abscess is a more common sequelae.

Reactivation of latent TB can occur as CD4 counts decline, and active TB is an AIDS-defining illness. Miliary TB and extrapulmonary TB of bones (Pott's disease), kidney, bladder, and epididymitis all may occur. Annual PPD testing is recommended for all HIV patients, and treatment of a positive PPD reaction is extended. Treatment of active TB in conjunction with ART can require adjustment of medication because of significant drug–drug interactions, and immune reconstitution syndrome can occur with TB.

HIV itself causes significant damage. Chronic infection and active viremia is debilitating, with weight loss, anorexia, malaise, and chronic diarrhea. The virus is neurotropic and can cause peripheral sensory neuropathy, muscle pain, and atrophy along with severe neuropathic pain. Advanced disease is associated with cognitive decline and dementia. Unexplained CNS decline in young adults should prompt HIV testing. Progressive multifocal leukoencephalopathy (PML) can be seen in advanced disease but is much less common with the advent of ART. Cancer is more common, especially lymphomas and anal cancer from HPV.

Differential Diagnosis

The differential diagnosis of acute retroviral syndrome includes infections that cause fever, fatigue, headache, pharyngitis, rash, and lymphadenopathy, such as Epstein-Barr virus, *Streptococcus* sp. influenza, and Lyme disease.

HIV Testing and Laboratory Studies

The indications for HIV testing have recently been broadened. The 2006 CDC guidelines now advocate HIV screening of any patient in a healthcare setting—regardless of risk—ages 13 to 64 years, as part of routine health maintenance. HIV testing is routine for all pregnant women and recommended to be offered regularly to patients with high-risk behavior history, "injection-drug users and their sex partners, persons who exchange sex for money or drugs, sex partners of HIV-infected persons, and MSM or heterosexual persons who themselves or whose sex partners have had more than one sex partner since their most recent HIV test." Other high-risk individuals are those on methadone maintenance, users of cocaine, crack, and crystal methamphetamine, those with multiple sexual partners, commercial sex workers, patients presenting with any new STD, those with newly diagnosed hepatitis B or C or active TB, and those individuals who may have received a blood transfusion, injection, or surgery in areas of high HIV prevalence or transfusion in the USA before 1985. HIV testing should also be considered for any young adult with pneumonia, herpes zoster involving several dermatomes, severe and extensive HPV or molluscum, and extensive oral hairy leukoplakia noticed on oral examination. To make HIV testing more a part of routine health care, recommendations now state that patients should be should be informed either orally or in writing that HIV testing is being performed and that they have the option not to have the testing performed, but no special consent is needed—termed opt-out screening.

HIV testing requires confirmatory testing for all positive results. Initial enzyme-linked immunosorbent assay (ELISA) tests are confirmed, either by duplicate ELISA,

Western blot, or nucleic acid amplification tests. There are now reasonable, rapid tests for urine, cheek swabs, and fingerstick blood, some of which are available for patients to use themselves. Rapid testing is useful for women in labor for whom HIV status is unknown, STD clinics in high-prevalence areas when follow-up is less likely, and for testing index cases to determine postexposure prophylaxis (PEP), such as occupational exposures to body fluids and rape victims. Consent and counseling should be obtained whenever feasible, but should not be an impediment to testing. Seroconversion to positive antibody status will occur within 3 weeks to 3 months of exposure. Negative test results within that time should be followed up at 3 months for confirmation. Passive maternal antibody transfer persists up to 18 months of life.

Virologic tests are used to quantify amount of virus in blood. Tests are polymerase chain reaction (PCR)-based double-stranded DNA (dsDNA) or RNA, and require frozen specimens. Thresholds of viral detectability vary from <20 to 500. They are used to detect newborn or recently acquired infection and to assess indication for, response to, and failure of ART.

Absolute CD4 counts are standard tests for staging illness, deciding when to start therapy, and measuring immune rebound or deterioration. CD4 fluctuates widely under normal circumstances and will temporarily decrease with vaccinations and intercurrent illnesses. The normal range for infants and children is nearly twice that for adults.

Laboratory studies to order for a new patient include absolute CD4 count and HIV viral load/quantitative PCR. Additionally, CBC, chemistry panel with LFTs, RPR, Hepatitis A, B, and C, and a Toxo IgG titer, along with fasting cholesterol and blood glucose, and PPD placement—repeated annually—are done.

Treatment of HIV Infection

ART to reduce viral burden is effective and halts disease progression, but it is not curative. The goal is to interrupt viral replication and reduce circulating virus to undetectable levels, increasing CD4 cells. Guidelines for initiating therapy advise treatment if there has been an AIDS-defining infection or when the CD4 count is less than 350 mm^3 CD4 cells and for pregnant women, those with HIV-associated nephropathy, and those infected with and undergoing treatment for Hepatitis B irrespective of the CD4 cell count. Evidence shows that at these values immune functioning is not severely impaired and can be reconstituted while delaying the cost and side effects of treatment until absolutely necessary. Treatment may also be advisable in patients with CD4 > 350 who have a rapid decline in cells (> 120 per year) or viral loads in excess of 100,000 copies per ml. The CD4 threshold for treatment has changed over the years and will continue to evolve (Table 10.4).

Continued suppression of viral load and CD4 stability is monitored quarterly. If viral replication occurs on medication with a decline in CD4 cells, then a regimen is failing and should be changed.

Table 10.4 lists antiretroviral medication currently available in the USA. ART is always a minimum three-drug regimen or "cocktail." Two of these are the nucleotide reverse transcriptase inhibitors (zidovudine, didanosine, zalcitabine, stavudine,

Table 10.4 Guidelines for Starting Therapy in HIV Infection, Dec 1, 2007

Clinical Condition/CD4 Cell Count	Recommendations
History of AIDS-defining illness (AI)	Initiate therapy
CD4 count <200 cells/mm³ (AI)	Initiate therapy
CD4 count 22 – 350 cells mm³ (AII)	Initiate therapy
Pregnant women (AI)	Initiate therapy
Those with HIV-associated nephropathy (AI)	Initiate therapy
Those treating for Hepatitis B coinfection (AI)	Initiate therapy
CD4 count > 350 cells/mm³	Defer therapy

Guidelines for the Use of Antiretroviral Agents in HIV - 1 Adults and Adolescents, Department of Health and Human Services, Dec 1, 2007.

Category	Definition
Rating Scheme for Treatment Recommendations	
A	Both strong evidence for efficacy and substantial clinical benefit support recommendations for use. Should always be recommended.
B	Moderate evidence for efficacy - or strong evidence for efficacy but only limited clinical benefit–support recommendation for use. Should generally be recommended.
C	Moderate evidence for efficacy is insufficient to support a recommendation for or against use. Or evidence for efficacy might not outweigh adverse consequences (e.g. drug toxicity, drug interactions) or cost of the treatment under consideration. Optional.
D	Moderate evidence for lack of efficacy or for adverse outcome supports a recommendation against use. Should generally not be offered.
E	Good evidence for l ack of efficacy or for adverse outcome supports a recommendation against use. Should never be offered.
Quality of evidence supporting the recommendation	
I.	Evidence from at least one properly designed randomized, controlled trial.
II.	Evidence from at least one well-designed clinical trial without randomization, from cohort or case-controlled analytic studies (preferably from more than one center), or from multiple time-series studies. Or dramatic results from uncontrolled experiments.
III.	Evidence from opinions of respected, authorities based on clinical experience, descriptive studies or reports of expert committees.

lamivudine, emtricitabine, abacavir, and tenofovir). A third drug from either the nonnucleotide reverse transcriptase inhibitors (efavirenz, nevirapine, delavirdine) or protease inhibitor class (saquinavir, ritonavir, indinavir, nelfinavir, lopinavir/riton, fosamprenavir, atazanavir, tipranivir, and darunavir) is then added, often using a low dose of ritonavir in conjunction with the first protease inhibitor to increase drug levels and prolong half-life. The primary protease inhibitor is the active ingredient, ritonavir serving as the "booster". Four separate medications are used, three of them constituting the active regimen. The nonnucleotide reverse transcriptase inhibitors and protease inhibitors can be combined. Newer classes of drugs includ-

Table 10.5 Antiviral medication available in the USA in 2007, with adult dosing

Nucleotide/side reverse transcriptase inhibitors (NRTI)	Nonnucleotide reverse transcriptase inhibitors (NNRTI)	Protease inhibitors (PI)
Zidovudine (AZT, Retrovir®) Nausea, macrocytosis 300 mg twice daily $149(generic)	Efavirenz (EFV, Sustiva®) Rash, CNS disturbances, Teratogen 600 mg daily $553	Saquinavir (SAQ, Invirase) GI intolerance 1,000 mg SAQ/100 mg RTV twice daily $869
Didanosine (DDI, Videx® EC) Neuropathy, wasting, pancreatitis 400 mg daily $320	Nevirapine (NVP, Viramune®) Rash, liver failure, lactic acidosis 200 mg twice daily/400 mg daily $479	Ritonavir (RTV, Norvir®) Poorly tolerated, drug–drug interactions 100 mg daily or twice daily, booster medicine $320
Zalcitabine (DDC, Hivid®) Pancreatitis, wasting, not used $267	Delaviridine (DLV, Rescriptor®) Rarely used 400 mg three times daily/600 mg twice daily $311	Indinivir (IND, Crixivan®) Nephrolithiasis, LFT increase 800 mg IND/100 mg RTV twice daily $577
Stavudine (D4T, Zerit®) Neuropathy, wasting 30 or 40 mg twice daily $409		Nelfinavir (NFV, Viracept®) Diarrhea > 40% 1,250 mg twice daily $760
Lamivudine (3TC, Epivir®) Well-tolerated 300 mg daily $411	**Combination Medications**	Lopinavir/riton (LPV/r, Kaletra®) GI intolerance, nausea, $759 200 mg LPV/50 mg RTV, 4 daily/2 twice daily
Emtricitabine (FTC, Emtriva®) Well tolerated 200 mg daily $384	Zidovudine/lamivudine (Combivir®) See components 300 mg AZT/150 mg 3TC twice daily $811	Fosamprenavir (FOS, Lexiva®) Rash, GI intolerance 1,400 mg daily with 200 mg RTV $659
Abacavir (ABC, Ziagen®) Hypersensitivity reaction 600 mg daily $523	Emtricitabine/Tenofovir (Truvada®) See components 200 mg FTC/300 mg TNV daily $900	Atazanavir (ATV, Reyataz®) Jaundice, PR prolong, no PPI 300 mg daily/100 mg RTV with TNV 400 mg daily without TNV $892
	Lamivudine/abacavir (Epzicom®) See components 300 mg 3TC/600 mg ABC daily $813	

(continued)

Table 10.5 (continued)

Nucleotide/side reverse transcriptase inhibitors (NRTI)	Nonnucleotide reverse transcriptase inhibitors (NNRTI)	Protease inhibitors (PI)
Tenofovir (TNV, Viread®) Renal insufficiency, nausea, 300 mg daily $610	Zidov/lamiv/abacavir (Trizivir®) See components, $1,361 300 mg AZT/150 mg 3TC/300 mg ABC twice daily	Tipranivir (TPV, Aptivus®) Rash, hepatotoxic, refrigerate 500 mg twice daily/200 mg RTV $1,117
	Emtricitabine/tenofovir/efavirenz (Atripla®) See components $1,150 200 mg FTC/300 mg TNV/600 mg EFV daily $1,577	Darunavir (DRV, Prezista®) GI intolerance 600 mg twice daily/100 mg RTV $969

Fusion Inhibitor

Enfuvirtide (T-20, Fuzeon®)
Injected, mix daily, site reactions 90 mg SQ twice daily $2,844

Entry Inhibitors

Maraviroc (Selzentry®)
CCR5 trophic virus only (special testing)
Liver abnormalities. 300 bid $1,500/month

Integrase Inhibitor
Raltegravir (Isentress®)
Headache/fever 400 bid $800

Retail prices for 30 days of therapy. LFT, liver function test; PR, ; PPI, ; SQ, subcutaneous (Guidelines for the Use of Antiretroviral Agents in HIV-1 Infected Adults and Adolescents DHHS Dec 1, 2007).

ing fusion, entry integrase inhibitors are now available but should only be used in treatment-experienced patients with expert consultation (Table 10.5).

Initial starting regimens have been recommended by numerous societies and are similar. Preferred regimens to initiate therapy are well tolerated, suppress virus for many years, and increase CD4 counts if adherence is maintained. The nonnucleotide-based regimen is 600 mg efavirenz daily plus 300 mg lamivudine **or** 200 mg emtricitabine daily plus 300 mg zidovudine twice daily **or** 300 mg tenofovir daily; a combination emtricitabine plus tenofovir plus efavirenz allows for one pill daily, marketed as Atripla™. Recommended protease inhibitor–based regimens for once-daily dosing all involve boosted ritonavir and the combination emtricitabine plus tenofovir, marketed as Truvada™. Numerous other regimens are detailed on www.aidsinfo.nih.gov. Regimens to avoid are mononucleotide or dual nucleotide therapy, triple nucleotide regimens in naïve patients, stavudine with zidovudine, zalcitabine, or didanosine; lamivudine with emtricitabine; efavirenz in the first trimester of pregnancy and nelfinavir during pregnancy.

Highly active ART (HAART) carries significant risk and serious side effects, there are numerous black box warnings. All HIV medications can cause liver abnormalities, hepatic damage with nevirapine occurs in 4% of all patients and up to 11% of women. Lactic acidosis is seen with stavudine, didanosine, and zidovudine; and pancreatitis is seen with didanosine and stavudine. Skin rash occurs with nonnucleotides, nevirapine more than efavirenz, and can include Stevens–Johnson syndrome and toxic epidermal necrolysis. Abacavir has an HLAB5701-related systemic hypersensitivity reaction in 2 to 7% of patients, which can be fatal on rechallenge. Indinavir is associated with nephrolithiasis, especially when boosted with ritonavir. Zidovudine is a bone marrow suppressant with obligatory macrocytosis. Ritonavir is tolerable at the lower doses used to boost drug levels for most of the protease class, but not as a solo protease inhibitor. It is responsible for many of the drug–drug interactions that plague ART. Long-term protease inhibitor complications include hyperlipidemia with increased cardiovascular risk, insulin resistance, diabetes, osteonecrosis, and a fat redistribution syndrome known as lipodystrophy.

GI intolerance is seen with zidovudine, didanosine, and all protease inhibitors, especially ritonavir. Peripheral neuropathy occurs with stavudine, didanosine, and zalcitabine, and can be painful and debilitating. Older nucleotides, especially stavudine, cause facial wasting, which, along with lipodystrophy, is extremely distressing to patients. African American patients report skin pigment changes. Initial efavirenz treatment has CNS side effects in 50% of patients. Notable drug–drug interactions are protease inhibitors—especially ritonavir—with lovastatin, simvastatin, rifampin, midazolam, triazolam, ergots, and some cardiac medications. Protease inhibitors are linked to hyperlipidemia and glucose intolerance. Many of the nucleotides require dosing adjustments for renal insufficiency, whereas protease inhibitors require adjustments for hepatic insufficiency.

Prophylactic treatment against OI is indicated for patients with low CD4 counts started on ART. CD4 counts < 200 require TMP/SMX DS daily to prevent PCP and CD4 counts < 50 require a macrolide, such as 1 g azithromycin weekly as prophylaxis against MAC/MAI. Daily fluconazole can be offered for those with severe esophagitis or thrush, and daily acyclovir for those with severe recurrent herpes. Once CD4 counts rebound for 3 months, prophylactic therapy can be stopped. Immune reconstitution syndrome, a paradoxical worsening, can occur with certain

OIs, especially CMV and TB, as rebounding CD4 cells generate immune response and does not represent treatment failure.

Suppression of viral replication depends on consistent levels of HAART. Treatment failure is directly connected to poor adherence. Inadequate drug levels from nonadherence increases selection pressure for mutations and causes resistance. Regimens lose effectiveness; the virus rebounds, and CD4 cells decline. Adherence to complicated and poorly tolerated therapy rife with side effects and complications is one of the most significant issues for patients and providers.

Development of Resistance and Treatment Failure

Effective therapy will suppress viral load to undetectable levels with an average CD4 cell increase of 150 cells within the first year; this can persist for many years with preferred regimens and good adherence. Viral load testing after 4 to 8 weeks of therapy should show a reduction in virus by one half to three quarters, and, by 6 months on therapy, be undetectable. Testing should be performed at least biannually to monitor viral suppression and CD4 stability, more often if a regimen is new or failing. Any time virus rebounds and/or CD4 cells decline, the regimen is losing effectiveness, most likely from development of resistance. Adherence issues should be addressed and CD4 count and viral load repeated. Side effects and toxicities necessitate modification of at least one drug in many patients. Occasional "blips" of viral detectability up to 1,000 copies/ml can occur and do not warrant changing a regimen if not reproducible. Failure to suppress virus to undetectable levels necessitates changing to another regimen and should be anticipated.

Resistance testing to check for specific mutations is used to guide therapy in changing regimens. It should be ordered for all failing regimens while on the medications or within 4 weeks of stopping, during pregnancy, and at the time of diagnosis. Genotypic testing to look for specific viral mutations that confer resistance is standard and requires careful analysis. Phenotypic analysis is more costly and time consuming but gives dose-specific information regarding resistance patterns. A computer-generated virtual phenotype test is available that translates genotype information into phenotypic patterns. Treatment-experienced patients can be expected to have multiple resistance mutations to complicate the choice of therapy.

Changing a failing regimen should involve substituting at least two active drugs by resistance testing, within new or different classes, if possible (Table 10.6). Adding a fourth drug to a failing regimen or changing only one of the components is not advised and fosters resistance. Successive treatment regimens are invariably less convenient for patients and involve administration that is more frequent. In patients with highly resistant virus, it may be impossible to fully suppress viral load to undetectable levels in which case, reduction in virus to the lowest possible levels remains the goal of treatment.

Effective ART has transformed HIV infection into a chronic disease. Life expectancies on medication approach normal. In addition to regular health care, patients require at

Table 10.6 Recommended regimens to start therapy (one choice from each column)

Column A		Column B
NNRTI or PI		NRTI backbone, 2 drugs
NNRTI	**PI**	
Efavirenz	Atazanavir/ritonavir	Tenofovir + emtricitabine
Lopinavir/ritonavir twice daily	Fosamprenavir/ritonavir (BID)	**OR**
		Zidovudine + lamivudine

Once-daily regimens for starting a patient on therapy:
1 pill Coformulated efavirenz/tenofovir/emtricitabine Atripla™:
600 mg efavirenz/300 mg tenofovir/200 mg emtricitabine
3 pills atazanavir + ritonavir + coformulated tenofovir/emtricitabine
(Truvada™) 300 mg atazanavir + 100 mg ritonavir + Truvada™
5 pills lopinavir/ritonavir + coformulated tenofovir/emtricitabine
Kaletra™ (200 mg lopinavir/50 mg ritonavir) 4 pills + Truvada™

5 pills fosamprenavir + ritonavir + coformulated tenofovir/emtric-
itabine 700 mg fosamprenavir 2 pills + 100 mg ritonavir 2 pills +
Truvada™

Twice-daily regimens for the bottom two options are preferable in terms of side effects and trough
levels of drug but outweighed by the convenience and increased adherence of once-daily regimens
in most patients (Guidelines for the use of antiretroviral drugs in HIV-infected adults and adolescents. Department of Health and Human Services. Dec 1, 2007).

least biannual visits to monitor CD4 count and viral load, and assess the long-term side
effects of therapy. Immunizations for HIV patients are Pneumovax at the time of
diagnosis, meningococcal, yearly influenza, hepatitis A and B updating, and regularly
scheduled tetanus boosters. HPV vaccine is advised for female patients and may be
considered for gay males. Oral poliovirus vaccine, varicella, and smallpox vaccine
should be avoided in all HIV patients; and measles, mumps, rubella vaccine avoided if
the CD4 count is <200 cells. Women require Papanicolaou testing annually, and atypical squamous cells of undetermined significance (ASCUS) requires immediate colposcopy. Gay males require annual rectal Papanicolaou testing.

Pregnancy in the HIV-Positive Patient

Virtual elimination of vertical transmission is the biggest success of HAART. HIV
infection is no longer a contraindication to child bearing; transmission is
25 to 33% without therapy, 10% with perinatal zidovudine, and <2% with zidovudine and C-section. Perinatology and Infectious Disease specialists should be
involved whenever possible. All HIV-positive pregnant women should be treated
with ART. Resistance assays should be done when pregnancy is initially diagnosed,
unless the woman is on a maximally suppressive regimen, i.e., viral load <1,000 CD4
cells/mm. Women who do not require treatment for their own health based on current recommendations (i.e., CD4 > 350) should be offered triple-drug therapy after
the first trimester. Women on suppressive regimens with no detectable viremia

should continue unless it contains efavirenz or nevirapine, in which case a ritona-vir-boosted protease should be substituted. Zidovudine monotherapy after 14 weeks is no longer recommended but may be considered in women with viral loads < 1,000 who are opposed to triple therapy. Zidovudine is administered IV to all HIV-positive women before delivery, starting with a 2 mg/kg bolus followed by infusion at 1 mg/kg/hr, along with continuation of any oral medications. All neo-nates born to HIV-positive mothers receive 2 mg/kg zidovudine orally every 6 hours for the first 6 weeks of life with dosing adjustments in prematurity. This is the only indication for monotherapy. At the time of rupture of membranes, 200 mg nevirapine with a 2 mg/kg nevirapine single dose for the infant is used in resource-poor settings.

ART should generally be avoided during the first trimester if it is not required for the mothers' health; efavirenz is pregnancy category D, a known teratogen and nevirapine is now avoided during pregnancy due to increased risk for hepatotoxicity. Women plan-ning to become pregnant should avoid these two as components of ART until childbear-ing is finished. Women who require treatment for infection and subsequently become pregnant should be treated with ART promptly, with resistance testing to guide optimal therapy. Regimens of 300 mg zidovudine twice daily and 300 mg lamivudine, and with either saquinavir 1,000 mg/rit 100 twice daily or the use of coformulated lopinavir/rito-navir 200/50 twice daily (with possible dosage increase during third trimester) have been most widely studied in pregnancy, are well-tolerated and safe. Viral load should be followed at least each trimester and again at 36 weeks in preparation for delivery. Liver function testing is advisable monthly during the last trimester to screen for NRTI-related hepatic dysfunction and possible HELLP(Hemolysis Elevated Liver enzymes and Low Platelets) syndrome development. Women on therapy who become pregnant while on ART should be continued on their present regimen—unless it contains efavi-renz or nevirapine, with modification to include zidovudine if possible, again guided by resistance testing. Women in labor with no previous therapy should receive IV zidovudine as a 2 mg/kg bolus/1 mg/kg infusion, as above.

Elective C-section at 38 weeks with perinatal zidovudine is the most widely used delivery mode in the USA for HIV-positive women. Zidovudine IV is begun 3 hours before surgery. If C-section is not desired or possible, vaginal delivery should be done in a timely fashion; oxytocin augmentation should be considered. Artificial or prolonged rupture of membranes, invasive monitoring, forceps, and vacuum extraction are avoided to reduce fetal exposure to maternal blood; methergine vasoconstriction is exagerated by proteases and efavirenz and its use should be minimized or avoided unless absolutely necessary. C-section after rup-ture of membranes offers no reduced infection benefit to the baby. If the viral load is < 1,000, transmission rates are low even for vaginal delivery. Breastfeeding is associated with up to 40% vertical transmission and is contraindicated.

Care of Infants and HIV-Positive Children

Routine HIV testing of all pregnant women will identify infants exposed to HIV in utero. Rapid HIV testing should be available for all laboring women with unknown HIV status. Postnatal 2 mg/kg zidovudine should be given to all infants whose mothers test positive as soon as possible and then every 6 hours. Infants of women who refuse HIV testing, have high-risk behavior practices, or evidence of illicit injection drug use by UDS, and those who are abandoned or in state custody should be considered at high risk for HIV exposure and treated with zidovudine while undergoing testing. HIV antibody testing in infants will not diagnose infection until 18 months of age because of passive maternal antibody transfer. Viral load is used for diagnosis; frozen PCR-RNA testing will be positive in 40% of infected infants at 2 days and 99% at 1 month.

Exposed infants should be viral load tested by 48 hours, 14 days, 1 to 2 months, and again at 3 to 6 months. Two negative virologic tests after 1 month exclude infection if the second test is done after 4 months. Two or more negative HIV antibody tests 1 month apart after 6 months of age also prove the infant is not infected. Persistent positive HIV antibody tests should be followed up to document loss of maternal antibody until the infant is 18 months old. If persistent by then, the child is infected. A single negative HIV IgG antibody test on a child older than 6 months of age when the antibody status of the mother is unknown, such as with foreign-born adoptees, is sufficient to exclude infection.

Staging and progression of disease in infants and young children is very different from adults. CD4 counts are two to three times higher in infants and decline to adult ranges at approximately age 5 years, with similarly elevated viral loads. Disease progression is fastest in the first year of life, with more than 15% developing AIDS or dying and 50% showing significant immunosuppression. Prophylactic daily TMP/SMX should be started in infants who show evidence of infection very early because they will have the fastest rate of progression. Infected infants younger than 6 months are treated with triple therapy. Older infants are followed closely and treated if they show significant immunosuppression or develop AIDS. A pediatric HIV specialist should manage these children because of the dosing difficulties. Primary care physicians should be aware of the medication regimen and side effects and vigilant about adherence issues with families and caregivers. HIV-infected infants and children have a higher rate of bacterial infections and bacteremia, and the threshold for antibiotics will be lower.

Postexposure Prophylaxis

Universal precautions in all patient encounters remain the standard of care and have greatly reduced occupational HIV exposures for all health care workers. The risk of HIV is 0.3% for percutaneous exposure and 0.09% for mucous membrane exposure. There have been no reported cases of occupational transmission from human bites or a source patient in the window of antibody formation. PEP with antiretroviral medication is recommended as soon as practical, preferably within 2 hours. To date, there have only been six health care professionals infected despite PEP, the last one infected in 2001.

Risk of transmission is proportional to amount of blood exposure; other fluids have lower risk, which increases if the fluid is bloody. Exposures to large amounts of blood, i.e., visible contamination, placing a hollow-bore needle directly into a vein or artery, and deep injuries carry the highest risk. Less risk of infection is conferred from closed and suture needles, mucous membrane "splash" exposure, and contact with vaginal secretions or semen. Healthcare workers should report to the closest facility, usually an emergency department, as soon as they become aware of an exposure, whenever possible.

If the source patient of unknown HIV status is available, testing should be done for HIV, with consent if possible. With a known HIV-positive source patient, viral load and resistance testing can be performed to further guide treatment. Table 10.7 shows recommendations for PEP ART choices. Expert consultation is advised for unknown source exposures, >24-hour delay in reporting, breastfeeding or pregnancy, known resistance of source virus, toxicity from PEP regimen, and extremely high-risk exposures. Patients should be followed up in 3 to 5 days to assess adherence and offer further emotional support.

Non-occupational exposures to HIV include victims of sexual assault or abuse—especially those with mucosal trauma or anal intercourse, unprotected homosexual intercourse, heterosexual HIV discordant couples, and needle sharing. PEP with ART as described above is advised only for high-risk exposures presenting within 72 hours, as depicted in Fig. 10.2. HIV antibody testing is done initially and symptoms of acute retroviral syndrome should be reviewed.

Table 10.7 Changing a failing regimen

Regimen class	Initial regimen	Recommended change with evidence level
NNRTI	2 NRTIs + NNRTI	2 NRTIs (based on resistance testing) + PI (±ritonavir boost) (AII)
PI	2 NRTIs + PI (±ritonavir boost)	2 NRTIs (based on resistance testing) + NNRTI (AII)
		2 NRTIs (based on resistance testing) + alternative PI (±ritonavir boost, based on resistance testing) (AII)
		NRTI (based on resistance testing) + NNRTI + Alternative PI (+ritonavir boost, based on resistance testing) (AII)
3 NRTI	3 nucleosides	2 NRTIs (based on resistance testing) + NNRTI **or** PI (±ritonavir boost) (AII)
		NRTI(s) (based on resistance testing) + NNRTI + PI (±ritonavir boost) (CII)
		NNRTI + PI (±ritonavir boost) (CIII)

Guidelines for the Use of Antiretroviral Agents in HIV-1 Infected Adults and Adolescents October 10, 2006 DHHS.

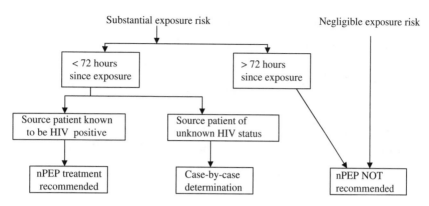

Fig. 10.1 Algorithm for treatment of possible non-occupational HIV exposures.

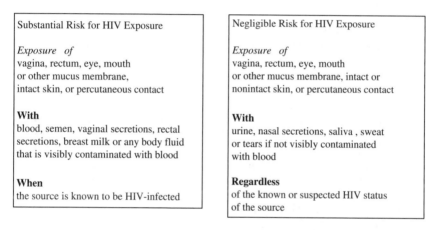

Fig. 10.2 Antiretroviral post-exposure prophylaxis after sexual, injection drug use or other non-occupational exposure to HIV in the United States. MMWR Jan 21, 2005; p 10.

The patient should get medical follow-up within 3 to 5 days for support and to assess adherence with further HIV antibody testing at 4 to 6 weeks, and 3 and 6 months. Bites, fights, community needlestick injuries, and playground incidents have minimal risk of infection unless there is significant blood exposure to a known HIV-positive individual, and the risks of PEP far outweigh any theoretical benefit in these situations.

Table 10.8 Exposure type and recommended prophylaxis

	Source Status	Regimen
Severe—higher risk for infection		
Involves exposure to blood/bloody fluids; semen, vaginal secretions, and pericardial, spinal, peritoneal, synovial, pleural, and amniotic fluids are all potentially infectious		
Percutaneous—Hollow-bore needle/deep/vein/art	Any HIV+ patient	3 drugs Atripla daily*
Percutaneous—Closed/suture needle/superficial	Sick HIV patient AIDS/VL >1,500	3 drugs As above
Mucous membrane/nonintact skin	Sick HIV patient AIDS/VL >1,500	3 drugs As above
Large volume blood splash/bloody fluid/semen/vaginal secretions. Concentrated virus in laboratory		
Non-occupational exposure—blood	Known HIV+	3 drugs If <72 hours
Rape victim—mucosal/anal trauma Unintended exposure—needle/sexual		
Fight/bite with significant trauma		
Non-occupational exposure—blood Rape victim—mucosal/anal trauma Unintended exposure-needle/sexual	Source status: ???	3 Drugs: ??? If <72 hours Individual basis Consider
Less severe—low risk for infection		
Percutaneous—Closed/suture needle/superficial	HIV + not sick Asymptomatic/VL <1,500	2 drugs Combivir twice daily Truvada daily
Mucous membrane/nonintact skin		
Large volume blood splash	HIV + not sick	2 drugs as above
Small volume blood/few drops	Sick HIV patient	2 drugs as above
Small volume blood/few drops	HIV+ not sick	2 drugs: optional
Any percutaneous exposure or large volume mucus membrane type	Source status: ???	2 drugs: optional if source with risk factors
Any percutaneous exposure or large volume mucus membrane type	Source is unknown Sharps disposal Major blood splash	2 drugs: optional if a setting with exposure to HIV+ patients
Minor—negligible risk of infection		
Small volume—few drops	Source status: ??? Source is unknown	PEP not indicated
Any occupational exposure	Source is HIV−	PEP not indicated
Any non-occupational exposure	>72 hours	PEP not indicated
Any exposure to nonbloody urine, saliva, sweat, tears, nasal secretions, vomitus, stool, or sputum	Any time	PEP not indicated

*Three-drug Atripla™, 1 pill daily is most convenient, other regimens are listed in Table 10.5 or can be found in the guidelines. (Antiretroviral post-exposure prophylaxis after sexual, injection drug use, or other non-occupational exposures to HIV in the US. MMWR Jan 21, 2005; 54(RR02):1–20).

Special Situations

Active TB warrants aggressive treatment in HIV-positive individuals, temporary modification of the ART regimen may be necessary because of drug–drug interactions, and reconstitution syndrome can occur; see CDC guidelines for treatment. Hepatitis C co-infection is common because of overlapping risk factors and will progress more rapidly; treatment times may be longer. ART therapy is now a risk factor for atherosclerotic disease. Addiction, psychiatric conditions, and chaotic social circumstances complicate the lives of many HIV patients and make adherence difficult. Primary care physicians are often their only source of treatment, know their comorbidities well, and are ideally suited to manage HIV infection as part of the entire care of the patient.

Resources for Consultation

Occupational and non-occupational exposure questions: PEPline; www.ucsf.edu/hivcntr/Hotlines/ PEPline; 1-888-448-4911.
Pregnancy in HIV patients: HIV Antiretroviral Pregnancy Registry; www.apregistry.com/index. htm; 1-800-258-4263.
HIV/AIDS treatment information: http://aidsinfo.nih.gov.

Bibliography

Panel on Antiretroviral Guidelines for Adults and Adolescents. Guidelines for the use of antiretroviral drugs in HIV-infected adults and adolescents. Department of Health and Human Services. Dec 1, 2007. Available at: http://www.aidsinfo.nih.gov//Contentfiles/AdultandAdolescentsGL. pdf.
Working Group on Antiretroviral Therapy and Medical Management of HIV-infected Children. Guidelines for the Use of Antiretroviral Agents in Pediatric HIV Infection. Oct 26, 2006; 1–126. Available at: http://www.aidsinfo.nih.gov/Contentfiles/PediatricGuidelines.pdf.
Perinatal HIV Guidelines Working Group.
Public Health Service Task Force Recommendations for the Use of Antiretroviral Drugs in Pregnant HIV-1 Infected Women for Maternal Health and Interventions to Reduce Perinatal HIV Transmission in the United States. Nov 2, 2007; 1–101. Available at: http://www.aidsinfo. nih.gov/Contentfiles/PerinatalGL/pdf.
Treating Opportunistic Infections Among HIV-1 Infected Adults and Adolescents. Recommendations from the CDC, the National Institutes of Health and the HIV Medicine

Association/Infectious Disease Society of America. December 17, 2004;1–135. Available at: http://www.aidsinfo.nih.gov/contentfiles/TreatmentofOI_AA.pdf.

2002 USPHS/ISDA Guidelines for Preventing Opportunistic Infections in Persons Infected with Human Immunodeficiency Virus. US Public Health Service and Infectious Disease Society of America guidelines for the prevention of opportunistic infections in persons infected with HIV. June 28, 2002;1–55. Accessed at: http://www.aidsinfo.nih.gov/Contentfiles/OipreventionGL/pdf.

Updated US Public Health Service Guidelines for the Management of Occupational Exposures to HIV and Recommendations for Post-Exposure Prophylaxis. MMWR Sept 30, 2005;54 (RR09):1–17.

Antiretroviral post-exposure prophylaxis after sexual, injection drug use, or other non-occupational exposures to HIV in the US. MMWR Jan 21, 2005;54(RR02):1–20.

Cases of HIV infection and AIDS in the United States and dependent areas 2005. Available at http://www.cdc.gov/hiv/topics/surveillance/basic.htm.

1993 Revised Classification System for HIV Infection and Expanded Surveillance Case Definition for AIDS Among Adolescents and Adults. MMWR Dec 18, 1992;41(RR 17). Available at: http://www.cdc.gov/mmwr/preview/mmwrhtml/00018871.htm. Guidelines for the use of anti-retroviral drugs in HIV-infected adults and adolescents. Department of Health and Human services. Dec 1, 2007.

Part IV
Skin, Bone, and Joint Infection

Chapter 11
Cellulitis and Skin Infections Associated with Bites

Steven Zinn and Judith A. O'Donnell

Introduction

Skin and soft tissue infections (SSTI) are common in primary care, representing 2 to 3% of all office visits. Although these infections can usually be accurately diagnosed and effectively treated, physicians must be capable of identifying the signs and symptoms of the various SSTI, along with differentiating them from the noninfectious conditions with a similar clinical presentation. It is important to accurately and efficiently identify invasive SSTI, such as necrotizing fasciitis or pyomyositis, which require management that is more aggressive.

Cellulitis and Erysipelas

Cellulitis is an acute, painful, spreading erythematous infection involving the dermis and subcutaneous tissues, with poorly demarcated borders. Erysipelas is a superficial skin infection usually limited to the upper dermis and lymphatics most commonly caused by Group A *Streptococcus*, and characterized by intense erythema and edema with a clearly demarcated, indurated border.

Pathophysiology

Intact skin in a normal host is generally impervious to infection. The skin is protected from infection by an active, intact immune system and the antimicrobial properties of the fatty acid layer. Many conditions, however, can compromise these defenses and allow for the introduction of potential pathogens and subsequent development of infection. Although cellulitis can occur in patients with apparently normal, intact skin, it is most common when there has been a breech of the skin in association with trauma, dermatitis, insect bites, tinea infections, chronic ulcers, or surgery. The hair follicle and periungual areas are frequent sites for invasion and

N.S. Skolnik (ed.), *Essential Infectious Disease Topics for Primary Care.*
© Humana Press, Totowa, NJ

proliferation of bacteria. The interdigital spaces, especially in patients with tinea pedis, are a common entry point for pathogens causing cellulitis in the lower extremity. Edema, poor hygiene, and excessive moisture and occlusion as occurs in body folds, also increase the risk for SSTI. Chronic arm lymphedema often presents after breast cancer surgery and may put a woman at risk for cellulitis of the upper extremity. Cellulitis infrequently occurs as a result of a primary bacteremia. Osteomyelitis may rarely cause a cellulitis in the overlying skin.

Bacteriology

Most cases of cellulitis are caused by Group A streptococci, other hemolytic streptococci, or *Staphylococcus aureus*. *S. aureus* is often the pathogen in the setting of illicit injection drug use, concomitant abscess formation, and in bullous impetigo. Many other pathogens can be implicated as the etiologic agents of SSTI in specific epidemiologic settings or in certain patient populations. Some of these pathogens are listed in Table 11.1.

Diabetic foot infections, which are discussed in a separate chapter, always involve multiple pathogens, including aerobic gram-negative bacilli and anaerobes in addition to the common gram-positive bacteria. Human and animal bites, reviewed in the next section, may be infected with either the oral flora of the biter and/or the skin flora of the victim. Lyme disease, which is caused by *Borrelia burgdorferi*, presents in its early stage with clinical manifestations that may be confused with cellulitis. Early Lyme disease may present with the bright red, circular, bull's eye, or target lesions of erythema migrans at the primary site of inoculation, and, in early disseminated Lyme disease, the patient will have secondary areas of skin involvement distant from the tick bite. Lyme disease is discussed in detail in its own chapter.

Methicillin-resistant *S. aureus* (MRSA) infections have been common in hospital settings for years, and MRSA has traditionally been considered a nosocomial pathogen. In contrast, most community-acquired staphylococcal infections have traditionally been caused by methicillin-susceptible *S. aureus* (MSSA), which are susceptible to semisynthetic penicillins, cephalosporins, and macrolides. Recently, novel community-acquired MRSA strains (CA-MRSA) have emerged as an important health issue. The CA-MRSA strains are distinct from the hospital-acquired MRSA strains, and have different virulence factors. Initial reports of community outbreaks of SSTI caused by CA-MRSA were first reported in children, athletes in contact sports, gay men, prisoners, and Native Americans. In many communities, CA-MRSA has now become the predominant *S. aureus* isolate and is a frequent pathogen in SSTI, even in patients without the traditionally reported risk factors for MRSA. These CA-MRSA infections continue to be reported commonly in children and young adults, though they are seen across the spectrum of age.

Table 11.1 Specific pathogens for skin structure infections in special settings

Pathogen	Epidemiologic risk factors	Clinical presentation	Treatment	Comment
Haemophilus influenzae type b	Infants and children between 1 and 24 months	Buccal cellulitis Fever, upper respiratory tract symptoms, and blue-purple discoloration of involved skin; patients often bacteremic	Ceftriaxone 1–2 g daily	Immunization with the conjugated *H. influenzae* vaccine has made this disease very uncommon
Group A β hemolytic streptococci (GABHS)	Children	Perianal cellulitis associated with pruritus, anal fissures, and erythema	40 mg/kg amoxicillin daily	
Vibrio vulnificus and other *Vibrio* spp.	Contact with salt water or brackish water, with trauma to skin, specifically along the Gulf coast of the United States; or skin contact with raw contaminated seafood	Cellulitis with hemorrhagic bullae; in patients with liver disease this infection can lead to bacteremia and sepsis, or necrotizing fasciitis	200 mg doxycycline intravenously initially, then 100–200 mg/day IV, or cefotaxime or ciprofloxacin	Patients with chronic liver disease should be advised not to eat raw or undercooked seafood
Aeromonas hydrophila	Contact with fresh waters, injury occurring while in fresh water; leech therapy	Cellulitis or infected wounds after local trauma while in fresh water	400 mg ciprofloxacin IV every 12 h, or ceftazidime + gentamicin	
Erysipelothrix rhusiopathiae	Fish handlers, butchers		500 mg amoxicillin every 8 h orally	
Borrelia burgdorferi	Contact with infected deer ticks	Erythema migrans	See Chap. 5	

Most CA-MRSA isolates contain genes encoding the Panton-Valentine leukocidin (PVL) toxin, which is a cytotoxin that causes leukocyte and tissue destruction. Currently, most CA-MRSA isolates are sensitive to tetracyclines, trimethoprim–sulfamethoxazole, vancomycin, linezolid, and daptomycin. Clindamycin susceptibility is more variable, because of the presence of inducible resistance mechanisms in some of these strains. The fluoroquinolones (ciprofloxacin, levofloxacin, gatifloxacin, or moxifloxacin), although often reported out by the standard laboratory tests as sensitive to MRSA isolates, should not be used in the treatment of such infections because there may be a rapid emergence of resistance during treatment when this class of antimicrobial is prescribed (Moellering 2006).

Clinical Appearance and Differential Diagnosis

Cellulitis presents as an acute, often rapidly spreading, area of poorly demarcated erythema, warmth, and edema. Regional lymphadenopathy is common in cellulitis, whereas lymphangitis occurs occasionally and then usually in association with infection caused by Group A β hemolytic streptococci (GABHS). Cellulitis involves the deeper dermis and subcutaneous tissues. Bullae, ecchymoses, petechiae, and local abscess formation may all be a part of the clinical signs of cellulitis.

Erysipelas is a more superficial infection than cellulitis, involving the upper dermis and lymphatics, and is characterized by its well-demarcated borders. Edema is prominent in erysipelas, because of lymphatic blockade, and may take weeks to completely resolve. The classic clinical finding in erysipelas is the edematous skin with a dimpled "peau d'orange" appearance in the involved area. Erysipelas is caused by B-hemolytic streptococci, most often GABHS, and less commonly caused by Groups B, C, or G streptococci. It is frequently seen in infants, young children, and the elderly, but can affect anyone with predisposing risk factors, such as diabetes, alcoholism, and chronic edema. The most common site for erysipelas used to be the face, but now it is most often diagnosed in the lower extremity. It is most likely to occur at sites of preexisting chronic edema. Lymphatic obstruction is a part of erysipelas and, as such, can lead to increased risk of recurrent infection.

Cellulitis and erysipelas may be associated with only mild systemic manifestations, or with high fever, chills, and, less commonly, systemic toxicity or sepsis.

Invasive SSTI

Physicians must be able distinguish typical cases of cellulitis from more serious infections invading fascial or muscle compartments. Patients with invasive infections are generally systemically ill, often toxic or septic, and always require hospitalization; further diagnostic imaging, including computed tomography (CT) scanning or magnetic resonance imaging (MRI); along with a multidisciplinary approach to management, including surgical and infectious disease consultations is warranted.

Although the initial presentation may be similar to typical cellulitis, suspicion of invasive infection should be aroused in the presence of *severe pain, rapid spread* with *systemic toxicity, skin necrosis* that may be preceded by ecchymosis, *cutaneous anesthesia, edema extending beyond the area of erythema*, or *gas in the soft tissues* on exam or imaging (Stevens 2005). Pain out of proportion to the physical examination findings is one well-described clinical clue to the possible diagnosis of necrotizing fasciitis, and should warrant further imaging and surgical evaluation in the toxic patient.

Necrotizing Fasciitis

In necrotizing fasciitis, the pathogens infect not only the dermis and subcutaneous tissues but also extend to the fascial plane. Once the bacteria infect the fascia, the infection can rapidly progress over hours, because the pathogens elaborate toxins and enzymes that induce rapid local tissue destruction. There are two types of bacteriology seen in patients with necrotizing fasciitis. Some patients will have a polymicrobial infection that includes gram-negative bacilli, anaerobes, streptococci, and possibly *S. aureus*; others will have a monomicrobial infection caused by GABHS.

In 80% of necrotizing fasciitis cases, the infection is an extension from a visible skin lesion, often in patients with diabetes, peripheral vascular, or venous disease. The remaining 20% of patients do not have an overlying skin lesion, and, in these individuals, the diagnosis can be particularly challenging. In these patients, pain out of proportion to physical examination findings can be most helpful. All patients with necrotizing fasciitis will appear toxic; on examination, the involved skin and subcutaneous tissues will feel hard and unyielding, and the underlying fascial planes will not be discernible. Cutaneous anesthesia is an ominous clinical sign, because this indicates vascular and nerve infarction. Patients with necrotizing fasciitis need rapid surgical incision and debridement, which is the cornerstone of appropriate management in these patients. In the operative suite, easy passage of a blunt probe to and through the fascia is diagnostic of fasciitis. Most patients require at least one second-look procedure after their initial incision and debridement. CT scanning of the affected area can be very helpful in confirmation of those cases in which the diagnosis is suspected, but not definitive, at the time of initial presentation.

Pyomyositis

Pyomyositis is a rare form of SSTI, because striated muscle is generally resistant to infection. Patients with pyomyositis have pus, and sometimes frank abscess formation within an individual muscle group, and experience localized tenderness, firmness, and muscle spasm on examination. The diagnosis is usually confirmed by diagnostic imaging, specifically, a CT scan of the involved anatomic site. Pyomyositis is most commonly caused by *S. aureus*, although other pathogens are occasionally implicated in the etiology of this unusual SSTI. Appropriate management includes drainage of all purulent material in conjunction with appropriate antimicrobial therapy.

Noninfectious Conditions with Similar Appearance

Cellulitis is usually a straightforward diagnosis in the majority of patients presenting with acute onset of an erythematous, hot, painful, and swollen area. However, there are times when noninfectious inflammatory conditions may present with a similar appearance, thus, presenting a diagnostic challenge. Physicians may have to consider alternative rheumatologic, dermatologic, or malignant conditions when patients present with atypical features or have minimal or no response to appropriate antibiotic therapy (Falagas 2005).

Contact Dermatitis, Fixed Drug Reaction, Insect Bites, and Stings

Contact dermatitis, fixed drug reaction, insect bites, and stings may present as an area of erythema or a well-demarcated plaque. Clinical history and the presence of pruritus help to distinguish these entities from cellulitis. Insect bites rarely develop into cellulitis.

Stasis Dermatitis

Stasis dermatitis, especially with rapid development of edema of the legs, may cause intense erythema, warmth, and tenderness, as in cellulitis. Bilateral presentation should suggest a noninfectious cause.

Wells Syndrome

Wells syndrome (eosinophilic cellulitis) presents with erythematous, urticarial-like plaques that evolve over several days and may resemble cellulitis.

Sweets Syndrome

Sweets syndrome is a steroid responsive dermatosis sometimes associated with malignancy and characterized by acute, tender erythematous plaques on the face and with fever and leukocytosis. Its appearance may suggest periorbital cellulitis.

Superficial Thrombophlebitis

Superficial thrombophlebitis will present with erythema and tenderness along a vein that has been catheterized or along a superficial leg vein. It can be identified by the linear nature of the inflammation and the usual presence of a palpable cord. Secondary infection at a catheter site may be suggested by extension of the inflammation beyond the vein.

Deep Venous Thrombosis

Deep venous thrombosis can present with erythema tenderness and swelling of an extremity. Venous Doppler may be necessary to distinguish the condition from cellulitis.

Acute Gouty Arthritis

Acute gouty arthritis is usually recognized by its characteristic joint inflammation in the first metacarpophalangeal joint or knee in a patient with history of gout or recurrent monoarticular inflammatory episodes. Fever, leukocytosis, and extension of erythema beyond the affected joint may be present and can mimic infection. Joint aspiration and identification of urate crystals will confirm the diagnosis, but inserting a needle through an area of suspected cellulitis is not advised.

Carcinoma Erysipelatoides

Carcinoma erysipelatoides (inflammatory carcinoma) is most commonly associated with breast cancer. The infiltration of metastatic cancer into cutaneous lymph vessels results in the appearance of an erythematous plaque on an enlarged breast, usually without fever or leukocytosis. Tissue biopsy confirms the diagnosis. Although rarely misdiagnosed as cellulitis, lymphoma and leukemia may present with erythematous skin manifestations.

Diagnostic Studies

Blood cultures are positive in < 5% of patients with cellulitis. Needle aspiration from involved skin can implicate a pathogen in 5 to 40% of cases, and punch biopsy culture in 20 to 30% of cases. One study demonstrated higher yield with aspiration from the area of maximal inflammation versus from the "leading edge" of infection. Because of low yield, except in the sickest patients, blood cultures generally are not indicated in uncomplicated cellulitis. Culture, particularly to identify resistant staphylococcus, is appropriate when there is abscess material available from an incision and debridement procedure, or when there is spontaneous drainage from a cutaneous lesion or abscess. Local cultures of wounds or abscesses may also be indicated in diabetic and immuno-compromised patients, in those with the specific epidemiologic exposures, and when infection progresses despite antibiotics.

White blood cell count (WBC) elevation is common, but nonspecific. Plain radiographs are indicated when osteomyelitis is suspected, however, MRI is the most sensitive diagnostic imaging study when osteomyelitis is on the differential diagnosis. As noted above, both CT scanning and MRI may confirm invasive infection when necrotizing fasciitis or pyomyositis is suspected.

Treatment

Healthy, nontoxic patients with cellulitis can be treated as outpatients, allowing for close follow-up and hospital admission for nonresponders. Elevation of an involved extremity will reduce edema and aid in healing. If an abscess is present, it must be drained and cultures of pus obtained where possible. Drainage of an abscess may be sufficient therapy in cases where peri-abscess cellulitis is minimal, but antibiotics are usually used.

Antibiotic therapy for cellulitis should be directed at streptococci and *S. aureus*. Additional coverage may be indicated when exposure history or occupation suggests the risk of an unusual organism (see Table 11.1), or in the case of the diabetic patient with a diabetic foot infection or cellulitis. When erysipelas of the lower extremity is the clear diagnosis, it is appropriate to treat with 1 to 2 million U of intravenous (IV) aqueous penicillin every 6 hours. When erysipelas is suspected on the face, antistaphylococcal coverage should also be provided, with vancomycin being used empirically until culture data are available. Treatment for the majority of all other cases of uncomplicated cellulitis in nondiabetic patients should be directed at both streptococcal and staphylococcal pathogens. Nafcillin, oxacillin, and cefazolin are appropriate IV antibiotic choices for patients who require hospitalization; oral dicloxacillin or oral cephalexin are outpatient alternatives. In the penicillin-allergic patient, IV vancomycin or clindamycin is usually prescribed when the patient requires hospitalization; in the outpatient treatment of such patients, oral clindamycin, erythromycin, clarithromycin, minocycline, and doxycycline, may all be used. In patients with possible risk factors for CA-MRSA, or in communities where there is frequent

CA-MRSA circulating, patients who have moderate to severe cellulitis significant enough to require hospitalization should receive vancomycin empirically.

Until very recently, physicians could reliably treat SSTI with first-generation cephalosporins, antistaphylococcal penicillins, erythromycin, or clindamycin. However, the emergence of CA-MRSA has presented new therapeutic challenges to clinicians. Patients with either traditional risk factors for MRSA or new risk factors for CA-MRSA, and who need inpatient management should receive IV vancomycin therapy. In the unusual setting of vancomycin allergy or intolerance to vancomycin, IV linezolid can be prescribed.

CA-MRSA has emerged as a possible pathogen responsible for a variety of SSTI. In a few small cases series, CA-MRSA has been cultured from patients presenting to emergency departments with skin infections, in particular, localized abscesses. Suspicion for CA-MRSA should be particularly high when patients present with SSTI with purulent drainage or frank abscesses. Patients who have recently received recent antibiotic therapy may also be at increased risk for CA-MRSA SSTI. The currently recommended oral treatment for CA-MRSA SSTI is oral trimethoprim–sulfamethoxazole. Alternatives include the tetracyclines, including doxycycline and minocycline, and linezolid. Clindamycin should not be used empirically for the treatment of CA-MRSA because of the potential for resistance. However, if susceptibilities are known, and the organism is sensitive to clindamycin, then this agent may be prescribed. Adequate drainage of abscesses is critical to resolution of these infections, and, in one study, antibiotic therapy had no additional benefit after appropriate incision and drainage had been performed. As noted above, any patient requiring hospitalization for an SSTI with suspected CA-MRSA should receive IV vancomycin.

Anti-MRSA agents should be first-line therapy in communities and settings where resistant staphylococcal infections are common, perhaps in combination with more traditional antistaphylococcal therapy. Physicians need to be cognizant of updated treatment guidelines and local trends in their communities as more is reported about the epidemiology and optimal therapy of this evolving pathogen.

Prevention of Recurrence

There are multifactorial explanations for recurrent SSTI. Some patients suffer from frequent episodes of cellulitis, particularly in a chronically edematous extremity. Controlling edema may reduce the frequency of infection in these individuals. In the subset of patients with recurrent streptococcal cellulitis, or erysipelas, some clinicians prescribe monthly prophylaxis with intramuscular benzathine penicillin G injections of 1.2 million U, or oral therapy with 1 g of oral penicillin V daily or 500 mg of erythromycin daily in the penicillin-allergic patient. In other patients, treating dermatologic conditions that cause maceration or cracking of the skin, in particular, tinea pedis, may be essential to limiting recurrent SSTI. Clinicians should carefully examine all patients who present with lower extremity cellulitis for the presence of tinea pedis, and when it is diagnosed, appropriate antifungal therapy should be prescribed. Individuals with chronic eczema or dermatitis should also have optimal management of these conditions to prevent recurrent cellulitis.

Nasal mupirocin has been used to control MRSA outbreaks in hospital settings. It is also occasionally recommended for monthly use in the subset of outpatients who suffer from recurrent furunculosis or boils, which are usually caused by *S. aureus*. Mupirocin ointment is applied intranasally, and the cream can be applied under fingernails and in the groin. In one study, when nasal mupirocin was applied for 5 days per month in outpatients, there was a reduction in nasal carriage of *S. aureus*, as well as a decrease in recurrent skin infections. Reports of mupirocin resistance in *S. aureus* have been published, in particular, in patients with chronic use of mupirocin, and in the hospital setting. Other management recommendations for prevention of recurrent furuncles include showering with Hibiclens daily for 3 consecutive days followed by three times per week use when showering. Early reports in the CA-MRSA outbreak investigations have suggested that nasal carriage of CA-MRSA may not precede clinical infection, therefore, it is not clear that nasal mupirocin will help reduce CA-MRSA recurrences or spread to family members. Interestingly, there have been reports that household pets may be reservoirs for CA-MRSA.

Skin Infections Associated with Bites

It has been estimated that 2 million mammalian bites occur in the United States annually. Bite wounds represent 1% of ER visits and 30 million dollars in health care costs. Dog bites are most common, representing 80 to 90% of bites, with 5 to 15% of bites inflicted by cats and 3 to 20% by humans.

Physicians caring for these injuries need to consider the microbiology and particular risks associated with the biting animal, the location of the bite, as well as the mechanism of injury. Infections associated with bites reflect both the presence of the usual skin bacteria and the polymicrobial oral flora of the biter.

Dog and Cat Bites

Dog Bites

Dog bites most commonly affect the upper extremity, although small children are at risk for scalp and facial injury. The powerful jaws of dogs can inflict crush injury, puncture wounds, avulsions, tears, and abrasions. Although dog bites do not commonly become infected (2–20%), the edema and inoculation of devitalized tissue can set the stage for serious infection.

Cat Bite

Cat bite injuries reflect the small sharp feline teeth that cause puncture wounds, usually on the hands. These penetrating wounds have a high incidence of infection (80%). Penetration to bone and joint structures may cause closed-space infections, septic tenosynovitis, or osteomyelitis.

Bacteriology

Dozens of aerobic and anaerobic bacteria have been isolated from animal bite infections, with an average of three isolates per wound. *Staphylococcus* spp. and *Streptococcus* spp. are isolated from 40% of dog bite wounds and *Pasteurella* (usually *canus*) species in 25% of cases. Common anaerobes include *Bacteroides* species, *Fusobacterium* spp., *Peptostreptococcus, Prevotella* spp., and *Porphyromonas* spp. Seventy-five percent of cat bites are infected with *Pasteurella multocida*, which can cause a rapidly developing cellulitis.

Capnocytophaga canimorsus is a rare, but potentially fatal, bacterial infection associated with dog bites. Infection usually presents with overwhelming sepsis, rash, cellulitis, and bacteremia. Most cases have been in patients with predisposing conditions, such as splenectomy, alcoholism, steroid therapy, or lymphoma.

Initial Wound Management

Wounds should be thoroughly examined and the involved extremity evaluated for compromise of nerve, vascular or motor function. The risk of infection can be lowered with meticulous attention to wound management principles. The wound should be irrigated with copious normal saline to lower bacterial contamination. Devitalized tissue should be cautiously tissue removed with care not to remove too much tissue in cosmetically sensitive areas.

There is no clear consensus on primary wound closure. Some clinicians recommend primary closure of low-risk, noninfected dog bites. It is generally accepted that infected wounds, those more than 24 hours old, and bite wounds to the hand should *not* be sutured. Wound edge approximation with adhesive closure, with reevaluation after 72 hours for possible secondary closure, may be a reasonable alternative. An attempt should generally be made to suture facial wounds. Complicated wounds, especially of the face, should be evaluated by a plastic surgeon and joint or significant hand injuries should be evaluated by an orthopedic or hand surgeon.

Antibiotics

Although often administered, the benefit of antibiotics in preventing infection has not been clearly established. Prophylactic antibiotics for low-risk, clinically uninfected, superficial dog bites are not recommended. Wounds presenting more than 24 hours after infliction, and with no sign of infection, can also be monitored without antibiotics. Three to 7 days of antibiotics should be given to immunocompromised patients, as well as to all patients with hand and facial wounds, crush or tearing wounds associated with edema and devitalized tissue, or with bites penetrating close to bones. All deep puncture wounds by cats should be treated with antibiotics because of the risk of rapidly progressing infection. Of particular concern are bite wounds involving the small compartments and structures of the hand.

Amoxicillin–clavulanate (500 mg/125 mg three times daily or 875 mg/125 mg twice daily) is considered the first-line choice for both prophylaxis and outpatient treatment of established infection after a dog or cat bite. Amoxicillin–clavulanate effectively covers skin flora and the oral flora of the biting animal, including *Pasteurella* species, gram-positive organisms, and anaerobes. In those patients who have been bitten by a cat and are penicillin allergic, 100 mg doxycycline twice daily or 500 mg cefuroxime axetil every 12 hours are alternative oral antibiotic regimens. Doxycycline should not be prescribed in children. In those patients who have been bitten by a dog and are penicillin allergic, 300 mg clindamycin four times daily plus either a fluoroquinolone (500 mg levofloxacin daily) in adults or trimethoprim–sulfamethoxazole in children may be used. The first-generation cephalosporins, macrolides, and penicillinase-resistant penicillins should not be prescribed for prophylaxis or treatment of infected animal bites, because they have poor activity against *Pasteurella multocida*.

Immunization

Tetanus Vaccination History

Tetanus vaccination history should be documented and immunization updated in the event of a bite wound according to American College of Immunization Practices

(ACIP) recommendations. Tetanus immune globulin and tetanus toxoid should be administered to patients who have had two or fewer primary immunizations. Tetanus toxoid alone can be given to those who have completed a primary immunization series but who have not received a booster for more than 5 years.

Rabies Prophylaxis

Bites from nonprovoked dogs or cats should increase concern of rabies exposure. Animal bites should be reported to the local department of health, which can be consulted regarding rabies risks and protocols. If the animal is not located, or if its owner cannot document vaccination and the animal cannot be reliably monitored for 10 days, then a rabies vaccine series and rabies immune globulin may need to be considered, depending on the local risk of rabies. Local health departments should be consulted to assess the local risk in the biting species.

Human Bites

Bacteriology

Human bites are often more serious than animal bites. Infections are a polymicrobial mix of aerobic and anaerobic oral flora, with an average of five organisms isolated per wound. Streptococci (especially the *viridans streptococci*) are recovered from 80% of wounds. Other common aerobic pathogens in human bites are *S. aureus, Haemophilus* spp., and *Eikenella corrodens*, which is part of the normal human oral flora, and present in 25% of wounds. *E. corrodens* is usually susceptible to penicillin, ampicillin, and quinolones, but resistant to clindamycin and semisynthetic penicillins. Anaerobic pathogens include *Fusobacterium spp.*, *Peptrostreptococci, Prevotella spp.*, and *Porphyromonas spp.* and *Bacteroides spp.* Transmission of herpes simplex virus, hepatitis B virus, or human immunodeficiency virus (HIV) is possible.

Wound Management and Antibiotics

Management, as outlined for animal bites, includes thorough cleansing, irrigation, debridement, and delayed suturing in most nonfacial injuries. All human bite wounds to the hand that occur when the hand was clenched (clenched fist injuries) should have a plain radiograph. *Prophylactic antibiotics should be prescribed for all human bite wounds.* Antibiotic therapy must include coverage for gram-positive organisms, oral anaerobes, and *E. corrodens.* Amoxicilli–clavulanate (875 mg/125 mg twice daily or 500 mg/125 mg three times daily) for 5 days should be prescribed for human bite wound prophylaxis. In the penicillin-allergic adult patient, 300 to 450 mg oral clindamycin four times daily plus a fluoroquinolone such as 500 mg ciprofloxacin twice daily or 500 mg levofloxacin daily should be used. In a pediatric patient with a penicillin allergy, trimethoprim–sulfamethoxazole can be substituted for the fluoroquinolone in this alternative regimen. Clinicians should consider additional prophylactic therapy for victims of human bites by individuals with known infection, or at high risk for, hepatitis B or HIV infection.

A common and particularly serious human bite is the clenched-fist wound or "fight bite" which occurs when a fist strikes another person's face (Clark 2003). Skin penetration by a tooth results in a small laceration on the dorsum of the hand overlying the metacarpophalangeal joint. In 75% of cases, there will be an associated fracture of the metacarpal or phalangeal bones or injury to the extensor tendons or joint capsule. All clenched-fist wounds should be x-rayed to evaluate for fracture, and the wound should be explored for tendon and joint injury. Antibiotic therapy has been shown to markedly reduce the incidence of infection in these high-risk injuries.

Some recommend hospital admission after wound exploration for all patients with clenched-fist injuries, however, reliable patients who can be assured of close follow-up may be considered for outpatient monitoring. Unfortunately, patients often ignore the seemingly minor initial injury and present with an established infection requiring hospitalization and parenteral antibiotics.

When a patient presents with a human bite wound that is already infected at the initial presentation, hospitalization and IV antibiotics are advised. Initial IV therapy with ampicillin–sulbactam (1.5 g/3 g every 6 hours) is the preferred regimen. Cefoxitin and piperacillin–tazobactam are other alternatives. In penicillin-allergic patients, IV clindamycin and a fluoroquinolone, as noted above, can be prescribed.

References and Further Reading

Brook I. "Microbiology and management of human and animal bite wound infections," *Primary Care Clinical Office Practice* 2003;30:25–39.
Clark D. "Common acute hand infections," *American Family Physician* 2003;68:2167–2176.
Deresinski S. "Methicillin-resistant Staphylococcus aureus: An evolutionary, epidemiologic, and therapeutic odyssey," *Clinical Infectious Diseases* 2005;40:562–573.
Elston DM. "Optimal antibacterial treatment of uncomplicated skin and skin structure infections: applying a novel treatment algorithm," *Journal of Drugs in Dermatology* 2005;4.6.
Falagas M, Vergidis PI. "Narrative review: diseases that masquerade as infectious cellulitis," *Annals Internal Medicine* 2005;142:47–55.
Fleisher GT. "The management of bite wounds," *New England Journal of Medicine* 1999;340.
Frazee BW, Lynn J, Charlebois ED, Lambert L, Lowery D, Perdreau-Remington F. "High prevalence of methicillin-resistant Staphylococcus aureus in emergency department skin and soft tissue infections." *Annals of Emergency Medicine* 2005;45:311–320.
Fridken SK. Methicillin-resistant Staphylococcus aureus disease in three communities. *New England Journal of Medicine* 2005;352:1436–1444.

Griego RD, et al. "Dog, cat, and human bites: A review," *American Academy of Dermatology* 1995;33:1019–1029.

Moellering R. "The growing menace of methicillin-resistant *Staphylococcus aureus*," *Annals of Internal Medicine* 144(2006):368–369.

Morgan M. "Review: Hospital management of animal and human bites," *Journal of Hospital Infection* 61(2005):1–10

Presutti J. "Prevention and treatment of dog bites," *American Family Physician* 2001;63:1567–1574.

Stevens DL, et al. "Practice guidelines for the diagnosis and management of skin and soft-tissue infections," *Clinical Infectious Diseases* 2005;41:1373–1406.

Stulberg DL, et al. "Common bacterial skin infections," *American Family Physician* 2002;66:119–124.

Swartz MN. "Cellulitis," *New England Journal of Medicine* 2004;350:904–912.

Talan D, et al. "Bacteriologic analysis of infected dog and cat bites," *New England Journal of Medicine* 1999;340:85–92.

Chapter 12
Diabetic Foot Infections

Thomas C. McGinley, Jr.

Introduction

In the United States, foot infection is the leading cause of diabetes-related hospitalizations and lower extremity amputations. Approximately 90,000 lower extremity amputations occur annually secondary to diabetes. With the estimated percentage of Americans with diabetes approaching 8.9% of the population by the year 2025, it is easy to see the enormity of the problem of diabetic foot infections and the need to develop proficiency in diagnosing and treating these infections. In addition, with the 5-year survival rate of unilateral diabetic amputees at approximately 50%, physicians must initiate prompt, thorough care to influence mortality as well as morbidity.

Several guidelines for treating diabetic foot infections have been published by organizations such as the American Pharmacology Association, the American College of Foot and Ankle Surgeons, and the Infectious Diseases Society of America (IDSA). While there are similarities among the various guidelines, this chapter focuses on those from the IDSA.

Pathophysiology

Many predisposing factors contribute to diabetic foot infections: trauma, neuropathy, peripheral vascular disease (PVD), biomechanical alterations, lower extremity edema, hyperglycemia, patient disabilities, maladaptive patient behaviors, and impaired immunity all contribute to diabetic foot ulcers and infections. Of note, 85% of all diabetic lower extremity amputations were preceded by ulceration, and one amputation or ulcer can cause biomechanical stresses that increase future risks for subsequent ulcerations and amputations. Thus, it is not surprising that 70% of patients with ulceration or amputation develop a new lesion within five years.

Minor trauma, such as repetitive pressure, can cause high plantar pressures resulting in pain, erythema, and callus. Callus formation has been shown to be a risk factor in approximately 30% of patients with diabetic foot ulcers. The callus can break down underlying dermis, causing an ulcer that may lead to infection.

N.S. Skolnik (ed.), *Essential Infectious Disease Topics for Primary Care.*
© Humana Press, Totowa, NJ

Diabetic neuropathy is the most prevalent diabetes-related complication increasing the risk of diabetic foot infections, mostly secondary to ulcer formation. More than 50% of diabetic patients of at least five years duration have some combination of sensory, motor and autonomic neuropathy. With sensory neuropathy, loss of light touch, vibration, and pressure sensations can lead to loss of protective sensation, causing harmful redistribution of pressure and ataxic gait. In contrast, motor neuropathy leads to muscle weakness and atrophy, leading to excess pressure in some areas and loss of joint stability. This ultimately can lead to foot deformities such as, clawed toes. Autonomic neuropathy causes vasomotor disturbance of blood vessels, with resultant decreased blood flow, endothelial dysfunction, and bacterial entry.

PVD is more prevalent and more aggressive in diabetic patients than nondiabetic patients. Anatomically, PVD occurs at more distal areas in diabetics, often involving tibial and peroneal vessels. This causes increased susceptibility to limb ischemia, with a decreased ability to heal wounds and ulcers and an increased risk of amputation. Smoking, hypertension, and dyslipidemia increase the risk of atherosclerosis in diabetic patients.

Abnormalities in foot biomechanics, more prevalent in diabetic patients, can lead to foot deformities. New pressure points created by deformities may lead to skin damage and inflammation, which provide breakdown areas for bacterial entry and subsequent infection. The triad of neuropathy, minor trauma, and foot deformity is found in 63% of patients with diabetic foot ulcers.

Persistent hyperglycemia leads to microvascular complications. It also interferes with wound healing, results in endothelial dysfunction, and increases the risk of sepsis. Several theories have been proposed to explain the effect of persistent uncontrolled hyperglycemia, including protein glycosylation, increased poly-ol pathway flux, negative nitrogen balance, increased activation of protein kinase C, and increased hexosamine pathway flux. It has also been shown that hyperglycemia interferes with adaptive responses of cells to hypoxia in patients with diabetes-related foot ulcers.

Diabetic patients possess impaired immune systems, with an impaired host response. Neutrophils do not function as well in diabetic patients as they do in nondiabetic patients. This results in impaired bacterial killing, phagocytosis, and chemotaxis. Correcting hyperglycemia has been shown to improve chemotaxis and cell-mediated immune responses.

Clinical Presentation

Patients with diabetic foot infections can present in a variety of ways, depending on the severity of the infection. Those with mild infections may have superficial skin lesions or even frank ulceration, but may have little or no pain because of neuropathy, and no systemic signs of infection. Those with potentially life-threatening infection may have signs of sepsis and inflammation, including fever or hypothermia, tachycardia, tachypnea, leukocytosis or leukopenia with elevated immature (band) forms, hyperglycemia, fasciitis, gangrene, and hypocapnea. The clinician must remember, however, that various studies reveal that 50 to 75% of patients with severe infection lack systemic signs or symptoms of infection.

History

It is imperative to obtain as complete a history as possible when evaluating the patient. Inquiring about trauma, punctures, or burns can help explain mechanism and depth of infection. If a wound is present, the clinician should ask about duration and chronicity (acute or chronic). Is the wound painful? Did the patient have previous wounds or ulcers? Did the patient receive previous treatment? If so, what was effective? The clinician should inquire about vascular status by asking about claudication and rest pain. Finally, the clinician must ask about immobility, emotional state, nutritional status, and available resources of the patient.

Physical Exam

A thorough examination should be performed on the patient with suspected infection. Assessing vital signs and metabolic state to evaluate systemic response to infection is crucial, especially in deciding whether to hospitalize the patient. Performing a psychological and cognitive assessment will likewise help with treatment decisions.

A complete examination of the vascular status and biomechanics should be performed. Vascular evaluation for PVD should include palpation of dorsalis pedis, posterior tibial, popliteal, and femoral pulses. Careful skill must be practiced because many clinicians mistake feeling their own pulses for those of the patient. Inspecting the feet and legs for lack of hair growth, atrophic skin, edema, dependent rubor, and dystrophic nails can reveal signs of vascular disease. The clinician should pay particular attention to these features when the patient complains of intermittent claudication, cramping, fatigue, cold feet, or rest pain.

Wound assessment should be systematic and include assessment of location, appearance, temperature, and odor of the wound. The depth, extent, and area of the wound should be recorded. A diabetic foot ulcer can be considered clinically infected if purulent discharge is present with at least two other signs of local inflammation (warmth, erythema, edema, pain, tunneling, lymphatic streaking, or lymphadenopathy). The presence of a foul-smelling discharge suggests mixed anaerobic infections. All wounds should be probed for bone penetration, sinus tracks, undermining, and abscesses. Abscesses may form in the various foot compartments or expand to the heel.

There are various wound classification systems available for clinician use. The Megitt–Wagner diabetic foot ulcer classification is the most commonly used system, using a scale from Grade 0 (preulcer lesion, healed ulcer, bony deformity present) to Grade 5 (gangrene over entire foot). However, this system does not address ischemia or infection specifically. It was developed for the "dysvascular" foot and it contains all infections within a single grade. The University of Texas wound classification system uses depth, presence of infection, and vascular impairment, and has been validated as a reliable predictor of amputation. What is more important than the system used is the thoroughness of the evaluation and documentation.

Neurologic examination for the loss of protective sensation should be performed. Loss of protective sensation is most easily detected with a Semmes–Weinstein 5.07 (10 g) monofilament pressed against any two of three sites on the foot (plantar surface of heel, metatarsal heads and arch, and tips of toes). Loss of vibratory sense can be detected with a standard tuning fork (128 cycles per second). Early signs of neuropathy should lead to daily self-examinations by the patient.

Approximately two thirds of patients with moderate to severe diabetic foot infections are likely to have an associated bone infection. It should be suspected in all patients with infected ulcers extending to the bone, in patients with radiographic evidence of bone destruction, or in patients with nonhealing chronic ulcers despite adequate therapy. The probe to bone test has a positive predictive value of 89% and a negative predictive value of 56%. It should be performed in all wounds. Therefore, any ulcer that reveals visible bone or in which bone can be palpated by a blunt, metal probe is likely to be complicated by osteomyelitis.

The severity of diabetic foot conditions can be judged based on the specific tissues involved, the adequacy of arterial perfusion, and the presence of systemic toxicity or metabolic instability. Categorization helps determine the degree of risk to the patient and the limb and, therefore, guides management. Wounds lacking purulence or inflammation are considered uninfected. Wounds with at least two manifestations of inflammation and erythema at least 2 cm around the lesion but no signs of systemic illness are considered mildly infected. Patients are considered to have moderately infected wounds who are systemically well but who have at least two of the following characteristics: cellulitis or erythema >2 cm, lymphangitic streaking, spread beneath superficial fascia, deep tissue abscess, gangrene, and involvement of muscle, tendon, joint, or bone. Severe infections are in patients with systemic toxicity or metabolic instability.

Laboratory Investigations and Tests

The American Diabetes Association (ADA) recommends considering ankle-brachial index (ABI) screening, with or without toe pressures, for all diabetic patients older than 50 years. If surgery is planned, transcutaneous oxygen ($TcpO_2$)

measurements can be taken, with < 30 mmHg indicative of a poorer prognosis for healing than pressures above 30 mmHg.

Diabetic infections are usually diagnosed on the basis of local signs and symptoms of inflammation. Laboratory investigations are of limited use for diagnosing infection, except in cases of osteomyelitis. If possible, the clinician should send appropriately obtained specimens for culture before starting empirical therapy. For mild and previously untreated infections, this recommendation is not necessary and may not be beneficial. Tissue specimens obtained by biopsy, ulcer curettage, or aspiration are preferred over wound swab specimens.

Imaging studies may help diagnose deep, soft-tissue collections (abscesses) or sinus tracks and are usually needed to identify pathological abnormalities of bone. Magnetic resonance imaging (MRI) is the most useful modality available today because it is the most sensitive and specific for diagnosing osteomyelitis. Plain radiographs are not considered sensitive enough to diagnose acute osteomyelitis but are usually obtained first because of cost and accessibility. Infected bone usually is radiolucent on radiography within five to seven days, but findings of demineralization, periosteal elevation, cortical irregularity, and sclerosis are usually not visible until 35 to 50% of bone mineral density is lost usually starting at two weeks of infection. Plain radiographs can also reveal soft-tissue swelling, gas in tissues, and foreign bodies. On the other hand, radiographs can be used two weeks after the initial diagnosis of osteomyelitis to assess the bone healing and response to therapy.

MRI is the preferred way to diagnose osteomyelitis, with nuclear medicine scans or immunoglobulin techniques being a second choice. Nuclear medicine scans are more sensitive in diagnosing osteomyelitis than radiography, but they are not specific since they are also positive in Charcot osteoarthropathy, fracture, tumor, arthritides, and postsurgical changes. The performance of various types of nuclear medicine scans vary, but the newer generation leukocyte scans have proven to be much better than technetium scans, which have low specificity. MRI shows the pathological changes of marrow edema and soft tissue disease but also has some false positive results from Charcot, foot, trauma, fracture, and avascular necrosis. Computed tomography (CT) scans and ultrasonography are also helpful, especially in those patients who cannot undergo MRI. If results of the imaging tests are negative, osteomyelitis is unlikely. If the results suggest osteomyelitis, the clinician must determine the need for bone biopsy.

Bone biopsy samples, obtained either operatively or percutaneously, are recommended if the diagnosis is still in doubt after imaging, or if etiologic agents or antibiotic susceptibilities are not predictable. Some clinicians would also obtain biopsy samples of mid- or hind-foot infections, because they are more difficult to treat and lead to higher rates of amputation. Percutaneous biopsy is accomplished under fluoroscopic or CT guidance. It is preferable to get two to three specimens from biopsy with at least one for culture and another for histology.

Serum chemistries to measure blood glucose, liver function, renal function, and thyroid function are useful in identifying metabolic problems and for choosing and dosing antibiotic treatments. Albumin and prealbumin are useful measurements of nutritional status. Poor nutritional status leads to poor wound healing. Complete blood counts can suggest infection, especially with a left shift and increased immature neutrophils. Erythrocyte sedimentation rate (ESR) and C-reactive protein (CRP) are markers of inflammation but are nonspecific for diagnosis. An ESR > 70 mm/hour may suggest osteomyelitis. Both ESR and CRP have some use in monitoring effectiveness of treatment. Wound cultures, as mentioned previously, have some use in moderate to severe infections, if collected properly. Culturing clinically uninfected lesions is unnecessary unless the wound does not heal or if the wound becomes chronic, especially over bony prominences. Blood cultures, on the other hand, should be performed, particularly for patients with severe infections.

Differential Diagnosis

The spectrum of disease with diabetic foot infections includes non-infected foot lesions, paronychia, superficial infections, cellulitis, deep tissue infections, abscesses, osteomyelitis, and gangrene. As mentioned previously on page 206, they are distinguished by clinical features with the occasional use of studies, especially when considering osteomyelitis.

Charcot neuro-osteoarthropathy demonstrates erythema, edema, warmth, and crepitus, just like osteomyelitis. However, osteomyelitis is often accompanied by fever or chills, elevated white blood cell count, a left shift, a positive blood culture, and an open wound. When in doubt, the clinician is encouraged to obtain a bone biopsy to help distinguish between the two.

Dry gangrene and wet gangrene can both result from tissue death caused by loss of blood supply. Dry gangrene is not infected, although it often appears grossly discolored. The end result of dry gangrene can be auto-amputation. Having dry gangrene does confer some risk of future infection for the patient and must be observed closely. The primary difference between dry gangrene and wet gangrene is a lack of discharge in dry gangrene that accompanies wet gangrene infections.

Treatment

Antibiotic treatment is not indicated for clinically uninfected wounds. Prophylaxis has not shown to be beneficial. Antibiotic therapy is necessary for all infected wounds, but alone is insufficient without proper wound care, off-loading, and management of ischemia.

Initial empiric antibiotic treatment should be based on the severity of the infection and the likely causative agent(s). Therapy directed toward aerobic gram-positive cocci is usually sufficient for mild to moderate infections in patients who have not recently received antibiotic therapy. Broad-spectrum antibiotic therapy is indicated for severe infections while awaiting culture and susceptibility results. The clinician must take into account local susceptibility data, particularly the prevalence of methicillin-resistant *Staphylococcus aureus* (MRSA) and other resistant organisms. Definitive therapy must take into account clinical response to empiric therapy as well as culture and susceptibility results.

There is limited evidence on which to make antibiotic choices for type and duration of treatment. Table 12.1 lists some treatment recommendations based on the level of severity of infection. The predominant pathogens are aerobic gram-positive cocci, especially *S. aureus*. Fluoroquinolones are generally discouraged as monotherapy but may be used in combination therapies. In some geographic areas, fluoroquinolone resistance has reached unacceptable levels. Unfortunately, the escalation of MRSA has necessitated the consideration of vancomycin or linezolid therapy.

Some moderate and almost all severe infections require parenteral therapy, at least initially. Highly bioavailable oral agents can be used in most mild and in many moderate infections, as well as in some cases of osteomyelitis.

Deep tissue infections require surgical debridement with appropriate antibiotic treatment. Patients with chronic wounds or patients who have recently received antibiotic therapy may be infected with gram-negative rods. Patients with wounds accompanied by ischemia or gangrene may have obligate anaerobes. Parenteral antibiotics are generally indicated (see Table 12.1).

Severe infections generally constitute surgical emergencies because they are limb- or life-threatening in nature. Antibiotic therapy is generally initiated after intraoperative cultures are obtained. The therapy is prolonged and determined by the severity of the infection (see Table 12.1).

Table 12.1 Common antibiotic choices for diabetic foot infections

Severity of infection	Antibiotic choices
Mild	Cephalexin (oral)
	Amoxicillin/clavulanate (oral)
	Clindamycin (oral)
	Trimethoprim–sulfamethizole (oral)
	Vancomycin (oral or i.v.)[a]
	Linezolid (oral or i.v.)[a]
Moderate (deep tissue)	Amoxicillin–sulbactam (i.v.)
	Ticarcillin–clavulanate (i.v.)
	Piperacillin–tazobactam (i.v.)
	Cefoxitin (i.v.)
	Cefepime (i.v.) and metronidazole (i.v.)
Severe	Imipenem–cilastatin (i.v.)
	Aztreonam (i.v.) and vancomycin OR
	Clindamycin (i.v.) and metronidazole (i.v.)
	Piperacillin–tazobactam (i.v.)
	Vancomycin and cefepime (i.v.)
	Meropenem (i.v.)

[a]For MRSA infections. i.v., intravenous.

Antibiotic therapy should be continued until there is evidence that the infection has resolved. The wound does not necessarily have to be healed. Suggestions for duration of therapy are: 1 to 2 weeks for mild infections (some require longer therapy), and 2 to 4 weeks for moderate and severe infections, depending on the structures involved, the adequacy of the debridement, the type of soft tissue wound cover, and wound vascularity. Osteomyelitis is generally treated for at least 4 to 6 weeks, but a shorter duration can be considered if the entire infected bone is removed. Longer durations may be necessary if the infected bone remains.

Infections in clinically stable patients that fail to respond to one or more antibiotic courses should be reevaluated. The clinician should consider discontinuing all antibiotics and obtaining proper cultures.

Surgical consultation should be obtained for deep tissue infections, extensive bone or joint involvement, crepitus, substantial necrosis or gangrene, or necrotizing fasciitis. Addressing arterial insufficiency by revascularization may be needed. Proper treatment may require removal of devitalized bone and soft tissue, and drainage of pus and sinus tracks. Some wounds may need to be packed and left open to close by secondary intention. Sometimes, delayed primary closures may be undertaken. When sharp debridement of supposedly superficial infections reveals pus, it is imperative that a surgeon perform more extensive debridement and drainage, usually in an operating room setting. Before closure of any wound, all devitalized tissue must be removed and wound edges must bleed freely when curetted.

General principles of treatment of diabetic foot infections must include wound bed preparation, which may include wound cleansing and debridement, appropriate antibiotic treatment, off-loading, maintenance of good metabolic control, and securing adequate blood supply to the wound. Off-loading requires patient compliance and may be particularly difficult to obtain. However, its importance should not be underestimated. Total contact casts or removable casts or dressings may help. Currently, there is insufficient evidence to recommend use of specific wound dressings or wound healing agents, but a key goal is to keep the wound bed moist and free of necrotic tissue to promote adequate healing.

Studies have not adequately defined the role of adjunctive therapies for diabetic foot infections, but systematic reviews suggest that granulocyte colony-stimulating factors and systemic hyperbaric oxygen therapy may prevent amputations. Hyperbaric oxygen therapy has value in treating diabetic foot ulcers and decreasing hospital stays. It has documented benefits in healing diabetic foot ulcers, refractory osteomyelitis, and necrotizing soft tissue infections. Negative pressure therapies such as vacuum wound drainage systems also seem promising. They decrease edema by removing interstitial fluid and increase blood flow to the wound bed. Skin substitutes and antimicrobial dressings have also been used to help heal diabetic wounds, with some benefit.

Patients with infected wounds require early and careful follow-up to ensure that the therapies are appropriate and effective. Use of multidisciplinary foot care teams have proven to be effective. The team should include or have access to an infectious disease specialist or a medical microbiologist. Additional members can include primary care physicians, surgeons, podiatrists, and other healthcare providers.

Expected Outcomes

The goals of treating diabetic foot infections include eradication of infection and avoidance of soft tissue loss, death, and amputations. Overall, 80 to 90% of mild to moderate infections and 60 to 80% of severe infections or osteomyelitis cases achieve a good clinical response. Relapses occur in approximately 20 to 30% of patients, especially those with osteomyelitis, presence of necrosis or gangrene, and a proximal location to their infection.

Overall, diabetic wounds should generally heal completely in 12 to 20 weeks. However, constant observation for continuing signs of improvement should occur. If no evidence of healing occurs within two weeks, the clinician should reevaluate, with particular focus on ischemia, infection, need for debridement, and off-loading.

Bibliography

Armstrong DG, Lipsky BA. Diabetic foot infections: stepwise medical and surgical management. *International Wound Journal*. 2004;1(2):123–132.

Frykberg RG. A summary of guidelines for managing the diabetic foot. *Advances in Skin and Wound Care*. 2005;18(4):209–214.

Lipsky BA, Berendt AR, Deery HG, Embil JM, Joseph WS, Karchmer AW, LeFrock JL, Lew DP, Mader JT, Norden C, Tan JS. Diagnosis and treatment of diabetic foot infections. *Clinical Infectious Diseases*. 2004;39:885–910.

Lavery LA, Armstrong DG, Wunderlich RP, Mohler MJ, Wendel CS, Lipsky BA. Risk factors for foot infections in individuals with diabetes. *Diabetic Care*. 2006;29(6) 1288–1293.

Rich P. Treatment of uncomplicated skin and skin structure infections in the diabetic patient. *Journal of Drugs in Dermatology*. 2005;4(6) Supplement:526–529.

Younes NA, Ahmad A. Diabetic foot disease. *Endocrine Practice*. 2006;12(5):583–592.

Zgonis T. A systemic approach to diabetic foot infections. *Advances in Therapy*. 2005;22(3): 244–262.

Chapter 13
Osteomyelitis

Kelly L. Gannon and Todd Braun

Introduction

Osteomyelitis is an infection of bone that poses significant diagnostic and therapeutic difficulty. This infection can be categorized as an acute or a chronic inflammatory process of the bone and surrounding structures secondary to infection with pyogenic organisms. The infection may be localized or it may spread through the periosteum, cortex, marrow, and cancellous tissue. The progressive infection results in inflammatory destruction of the bone, which leads to bone necrosis, and inhibits new bone formation. Without prompt treatment, acute osteomyelitis can become chronic, possibly leading to decreased range of motion, physical deformity, or amputation. Cases are classified based on the causative agent, route of inoculation, duration of symptoms, location of infection, and host immune factors.

In 1970, Waldvogel devised a classification system for osteomyelitis, which included hematogenous, contiguous focus, or chronic.[1] In 1985, an additional classification, the Cierny–Mader system was created. This system stages osteomyelitis in a dynamic manner, allowing for alterations caused by any changes in the medical condition of the patient, successful antibiotic therapy, or other treatment.[2]

Pathophysiology

Staphylococcus aureus is the most common organism identified as a pathogen in cases of osteomyelitis. Other isolated organisms include *Staphylococcus epidermidis, Pseudomonas aeruginosa, Serratia marcescens*, and *Eschericia coli*. Predisposing factors to infection include diabetes mellitus, sickle cell disease, AIDS, intravenous drug use, alcoholism, chronic steroid use, immunosuppression, chronic joint disease, and rheumatoid arthritis. In addition, patients who have a prosthetic orthopedic device, recent orthopedic surgery, or an open fracture are at an increased risk.

When a microbe invades the bone, it must evade the immune system. *S. aureus* adheres to bone by expressing receptors (adhesins) for components of bone matrix,

N.S. Skolnik (ed.), *Essential Infectious Disease Topics for Primary Care.*
© Humana Press, Totowa, NJ

such as fibronectin, laminin, collagen, and bone sialoglycoprotein. Not only is the bone infected, but the bacteria can cause expression of collagen-binding adhesins, which allow attachment of the pathogen to cartilage as well. When *S. aureus* is ingested by osteoblasts, the bacteria can survive intracellularly, and a biofilm is produced. This also allows for the persistence of infection. The taxing rate of treatment failure may be explained by the microbes expressing phenotypic resistance to antimicrobials once they adhere to the bone.

During infection, phagocytes attempt to contain the pathogen by generating toxic oxygen radicals that release proteolytic enzymes that lyse surrounding tissue. Pus spreads through vascular channels, which raises intraosseous pressure and impairs blood flow. Ischemic necrosis occurs and separates the devascularized fragments, creating a sequestrum, which is a segment of bone separated from viable bone by granulation tissue and impervious to antibiotics.

Acute Osteomyelitis

Acute osteomyelitis can be classified based on the mechanism of infection; either by hematogenous spread or from a contiguous focus of infection. Hematogenous osteomyelitis often originates from a remote source and is predominantly a disease of childhood. This form of osteomyelitis generally occurs in bones with rich blood supply, such as long bones in children and the vertebral bodies in adults. In children, hematogenous osteomyelitis usually involves the metaphyseal area of the tibia, femur, or humerus.

Vertebral osteomyelitis is generally seen in adults, particularly in patients with diabetes mellitus, on hemodialysis, and abusing intravenous drugs. The bacteria tend to seed the intervertebral disc space and spread to the neighboring vertebrae on either side of the disc. Typically, vertebral osteomyelitis presents with severe back pain, especially at night. In these patients, a spinal epidural abscess may evolve suddenly or over several weeks and present with severe acute back pain, often with fever, followed by radicular pain and subsequent weakness below the affected spinal cord level. Irreversible paralysis may result from failure to recognize an epidural abscess before development of neurological deficits.

Unusual cases of hematogenous osteomyelitis include disseminated histoplasmosis, coccidiomycosis, and blastomycosis in endemic areas. Atypical mycobacteria, *Candida, Cryptococcus*, or *Aspergillus* may rarely be isolated from immunocompromised patients.

Osteomyelitis from a contiguous focus of infection is the most prevalent type and can be separated into those related to adjacent infection (including postoperative and posttraumatic infection) and those related to vascular compromise (such as diabetes or peripheral vascular disease). Posttraumatic infections can originate from open fractures or from internal fixation devices that introduce bacteria into the bone.

Table 13.1 Common bacterial causes of acute hematogenous osteomyelitis

Newborn (<4 months old)	*S. aureus, Enterobacter* species, *E. coli*, and group A and B *Streptococcus* species
Children (4 months–4 years)	*S. aureus*, group A *Streptococcus* species, *H. influenzae*, and *Enterobacter* species
Children/adolescents (4 years–adult)	*S. aureus*, group A *Streptococcus* species, *H. influenzae*, and *Enterobacter* species
Adult	*S. aureus* and occasionally *Enterobacter* or *Streptococcus* species

Osteomyelitis associated with diabetes is the most common presentation worldwide. Diabetic neuropathy and vascular insufficiency play key roles in the etiology. In diabetic foot ulcers, the diagnosis is often missed because of two major factors: most cases occur in ulcers without exposed bone, and many have no evidence of inflammation on physical examination. In addition to those with exposed bone, osteomyelitis should be suspected in patients who have a chronic ulcer that remains unhealed after appropriate therapy or if the ulcer is larger than 2 cm by 2 cm. The palpation of bone in foot ulcers strongly correlates with underlying osteomyelitis (85% specificity; 89% positive predictive value).[3]

Chronic Osteomyelitis

Chronic osteomyelitis is an infection of the bone that persists or recurs regardless of the primary cause and sometimes despite aggressive intervention. The risk of developing chronic osteomyelitis is significantly higher in patients with peripheral vascular disease or diabetes. Typically, the patients are asymptomatic, but they may have a draining sinus. Necrotic bone (sequestrum) surrounded by reactive bone (involcrum) may also be seen. Regardless of appropriate treatment, relapse is common.

Diagnosis

The diagnosis of osteomyelitis is established principally on the clinical assessment, with data from the initial history, physical evaluation, and laboratory tests. Symptoms will differ based on many variables: duration of illness, mechanism of infection, affected area, physiologic status of the host, and presence of orthopedic hardware. A complete history and thorough physical examination are of key importance when determining whether a patient may have osteomyelitis.

Acute hematogenous osteomyelitis develops rapidly and worsens over several days to a week. Symptoms and signs include bone pain, tenderness, warmth, and swelling. The patient may appear septic with fever, rigors, nausea, and malaise. In hematogenous osteomyelitis, 50% of cases have accompanying bacteremia.

Contiguous osteomyelitis usually presents with little or no fever. Patients may present with a painful, unstable joint on physical exam or as a finding on a routine radiograph after surgery.

Physicians must differentiate osteomyelitis from other medical conditions with similar clinical presentations. Cancer, degenerative diseases, and many inflammatory diseases affecting the bone may appear with symptoms that parallel those of osteomyelitis. In diabetic patients, osteomyelitis and diabetic osteoarthropathy may be indistinguishable clinically and radiographically.

Laboratory Tests

A specific microbiologic diagnosis is of great importance in treating osteomyelitis. This allows the physician to tailor antimicrobial therapy based on the identification and susceptibility of the organism. Proper specimen collection is important to increase the likelihood of obtaining a culture from which a pathogen may be isolated. Use of antimicrobials before culture collection decreases the sensitivity of the test; therefore, treatment may need to be withheld until a culture can be obtained, unless the patient has systemic signs of infection or limb compromise. Bone biopsy cultures and pathology are optimal for diagnosing osteomyelitis and helping to guide appropriate treatment. Deep surgical cultures are the best choice, if possible, because there is poor correlation between superficial and deep cultures. In a prospective study of 100 patients with chronic osteomyelitis, excluding diabetic foot infections and decubitus ulcers, positive cultures were obtained in 94% from first biopsy. Cultures of nonbone specimens agreed with the bone culture in only 30% of the cases.[4] Aerobic and anaerobic cultures should be ordered on all specimens, and cultures for fungi, mycobacteria, mycoplasma, or *Brucella* species can be collected as necessary based on the patient's history and clinical exam. Blood cultures should be collected when systemic infection is evident.

Table 13.2 Laboratory tests for osteomyelitis

Laboratory test	Clinical role	Other
ESR, CRP, WBC	Inflammatory markers	Useful in monitoring response
Blood cultures	Identify causative organism	
Joint aspirate	Identify causative organism, exclude other disorders with similar presentation	
Operative sample	Culture and histopathology to exclude disorders with similar presentation	Gold standard for diagnosing osteomyelitis

Although a sample taken from a sinus tract or wound drainage is simple to obtain, the results are often misleading. In a study by Mackowiak et al., when sinus tract cultures were compared with operative specimen cultures, only 44% of sinus tract cultures contained the true pathogen. However, isolation of *S. aureus* from a sinus tract often correlated with the presence of *S. aureus* in the operative specimen.[5]

Radiology

Although microbiology and pathology may be the most significant tests for determining treatment, radiographic examination provides a clue to the presence of osteomyelitis. Plain radiographs may reveal osteolysis, periosteal reaction, and sequestra, but these findings may not be evident until 14 to 21 days after the onset of infection. Scintigraphic studies, such as three-phase bone scan, indium-labeled leukocyte scan, bone marrow scan, or dual tracer scans may complement other radiographic studies, but should not be used as the sole criterion for diagnosing osteomyelitis because of their poor specificity.

Both CT and MRI have excellent resolution and can reveal edema and the destruction of bone, as well as any periosteal reaction, cortical destruction, articular damage, and soft tissue involvement before abnormal plain radiograph results. A CT scan is prone to degradation because of artifacts from bone or metal, but is very useful for guided needle biopsy. MRI may detect bone marrow involvement earlier than scintigraphy. MRI is the imaging procedure of choice for osteomyelitis in diabetic foot ulcers.

Table 13.3 Radiologic tests for osteomyelitis

Radiologic test	Diagnostic findings	Other significance
Radiographs	Soft tissue swelling, effusion, bone destruction, periosteal reaction, fracture/tumor exclusion	Inexpensive; if positive, may obviate need for CT or MRI
Bone scan	Osteoblastic reaction to bone pathology; may differentiate cellulitis from osteomyelitis	Suffers from poor specificity
MRI	Intraosseous and soft tissue edema, cortical destruction, abscess, paraspinal soft tissue edema or abscess, extent of bone marrow and bone involvement	Operative planning; image of choice for diabetic foot ulcer and vertebral infections
CT	Periosteal reaction, cortical destruction, articular damage, soft tissue edema	Image may degrade because of artifacts from bone and metal; useful for guided biopsy

Treatment

Treatment generally involves clinical assessment, staging, determination of microbial etiology and susceptibilities, antimicrobial course, and, if required, debridement, dead-space management, and stabilization of bone. The goal of treatment is to eliminate the infection and prevent it from advancing. Most patients with osteomyelitis require hospitalization for initial therapy. This is especially necessary when surgical intervention or parenteral antimicrobial therapy is planned. The recommended management includes a combination of surgical, medical, and adjunct therapies. Additionally, hospital-based therapy may be necessary if patients have soft tissue infection, such as cellulitis or abscess, or if they show any sign of sepsis syndrome. Consultation with infectious disease and orthopedic surgery specialists is recommended in cases of osteomyelitis. Specific recommendations can also include consultation from vascular surgery, cardiothoracic surgery, neurosurgery, and plastic surgery.

Surgical Therapy

Surgical intervention should be considered in cases of chronic osteomyelitis, contiguous focus osteomyelitis, and orthopedic implant associated osteomyelitis. In addition, the necessity of surgery should be contemplated when there is involvement of the femoral head, failure to make a specific diagnosis with noninvasive techniques, neurological complication, and failure to improve with appropriate antimicrobial therapy. Operative approaches that join the skills of orthopedic, plastic, and vascular surgeons should be used to allow more rapid growth of new bone. Complete drainage and debridement of all infected and necrotic soft tissue and bone is required. Debridement decreases the bacterial load and allows for a more thorough examination of the area. Any foreign bodies found at this time should be removed if possible, and blood supply should be restored.

Patients with orthopedic implant-related osteomyelitis should be managed individually, weighing the risk of recurrence against the functional outcome if the implant were removed. Failure to remove orthopedic implants sometimes allows microorganisms to form a biofilm and to escape antibiotics. Ideally, all orthopedic hardware should be removed at the time of bone debridement to allow for cure of infection. However, this is not possible in patients whose fractures have not developed union, because an infected union fracture is easier to deal with than an infected nonunion. In these cases, prolonged antibiotics while the fracture heals may be necessary, followed by removal of the hardware at a later date, in an attempt to fully cure the infection. In some patients with acute implant-related osteomyelitis, with < 1-month duration of symptoms, debridement and retention of hardware, followed by 3 to 6 months of a combined quinolone and rifampin regimen may provide a cure. Additionally, if a foreign body is not able to be removed, and the pathogen is identified to be *S. aureus*, one should consider an antimicrobial regimen using rifampin along with an additional antistaphylococcal agent for 3 to 6 months.[6] When debridement, reconstructive surgery, or vascular integrity cannot be restored, other options, such as limb amputation or chronic antimicrobial suppression, may be necessary.

Medical Therapy

Medical management is predominantly directed toward any metastatic foci of infection and at microfoci of osteomyelitis that remain after surgical debridement. This almost always includes parenteral antimicrobial medications.

Table 13.4 Organism-directed antibiotic regimens for acute osteomyelitis for adults

Osteomyelitis type	First-line antibiotic(s)	Alternative antibiotic(s)
S. aureus		
Penicillin sensitive	4 million U penicillin G every 4–6 h	2 g cefazolin every 8 h, or 600 mg clindamycin every 6–8 h, or 1 g vancomycin every 12 h
Penicillin resistant	2 g nafcillin every 4 h	2 g cefazolin every 8 h, or 600 mg clindamycin every 6–8 h, or 1 g vancomycin every 12 h
Methicillin resistant	1 g vancomycin every 12 h	600 mg linezolid every 12 h, or 500–750 mg Levaquin every 24 h plus 600–900 mg rifampin every 24 h
Streptococcus	4 million U penicillin G every 4–6 h	600 mg clindamycin every 6–8 h, or 1 g vancomycin every 12 h OR 2 g ceftriaxone every 24 h
Enterococcus		
Ampicillin sensitive	2 g ampicillin every 4 h	1 g vancomycin every 12 h
Vancomycin resistant	600 mg linezolid every 12 h	6 mg/kg daptomycin every 24 h
Enteric gram-negative rods	750 mg ciprofloxacin every 12 h	2 g ceftriaxone every 24 h
Pseudomonas aeruginosa	2 g ceftazidime every 8 h and an aminoglycoside OR 500–750 mg oral ciprofloxacin every 12 h	500 mg imipenem every 6 h, or 4 g piperacillin/0.5 g tazobactam every 6–8 h OR 2 g cefepime every 12 h (given with an aminoglycoside)
Anaerobes	600 mg clindamycin every 6 h	3 g ampicillin–sulbactam every 8 h, or 500 mg metronidazole every 8 h
Mixed aerobic and anaerobic organisms	4 g piperacillin–0.5 g tazobactam every 6–8 h	500 mg imipenem every 6 h

The Infectious Diseases Society of America recommends that parenteral antibiotics be started in a controlled setting, preferably inpatient, to carefully monitor for any serious side effects. Antimicrobial drug levels should be monitored, when indicated, to maximize efficacy and minimize toxicity. In acute hematogenous osteomyelitis, antibiotics may be the only intervention required. In the many cases, after 7 to 10 days of intravenous antibiotic therapy, the patient may be changed to an oral agent for 3 to 4 additional weeks. In adults with uncomplicated vertebral osteomyelitis, at least 4 to 6 weeks of antimicrobial therapy are necessary. In patients with chronic or contiguous focus osteomyelitis, antibiotic therapy should be continued for at least 4 to 6 weeks.

In patients with implant-associated osteomyelitis, the duration of antibiotic therapy should be adjusted according to the surgical modality. Typically, all infected hardware is removed, and the involved bone is debrided, followed by 4 to 6 weeks of effective antimicrobial therapy. This antibiotic regimen will allow time for the debrided bone to be covered by vascularized soft tissue. This has been shown to reduce the relapse rate by 20%.[7] To further decrease the chance of recurrence, local antibiotics may be instilled by way of antimicrobial coated spacers and beads. This allows for a higher level of antimicrobial medication in the local area.

Hyperbaric Oxygen Therapy

Although antimicrobial therapy and surgery are the cornerstones of treatment, adjunct modalities are available. Hyperbaric oxygen can be used in combination with antibiotics and surgery when treating patients with recurrent posttraumatic or chronic osteomyelitis. The hyperbaric oxygen increases the oxygen tension in infected tissue, including bone. This has a direct bacteriostatic as well as a bactericidal effect on anaerobic organisms. The patient must undergo 90 to 120 minutes daily for 15 to 20 separate sessions. In a randomized trial, patients with significant infected lower extremity ulcers treated with hyperbaric oxygen had a significantly lower amputation rate.[8] However, the study included patients with and without osteomyelitis.

Follow-Up

After patients are discharged from the hospital, it is important for care to be continued as an outpatient. Many of these patients will receive antibiotic therapy intravenously for several weeks after discharge. The patients should be asked about the persistence of pain, recurrence of symptoms, presence of fever, discharge from any surgical site, and medication side effects. The physical exam should include temperature, examination of the site, and inspection of any intravenous access. Early postoperative wound healing problems and infection have been associated with subsequent deep, surgical site infections.[9]

Laboratory data can be extremely helpful during treatment. A persistently elevated C-reactive protein level (CRP) or erythrocyte sedimentation rate (ESR) may convey a poor response to therapy. A decrease of >50% in the ESR is rarely associated with treatment failure in patients with vertebral osteomyelitis.[10] An elevated or decreased white blood count (WBC) can indicate therapy failure as well. Therapeutic drug levels and toxicity can be measured weekly through serum assays. The drug level should be measured to ensure adequacy of treatment. Subtherapeutic antimicrobial blood levels may be associated with levels that are below the minimal inhibitory concentration of selected organisms, and can lead to clinical failure or the emergence of resistance.[11] Serum creatinine can monitor for any drug-related nephrotoxicity, and assist in altering the dose of some antimicrobials.

Radiological reevaluation may be done at any time if there are signs of treatment failure. In a patient who is progressing well, plain radiographs should be rechecked after 8 to 12 weeks from therapy initiation to assess for bony fusion in infected nonunion sites. In addition, a repeat MRI may be done after 4 to 8 weeks of antibiotic therapy to assess risk of treatment failure in vertebral osteomyelitis. One study of eight patients treated medically for pyogenic vertebral osteomyelitis showed that six patients had evidence of progressive disease on MRI performed within 6 weeks, despite their clinical improvement.[12]

Prognosis

When appropriate treatment is received promptly for acute osteomyelitis, the outcome is usually good. <5% of cases of the acute hematogenous form will progress to chronic osteomyelitis. Chronic osteomyelitis is more likely to develop in the contiguous focus patient, especially if there is a foreign body present.

The prognosis is worse for chronic osteomyelitis. Even with appropriate medical and surgical treatment, and meticulous follow up, relapse is common. Chronic osteomyelitis imparts a massive economic burden and has a significant impact on quality of life. Amputation may be necessary, especially in diabetic patients and patients with peripheral vascular disease. The outlook is guarded in patients who have an infection of a prosthetic device.

In all cases, patient compliance is one of the most important prognostic indicators. Each patient should know about the natural history and management of osteomyelitis. They should be clearly informed about the pathophysiology, symptoms, therapy, and prognosis. The different modalities of treatment should be discussed with the patient.

Prevention

Prevention of osteomyelitis is critical. Delay elective orthopedic surgical procedures if the patient has a current or recent history of infection. During orthopedic surgery, careful attention is paid to sterile techniques and to practices that reduce bone contamination. Prophylactic antibiotic therapy can be administered at the time of surgery and for 24 hours postoperatively to achieve adequate tissue levels. The incidence of hematogenous distribution of infection can be decreased if urinary catheters and drains are removed as soon as possible.

Treatment of localized infections diminishes hematogenous spread. Proper wound care reduces the occurrence of superficial infections and osteomyelitis. Prompt management of soft tissue infections reduces expansion of infection to the bone. In patients with open contaminated fractures involving extensive injury or loss of soft tissue, periosteal stripping, and bone exposure, administer antimicrobial prophylaxis and perform surgical debridement and delayed wound closure. In one study involving 1,102 open fractures, the infection rate was 24% in patients receiving no prophylactic antibiotics, whereas the infection rate was 4.5% in the patients receiving prophylactic antibiotics.[13] Prophylactic antibiotics are frequently recommended when patients with joint replacements undergo dental procedures or other invasive procedures.

Patients with diabetes or peripheral vascular disease should be instructed on proper foot care. Patients should perform daily foot inspection, have an annual foot exam by a physician, and accommodate any foot deformities with custom-made footwear. They should use gentle soap and water to cleanse their feet and apply moisturizer afterwards. Two studies that used a multiple intervention program, including footwear, showed reduced rates of repeat ulceration in patients with a history of ulceration.[14]

Conclusion

Although diagnosis and management may be difficult in osteomyelitis, the prognosis is much better for patients when proper steps are taken. The diagnosis of bone and joint infection should be carefully considered in appropriate presentations. Careful microbiological specimen collection to direct antibiotic therapy is imperative. In addition, excellent surgical judgment and technique is necessary.

The primary care physician plays a key role in coordinating care and managing comorbidities, polypharmacy, psychologic issues, and physical therapy. A good relationship between the primary physician and consultants is imperative. In addition, collaboration between the patient and physician is crucial in the treatment of this disease.

References

1. Waldvogel FA, Medoff G, Swartz MN. *Osteomyelitis: a review of clinical features, therapeutic considerations and unusual aspects (first of three parts).* N Engl J Med. 1970;282:198–206.
2. Cierny G, Mader JT, Pennick JJ. *A clinical staging system for adult osteomyelitis.* Contemp Orthop. 1985;10:17–37.

3. Newman LG, Waller J, Palestro CJ, et al. *Unsuspected osteomyelitis in diabetic foot ulcers: diagnosis and monitoring by leukocyte scanning with indium In 111 oxyquinoline.* JAMA. 1991;266(9):1246–1251.

4. Zuluaga AF, Galvis W, Saldarriaga JG, Agudelo M, Salazar BE, Vesga O. *Etiologic diagnosis of chronic osteomyelitis: a prospective study.* Arch Intern Med. 2006;166:95–100.

5. Mackowiak PA, Jones SR, Smith JW. *Diagnostic value of sinus-tract cultures in chronic osteomyelitis.* JAMA. 1978;239:2772–2775.

6. Black J, Hunt TL, Godley PJ, Matthew E. *Oral antimicrobial therapy for adults with osteomyelitis or septic arthritis.* J Infect Dis. 1987;155:968–972.

7. Hanssen AD, Rand JA, Osmon DR. *Treatment of the infected total knee arthroplasty with insertion of another prosthesis. The effect of antibiotic-impregnated bone cement.* Clin Orthop. 1994;309:44–55.

8. Morrey BF, Dunn JM, Heimbach RD, Davis J. *Hyperbaric oxygen and chronic osteomyelitis.* Clin Orthop. 1979;144;121–127.

9. Berbari EF, Hanssen AD, Duffy MC, Steckelberg JM, Ilstrup DM, Harmsen WS, et al. *Risk factors for prosthetic joint infection: case-control study.* Clin Infect Dis. 1998;27:1247–1254.

10. Carragee EJ. *Pyogenic vertebral osteomyelitis.* J Bone Joint Surg Am. 1997;79:874–880.

11. Jordan GW, Kawachi MM. *Analysis of serum bactericidal activity in endocarditis, osteomyelitis, and other bacterial infections.* Medicine (Baltimore). 1981;60:44–49.

12. Carragee EJ. *The clinical use of magnetic resonance imaging in pyogenic vertebral osteomyelitis.* Spine. 1997;22:2089–2093.

13. Patzakis MJ, Wilkins J, Moore TM. *Use of antibiotics in open tibial fractures.* Clin Orthop. 1983;178:31–35.

14. Faglia E, Favales F, Morabito A. *New ulceration, new major amputation, and survival rates in diabetic subjects hospitalized for foot ulceration from 1990 to 1993: a 6.5-year follow-up.* Diabetes Care. 2001;24:78–83.

Chapter 14
Septic Arthritis and Infectious Bursitis

Gene Hong and Nirandra Mahamitra

Introduction

Septic arthritis is a medical emergency which warrants prompt investigation. The incidence of septic arthritis in the general population ranges from 2 to 10 per 100,000 in the general population and 30 to 70 per 100,000 in patients with rheumatoid arthritis and joint prostheses. Twenty-five to 50% of patients may develop irreversible loss of joint function.[1]

Many different organisms may infect the joint, and any joint may be affected. Unfortunately, diagnosis at presentation may be difficult. The most important initial step is a thorough history and physical examination, because laboratory studies may prove to be only supportive of the diagnosis.

This chapter outlines the extent, pathogenesis, presentation, diagnosis, and treatment of septic arthritis. This chapter also describes the clinical signs and methods of diagnosis and treatment of infectious bursitis. Common sites of infectious bursitis include the prepatellar and olecranon bursa; although usually not as potentially devastating as an infected joint, timely diagnosis and management of infected bursa can improve outcomes and shorten the course of illness.

Background

Infection is one of the most important causes of acute monoarthritis. Rapid diagnosis, often by arthrocentesis, is important because of its devastating course. The most important risk factors for septic arthritis are an impaired immune system, including rheumatoid arthritis, diabetes mellitus, malignancies, liver disease, renal disease, and organ transplantation. Other predisposing factors include prosthetic joints, joint surgery, advanced age beyond 80 years, large vein catheterization, and intravenous drug use (Table 14.1).

Nongonococcal infections are typically the most severe joint infections. Any joint may be involved, but most frequently large joints, such as the knee or hip, are affected. Less frequently affected joints may include the sternoclavicular joint in

N.S. Skolnik (ed.), *Essential Infectious Disease Topics for Primary Care.*
© Humana Press, Totowa, NJ

intravenous drug users. The majority of nongoncoccal infections are monarticular. However, polyarticular involvement is more common in the setting of rheumatoid arthritis. The vast majority of nongonococcal infections are caused by *Staphylococcus aureus*. Other commonly involved organisms include non-group A, β hemolytic streptococci, and *Streptococcus pneumoniae*. Anaerobes and gram-negative bacteria are increasing in frequency because of drug use and the increasing number of immunocompromised hosts.[2]

Pathogenesis

Bacteremia secondary to joint infections typically occurs via hematogenous seeding of the synovial membrane. Direct introduction has increasingly occurred with knee and hip arthroplasties. Rare causes may arise from local corticosteroid joint injections or from joint aspirations. It is estimated that there is a 0.01% risk (or 1 in 10,000) of causing an iatrogenic joint infection after an intra-articular knee injection; other studies have found joint infections to occur in 0.002% of all injections.[3] Secondary causes of bacterial infection include penetrating trauma (human or animal bite, or nail puncture) or after blunt joint trauma.[4]

The synovium is highly vascular and is vulnerable to bacteremic seeding because of its lack of a protective membrane. Therefore, blood contents have easy access to the synovial space. Bacteria produce an acute inflammatory response once they enter the enclosed joint space. There is an influx of acute and chronic inflammatory cells when the synovial membrane reacts with a proliferative lining cell hyperplasia. This creates the acute, purulent joint infection. Furthermore, cartilage degradation, inhibition of cartilage synthesis, and bone loss occur as the inflammatory cells release cytokines and proteases.

Table 14.1 Risk factors in septic arthritis

Systemic diseases
Rheumatoid arthritis
Diabetes mellitus
Malignancies
Liver disease
Renal disease
Organ transplantation
Individual factors
Prosthetic joints
Joint surgery
Advanced age beyond older than 80 years
Large vein catheterization
Intravenous drug abuse
Drug treatment with immunosuppressants or steroids

During joint surgery, physicians may encounter septic joints caused by previous surgery or caused by trauma. Arthroplasty of the knee has become a reliable procedure, however, infection is a major source of failure. Infection may be caused by a variety of factors. Extensive soft tissue scarring, poor vascular supply, repeated trauma, and multiple incisions from previous surgeries may devascularize the skin and cause poor wound healing. These causes may also lead to poor exposure during surgery, thus, resulting in soft tissue dissection, which may, in turn, lead to potential dead spaces. However, the rate of infection may be minimized when antibiotic-impregnated cement is used in patients with previous sepsis around the knee.[5] Foreign bodies or penetrating injuries may be present. Late infections of prosthetic joints may occur secondary to introduction of bacteria at the time of the previous procedure or from bacterial seeding from transient bacteremia. Late infection is defined by a period longer than 1 year after the initial joint surgery.

Presentation

Patients may present to the physician with a variety of symptoms including joint pain, swelling, tenderness, and fever (Table 14.2). High-grade fever is only present in 58% of patients, whereas 90% have at least low-grade fever. Joint pain may be blunted in the immunocompromised patient, leading to a delay in diagnosis. The immunocompromised host may not respond to an infection in a timely or appropriate manner because of physiological limitations. The immunocompromised patient may present with indolent sepsis for an extended period of time before evaluation by a physician.[6] Steroid therapy and impaired bone marrow function may decrease signs of inflammation, such as pain, swelling, and effusion.[7]

When a patient complains of joint pain, it is imperative to determine whether symptoms are truly originating from the joint or from a soft tissue structure, such as a bursa or tendon. True intra-articular problems may cause restriction of both active and passive range of motion. Peri-articular problems may be more restrictive for active rather than passive range of motions. A septic joint may be more likely

Table 14.2 Presentation of septic arthritis

Symptoms
Joint pain
Swelling
Tenderness
Fever
Immunosuppressed patients: decreased systemic signs
Signs
Usually monarticular
Swollen, erythematous and warm joint
Possible fever

to cause pain with both active and passive range of motion on exam, in contrast to an aseptic non-inflammatory joint, such as in the setting of osteoarthritis.

Joint effusions may not be visible to the eye. Certain tests, such as the "bulge sign" in the knee joint or anterior palpation on the ankle may help make the correct diagnosis. Additionally, a thorough physical exam may provide clues regarding the diagnosis. Tachycardia and fever may represent infection. Other signs, such as a rash, may be present in gonococcal infection; the skin lesion may be a nonspecific dermatitis, maculopapular or even pustular in appearance.[8]

Infectious bursitis is a condition that commonly affects the olecranon and the prepatellar bursa. These are common sites because of their predisposition to trauma and relatively superficial bursa location. Housemaid's bursitis is named for the position that a housemaid may take while scrubbing the floor, thus, placing pressure on the prepatellar bursa. Patients who frequently lean forward and place their elbows on a hard surface may predispose themselves to olecranon bursitis.

Most patients will report pain, and on exam have tenderness, erythema, and warmth over an infected bursa. They may also complain of a fever.[9] Diagnosis is made by a thorough history and physical examination. As stated previously, many patients will recall some type of trauma, however minor. Aspiration of the bursa should be considered with the aspirate sent for Gram stain and culture. The fluid may appear purulent, turbid, or hemorrhagic. White blood cell counts of 20,000 cells/mm³ or greater may indicate an infection in the setting of clinically suspected infectious bursitis.

Diagnosis

Aspiration of synovial fluid is a frequently used procedure used in the outpatient setting. Approximately 90% of family physicians reported performing joint aspiration and injection at least once per month.[10]

Septic arthritis is a medical emergency. If suspected, synovial fluid analysis should be performed. By performing an aspiration, a physician may limit joint damage, provide relief from an effusion, facilitate the diagnosis, and begin the appropriate management, i.e., that of draining the infection.

Initially, when performing arthrocentesis, the joint line should be identified. The skin is then cleansed with sterile technique and a needle is inserted; both Betadine and alcohol may be considered for skin preparation when aspirating a possible infected joint. A more detailed description of joint aspiration technique has been described elsewhere, and is beyond the scope of this chapter. If the initial withdrawn fluid is bloody, rather than becoming bloody during aspiration, previous hemarthrosis should be suspected. Overlying cellulitis is a relative contraindication to arthrocentesis; however, if the clinical need for aspiration outweighs the risk, the use of the smallest possible needle is recommended.

Aspiration of large amounts of fluid may be difficult if the fluid is loculated. Gently massaging the joint may be helpful in increasing the amount of fluid obtained. Intravenous antibiotics should be started immediately after aspiration if infection is suspected, and this should be done before receiving results of the culture. Urgent arthroscopic or surgical drainage may be necessary if needle drainage is not effective.[11]

The most important synovial fluid studies include its physical characteristics (i.e., color, clarity, and viscosity), white blood cell count with differential, presence of crystals, and microbiology.[12] All of these studies may be done with as little as 1 to 2 ml of fluid. If the available amount of joint aspirate is 2 ml or less, culture may be done using blood culture bottles as opposed to solid media. A differential diagnosis then can be established based on the results of synovial fluid analysis. Studies for Lyme disease or viral etiologies may also be sent, depending on the clinical setting.

Gram staining of the aspirate, if positive, can be helpful, but Gram staining alone is insufficient to exclude a septic joint. Gram stains can be positive in two thirds of gram-positive septic arthritis, and only positive in half of the cases of gram-negative septic arthritis.

Normally synovial fluid contains mostly mononuclear cells (usually < 180 cells/cm^3). Noninflammatory synovial fluids usually have fewer than 2000 cells/cm^3. An inflammatory process is more likely with a sample with > 2000 leukocytes/cm^3 (see Table 14.3). As a guideline, effusions containing more than 100,000 leukocytes/cm^3 are septic.[13] It should be noted, however, that one study found that one third of septic joints had WBC counts of $<50,000$/cm^3.[14]

Compared with cerebral spinal fluid analysis, analysis of the aspirate for additional chemistries, such as glucose or protein, is not as useful when evaluating a possible septic joint. Joint fluid should be analyzed for the presence of crystals. Additional studies that should be performed include serology for complete blood count with differential, erythrocyte sedimentation rate, and blood cultures, as well as plain radiographs. Blood cultures are positive in approximately 50% of nongonococcal joint infections, but are less frequently positive in gonococcal joint infections (10%). If a gonococcal infection is suspected, pharyngeal, urethral, and rectal swabs should be obtained.[15] Plain film radiographs are indicated in patients who present with trauma or with symptoms that have lasted for several weeks. The plain films may detect joint destruction or bony changes consistent with osteomyelitis or malignancy. In addition, bone scan may be helpful when considering a chronic joint infection after a history of joint arthroplasty.

Table 14.3 Synovial fluid categories with differential diagnoses[21]

Noninflammatory: $<2,000$ WBC/cm^3	Inflammatory: $>2,000$ WBC/cm^3
Osteoarthritis	Septic arthritis
Trauma	Crystal-induced monoarthritis
Avascular necrosis	Rheumatoid arthritis
Charcot arthropathy	Spondyloarthropathy
Hemochromatosis	Systemic lupus erythematosus
Pigmented villonodular synovitis	Juvenile rheumatoid arthritis, Lyme Disease

In cases of suspected infectious bursitis, if the diagnosis is clinically suspected on the history and exam, an aspiration should be considered. The cell count and Gram stain can be helpful in management, but should not be the sole basis for management; the risks and benefits of initiating empiric antibiotic therapy need to be weighed on a case-by-case basis. As mentioned earlier, if a culture is negative, this does not exclude an infection.

Bacteriology

Septic arthritis can be caused by bacteria, mycobacteria, viruses, and fungi. The bacterial pathogens are the most severe because of their rapidly destructive nature. Thus, this chapter primarily focuses on bacterial causes (see Table 14.4).

There are two classes of bacterial arthritis: gonococcal and non-gonococcal. *Neisseria gonorrhea* was previously the most common cause of septic arthritis in the United States, but its incidence has decreased recently. *S. aureus is now the most common cause of septic arthritis.*

S. aureus currently accounts for 44% of septic arthritis, and, of these, only 46% have an underlying cause such as cellulitis. The remaining cases of *S. aureus* arthritis originate from transient bacteria sources such as the skin or mucous membranes. With *S. aureus*, mortality ranges from 7 to 18%, and osteomyelitis or loss of joint function may occur in up to 27 to 46% of cases.[14]

Studies have shown an increasing incidence of methicillin-resistant *S. aureus* (MRSA) causing pathologic infection.[16] This increase in MRSA has greatly affected the clinical approach to suspected staphylococcal infections. There should now be a low threshold in obtaining cultures to document MRSA. Additionally, patients who are hospitalized for suspected MRSA infection should be treated appropriately; intravenous vancomycin is currently the preferred antibiotic for empiric therapy.[17] Risk factors for MRSA infection include a patient who is infected after institutionalization, recent hospitalizations, immunocompromised states, and, possibly, involvement in organized athletic settings.

Group A β-hemolytic streptococci are the next most common organism found in septic joints. Group B, C, and G streptococci are often found in compromised hosts or in patients with genitourinary or gastrointestinal infections.[18] Gram-negative

Table 14.4 Organisms causing septic arthritis

Gram-positive aerobes
S. Aureus
Streptococci
S. Pneumoniae
Gram-negative bacilli
H. influenza
E. Coli
Neisseria gonorrhea

bacilli are a common cause of septic arthritis in intravenous drug abusers, the elderly, and patients who are immunocompromised. In newborns and in children younger than the age of 5 years, *Haemophilus influenza* and gram-negative bacilli are the most common agents. However, the incidence of septic arthritis secondary to *H. influenza* is now less common because of vaccination against *H. influenza*. The incidence of *H. influenza* among children younger than the age of 5 years has decreased by 70 to 80% with the use of *H. influenza* type b conjugate vaccines.

Neisseria gonorrhea is the most common sexually transmitted disease to cause septic arthritis, and, in the 1970s and 1980s, was the most common cause of all septic arthritis in the United States. The clinical features of gonococcal arthritis are classified into two stages: a bacteremic stage and a joint-localized stage with suppurative arthritis. During the bacteremic stage, patients typically have fever and rigors. Polyarthralgia and skin lesions are also common during this stage. The joints most often affected include the knees, elbows, and the more distal joints. The axial skeleton is often spared. Skin lesions occur in 75% of patients. These lesions often number between 5 and 40 and are usually painless. Papules are the most common lesions, followed by pustules.

Suppurative gonococcal arthritis usually involves one or two joints. This type of arthritis may occur without the signs and symptoms of the bacteremic stage. Many patients who develop gonococcal suppurative arthritis present without previous joint pain and skin lesions. Because this type of arthritis may occur without the bacteremic syndrome, it is thought that these may be two separate syndromes.

The most common organism causing infectious bursitis is *S. aureus*, accounting for an estimated 80% of cases. Other organisms include the β hemolytic streptococcus, coagulase negative staphylococci, enterococci, *Escherichia coli*, and *Pseudomonas aeruginosa*.[19]

Treatment

As noted above, clinical exam, the Gram stain, cell count, and peripheral and joint culture results all contribute to making a diagnosis in a patient presenting with joint pain. It is important that the clinician have a high index of suspicion for the diagnosis, and a low threshold to start antibiotics empirically, because of the potentially rapid and devastating consequences of untreated infection. If an infected joint is suspected, one should begin broad-spectrum intravenous antibiotics. Once culture results are available, antibiotic choices can be narrowed. Initial selection is based on the clinical setting: for example, a broad-spectrum second- or third-generation cephalosporin such as cefepime can be used to cover gram-negative bacilli more likely in the elderly or immunocompromised; antipseudomonal agents such as an antipseudomonal β-lactam with or without an aminoglycoside should be used if pseudomonas is a possible infectious agent; ampicillin with sulbactam should be used especially if human or animal bites are involved; and vancomycin should be used if MRSA coverage is indicated (see Table 14.5).[14] Combination therapy is indicated for seriously ill patients presenting with an infected joint.

Table 14.5 Initial empiric antibiotic therapy

Gram stain results	
Gram-positive cocci	2 g cefazolin IV every 8 hours
If MRSA risk	1 g vancomycin IV every 12 hours
Gram-negative cocci	1 g ceftriaxone IV every 24 hours
Gram-negative rods	2 g cefepime IV every 8 hours or 4.5 g piperacillin/tazobactam IV every 6 hours
No organisms on Gram stain	2 g cefazolin IV every 8 hours or 4.5 g piperacillin/tazobactam IV every 6 hours
Low MRSA risk	Or 2 g nafcillin IV every 4 hours and ceftriaxone
MRSA risk	Vancomycin and either cefepime or piperacillin/tazobactam
Other considerations	
Human bites	Ampicillin–sulbactam (pseudomonas not covered)
Narrow therapy when and if a specific organism and sensitivities are identified	
Consider addition of aminoglycoside if pseudomonas is being treated	

For gonococcal arthritis, ceftriaxone is the treatment of choice. Patients should also be tested for *Chlamydia trachomatis* from urine or from genital secretions. Treatment with ceftriaxone should be continued until a minimum of 24 to 48 hours after clinical improvement begins; at this stage, treatment may be able to be switched to an oral agent, such as cefixime. Alternatively, at least 2 weeks of continuous intravenous ceftriaxone may be used to treat gonococcal septic arthritis. Before using a fluoroquinolone, culture sensitivities must be available, because gonococcal resistance to fluoroquinolones has increased in the United States to the point that more than 30% of some populations have resistant infections, leading the CDC to recommend that fluoroquinolones no longer be used as first-line treatment for gonococcal infections. Patients can also receive a single oral dose of 1 g of azithromycin or 100 mg doxycycline twice daily for 1 week to treat a possible co-infection with chlamydia.[20]

Duration of antibiotic therapy is controversial; it can range from 3 to 6 weeks, including intravenous and oral medication. Drainage of the joint infection, whether by repetitive arthrocentesis or surgical intervention, is also indicated in septic arthritis management. Surgical drainage may be considered in infections involving the hip, if no clinical improvement is seen after 5 days of non-operative treatment, and if the infection extends into the surrounding soft tissue. There are no randomized prospective clinical studies comparing repetitive arthrocentesis and surgical drainage in improving clinical outcomes; previous retrospective studies are controversial in demonstrating preference for one intervention over another. Early mobilization with physical therapy and rehabilitation is also indicated, and should be part of the appropriate management for septic arthritis.

As mentioned previously, after the initial presentation, the further evaluation and management of septic arthritis can involve, but not be limited to, consultation with specialists from infectious disease, orthopedic surgery, and physical therapy, depending on the clinical situation, clinician comfort, and available resources.

Treatment for infectious bursitis is typically more straightforward than that of joint infections. If the patient is not seriously ill with systemic signs and does not require a hospitalization, oral antibiotics can be started empirically, pending culture results of the aspirate. If infectious bursitis is a possibility, then corticosteroids should not be injected into the bursa after the aspiration. Oral cephalexin or dicloxacillin can be used to cover gram-positive skin flora. If MRSA is a concern, and oral therapy is indicated, one can consider trimethoprim–sulfamethoxazole, clindamycin, or tetracycline, depending on local resistance patterns. If the culture is negative and yet the clinical suspicion still remains high, it is appropriate to continue the oral antibiotics for the full course rather than stopping them prematurely. If the patient fails to respond to aspiration and oral antibiotics, then intravenous antibiotics and hospitalization may be appropriate; in cases of failed non-operative treatment, surgical consultation may be considered for operative drainage or bursectomy.

Conclusion

Septic arthritis is a medical emergency that may be managed with improved outcomes when the provider has a high clinical suspicion, uses rapid diagnosis via arthrocentesis, and promptly uses appropriate intravenous antibiotics. Physicians should have a higher clinical suspicion in those with an impaired immune system, such as in rheumatoid arthritis, diabetes mellitus, malignancies, liver disease, renal disease, and organ transplantation. Physicians must also be aware of the increasing incidence of MRSA. To avoid permanent joint damage and potentially life-threatening consequences, the family physician should include septic arthritis within the differential diagnosis of any patient presenting with joint pain.

Infected bursitis is a more common condition, with usually less significant consequences; nonetheless, the clinical outcome and overall course can be improved with the same principles as in septic joint evaluation: high clinical suspicion, appropriate use of further studies, including aspiration, and judicious use of early treatment and appropriate management.

References

1. Goldenberg D. Septic Arthritis. The Lancet. January 17, 1998;351:197–202.
2. Baker D and Shumacher H. Acute Monoarthritis. The New England Journal of Medicine. September 30, 1993;329:1013–1020.
3. Garcia-De La Torre I. Advances in the Management of Septic Arthritis. Rheumatic Disease Clinics of North America. 2003;29:61–75.

4. Shirtliff M and Mader J. Acute Septic Arthritis. Clinical Microbiology Reviews. October 2002;15:527–544.
5. Lee G, Pagnano M, Hanssen A. Total Knee Arthroplasty After Prior Bone or Joint Sepsis About the Knee. Clinical Orthopaedics and Related Research. November 2002;404: 226–231.
6. Sauer S, Farrell E, Geller E, Pizzutillo. Septic Arthritis in a Patient with Juvenile Rheumatoid Arthritis. Clinical Orthopaedics and Related Research. January 2004;418:219–221.
7. Edwards SA, Cranfield T, Clarke HJ. Atypical presentation of Septic Arthritis in the Immunocompromised Patient. Orthopedics. October 2002;25:1089–1090.
8. Siva C, Velazquez C, Mody A, Brasington R. Diagnosing Acute Monoarthritis in Adults: A Practical Approach for the Family Physician. American Family Physician. July 1, 2003; 68: 83–90.
9. Stell I, Gransden W. Simple Tests For Septic Bursitis: Comparative Study. BMJ. 1998;316: 1877–1880.
10. Carek PJ, King DE, Abercrombie S. Does Community or University Based Residency Sponsorship Affect Future Practice Profiles. Family Medicine. 2002;34:592–597.
11. Siva C, Velazquez C, Mody A, Brasington R. Diagnosing Acute Monoarthritis in Adults: A Practical Approach for the Family Physician. American Family Physician. 2003;68:83–90.
12. Carek P, Hunter M. Joint and Soft Tissue Injections in Primary Care. Clinics in Family Practice. 2005;2:359–378.
13. Baker D, Schumacher H. Acute Monoarthritis. The New England Journal of Medicine. September 30, 1993;329:1013–1020.
14. Ross J. Septic Arthritis. Infectious Disease Clinics of North America. 2005;19:799–817.
15. Cucurull E, Espinoza L. Gonococcal Arthritis. Rheumatic Diseases of North America. 1998; 24:05–322.
16. Dubost J, Soubrier M, De Champs C, Ristori J, Bussiere J, Sauvezie. No Changes in the Distribution of Organisms Responsible for Septic Arthritis Over A 20 Year Period. Annal of Rheumatological Disease. 2002;61:267–269.
17. Chambers H. Community Associated MRSA- Resistence and Virulence Converge. The New England Journal of Medicine. April 7, 2005;352:1485–1487.
18. Goldenberg, D. Septic Arthritis. The Lancet. January 17, 1998;351:197–202.
19. Cea-Pereiro J, Mera-Vareal A, Gomez-Reino J. A Comparison Between Septic Bursitis Caused By Staphylococcus Aureus and Those Caused by Other Organisms. Clinical Rheumatology. 2001;20:10–14.
20. Rice P. Infectious Gonococcal Arthritis (Disseminated Gonococcal Infection). Infectious Disease Clinics of North America. 2005;19:853–861.
21. Siva C, Velazquez C, Mody A, Brasington R. Diagnosing Acute Monoarthritis in Adults: A Practical Approach for the Family Physician. American Family Physician. 2003;68:83–90.

Chapter 15
Lyme Disease Prevention, Diagnosis, and Treatment

Ross H. Albert and Neil S. Skolnik

Lyme disease is a multisystem disease caused by the tick borne pathogen, *Borrelia burgdorferi*. *B. burgdorferi* is a spirochete—a long, helically shaped bacteria. The course of infection begins with ingestion of the bacteria by the vector species, *Ixodes* ticks, through the blood of its "reservoir" animal (i.e., deer). After this ingestion, the bacteria can be transmitted to humans via a bite from the *Ixodes* tick. Lyme disease is a highly variable infection, presenting with many different initial signs and symptoms, which can appear at various stages of the disease process.

The presentation of the infection often depends on the stage of the disease. Lyme disease is classically divided into three phases—early localized, early disseminated, and late or chronic disease. Early Lyme disease typically presents with the classic erythema migrans (EM) rash. The rash is not essential for diagnosis, however, and only approximately 30% of patients will recall such a rash.[1] Early disease typically occurs within 1 month after the tick bite. It can present with associated symptoms such as fevers, arthralgias, headache, and malaise. Early disseminated disease can occur within days to almost 1 year after a tick bite. Early disseminated disease includes processes such as carditis, neurological disease (neuropathies, encephalitis), skin changes, and liver and kidney disease. Finally, occurring months to years after the tick bite, late Lyme disease includes complications such as chronic arthritis and chronic neurological disorders.[2]

The Infectious Diseases Society of America (ISDA) released guidelines for the diagnosis and treatment of Lyme disease in 2006.[3] The guidelines address primary prevention, diagnosis methods, antibiotic prophylaxis, and antibiotic treatment regimens for the various stages of the disease. This chapter reviews the ISDA guidelines and summarizes the essential points that relate to the management of Lyme disease by the primary care physician.

Prevention and Prophylaxis

The ISDA guidelines discuss methods of prevention of Lyme disease as well as a regimen for antibiotic prophylaxis in the event of a tick bite. The simplest and likely most effective measure to prevent Lyme disease is the avoidance of tick-infested

N.S. Skolnik (ed.), *Essential Infectious Disease Topics for Primary Care.*
© Humana Press, Totowa, NJ

areas. Frequent skin inspection during outdoor activities as well as after leaving tick infested areas is a key component of prevention. Protective, light colored clothing also may allow prompt tick removal. Tick repellents containing *N,N*-diethyl-3-methyylbenzamide (DEET) and permethrin are effective, but must be used with caution on children. It is noted in the guidelines that though these preventative measures are recommended, none has been proven to decrease the number of human Lyme disease cases.

Routine prophylaxis is *not* recommended after a bite. However, when very specific criteria are met, antibiotic prophylaxis may be considered—the tick must be clearly identified as an *Ixodes* tick that has been attached for at least 36 hours; the local rate of infection of ticks with *B. burgdorferi* is at least 20% (this rate of infections occurs in parts of New England, parts of the mid-Atlantic States, and in parts of Minnesota and Wisconsin, but seldom in most other locations in the United States); treatment must begin within 72 hours from when the tick was removed; and doxycycline must not be contraindicated for the patient (contraindications are pregnancy and age younger than 8 years old). Doxycycline is the only recommended medication for the prophylactic treatment of Lyme disease. The dosing of doxycycline for this specific use is 200 mg, in one single dose for adults, and 4 mg/kg in one single dose for children (maximum, 200 mg). Implicit in this recommendation is that physicians become facile in the identification of *Ixodes* ticks at various time points after attachment.

Required criteria for Lyme disease prophylaxis after a tick bite:

- Tick must be clearly identified as an *Ixodes* tick
- Tick must be attached for at least 36 hours
- Local rate of infection with the *Ixodes* ticks must be at least 20%
- Treatment must begin within 72 hours from when the tick was removed
- Doxycycline must not be contraindicated for the patient

Diagnosis

The diagnosis of Lyme disease can be made clinically or serologically. In early Lyme disease, when the EM rash is apparent, serological tests often have not yet turned positive, so there is little value in obtaining serologic testing when deciding whether or not to treat early Lyme disease. The diagnosis of early Lyme disease is a clinical diagnosis.

When serological testing is warranted, enzyme-linked immunosorbent assay (ELISA), Western blot, and polymerase chain reaction (PCR) tests are available. It is important to note that, although serologic testing is useful in supporting the clinical diagnosis of Lyme disease, *laboratory confirmation is not a necessary requirement for the diagnosis*. Typically, a polyvalent ELISA is carried out as the first-line test. Although validated PCR tests are available, the ISDA guidelines state that these tests are likely too expensive and cumbersome to be used routinely. They also stress that only validated, Centers for Disease Control and Prevention (CDC)-approved tests should be used in the diagnosis of Lyme disease. Lyme disease titers suffer from a lack of specificity and can remain seropositive long after infection. In patients with a low clinical likelihood of illness, the clinician should be cautious in ordering Lyme disease serology, because a positive test in that setting most likely represents a false positive or is a reflection of previous, not current, disease.

Treatment of Early Lyme Disease

The treatment of early Lyme disease with no central nervous system (CNS) or cardiac involvement is with oral antibiotics only. The first-line treatment choices for early Lyme disease are 14 days of 100 mg doxycycline twice per day, 500 mg amoxicillin three times per day, or 500 mg cefuroxime twice per day. Recommended dosing for children is 14 days of 50 mg/kg amoxicillin daily in three divided doses (maximum, 500 mg per dose), 30 mg/kg cefuroxime daily in two divided doses (maximum, 500 mg/dose), or, if the child is older than 8 years old, 4 mg/kg doxycycline daily in two divided doses (maximum 100 mg/dose). For patients unable to tolerate the above regimens because of drug allergies or intolerances, second-line treatment options include azithromycin, clarithromycin, or erythromycin.

The ISDA guidelines recommend against the use of first-generation cephalosporins, such as cephalexin, in the treatment of Lyme disease. Because an EM rash can, at times, mimic skin manifestations of cellulitis, the guidelines recommend the use of cefuroxime or amoxicillin–clavulanic acid when the differential diagnosis of a rash includes Lyme disease. Intravenous ceftriaxone, which is effective in the treatment of Lyme disease, is not recommended for the routine treatment of early Lyme disease because of its higher risk of side effects, relative to oral agents.

Lyme Meningitis and Other Manifestations of Early Neurologic Lyme Disease

The treatment of disseminated Lyme disease with neurological or cardiac effects differs from that of early Lyme disease. *Intravenous antibiotic therapy should be used when symptoms of radiculopathy or meningitis are present.* Therapy with 14 days of 2 g ceftriaxone once per day, 2 g cefotaxime every 8 hours, or 18 to 24 million U penicillin G per day, divided every 4 hours, are appropriate. In pediatric patients, dosing of ceftriaxone is 50 to 75 mg/kg given once per day (maximum, 2 g), dosing of cefotaxime is 150 to 200 mg/kg/day divided three to four doses/day, and dosing of penicillin G is 200,000 to 400,000 U/kg/day divided every 4 hours (maximum, 18–24 million U/day).

Special consideration should be given to patients presenting with Lyme disease associated with isolated cranial nerve palsies but no other CNS findings.

There is debate regarding the management of these patients. Some ISDA panel members advocate cerebrospinal fluid (CSF) examination in these patients because of the frequent CSF pleocytosis associated with cranial nerve palsies. Others recommend against CSF analysis if there are no other signs of CNS involvement (i.e., headache, lethargy, meningismus), because these patients can often be treated successfully with oral courses of antibiotics using dosing regimens for early Lyme disease. CSF evaluation should be conducted whenever CNS involvement is suspected.

Patients with normal CSF examination findings and patients who do not need a lumbar puncture because of lack of clinical signs of CSF involvement can be treated with a 14-day course (range, 14–21 days) of the same antibiotics used for patients with EM.

The guidelines note that children older than the age of 8 years old with disseminated Lyme disease have been effectively treated with oral doxycycline in clinical studies. Doses used in these studies were 4 to 8 mg/kg/day in two divided doses (maximum, 100–200 mg/dose)—approximately twice the dose used for early Lyme disease.

Early disseminated Lyme disease can also cause cardiac manifestations, such as arrhythmias and heart block. Patients with cardiac manifestations of Lyme disease may be treated with oral or intravenous therapy. Symptomatic patients may be hospitalized as indicated for cardiac monitoring, and intravenous antibiotics should initially be started at doses shown below in table 15.1 for Lyme disease affecting the CNS. A temporary pacemaker may need to be placed if heart block is life threatening. Antibiotic therapy can be changed from intravenous to oral agents if conduction deficits resolve, to complete the patients' course of treatment outside of the hospital.

Table 15.1 Adult treatment regimens for the stages of Lyme disease

Early disease—oral treatment for 14 days	Early disease with CNS or cardiac manifestations	Late disease—oral treatment for 28 days
Preferred regimens	Preferred regimen	Preferred regimens
100 mg doxycycline twice daily	2 g ceftriaxone daily	100 mg doxycycline twice daily
500 mg amoxicillin three times daily		500 mg amoxicillin three times daily
500 mg cefuroxime twice daily		500 mg cefuroxime twice daily
Alternative regimens	Alternative regimens	Alternative regimens
Selected macrolides	2 g cefotaxime every 8 hours 18–24 million U/day penicillin G, divided every 4 hours	2 g ceftriaxone daily, intravenously

Treatment of Late Lyme Disease

Late symptoms of Lyme disease, such as arthritis, joint swelling, and neurological changes, can occur months to years after an initial tick bite. Lyme arthritis can be treated with oral antibiotics, at doses listed above in the "Treatment of Early Lyme Disease" section. A 28-day course of therapy is recommended for treatment of late disease, instead of the 14-day courses for early Lyme disease. This 28-day regimen can also be used for patients with persistent or recurrent joint swelling. The ISDA supports the use of intravenous ceftriaxone if a 28-day oral antibiotic regimen is ineffective. The guidelines suggest waiting several months before initiating these 28 day courses of treatment, however, because the inflammation associated with Lyme disease can often be slow to resolve (See Table 15.1).

Post-Lyme Disease Syndromes

The guidelines also comment on the phenomena of post-Lyme disease syndromes. The ISDA states "there is no convincing evidence of symptomatic chronic…infection among patients after receipt of recommended treatment regimens for Lyme disease. *Antibiotic therapy has not been proven to be useful and is not recommended for patients with chronic subjective symptoms.*"

Summary and Recommendations

Lyme disease can present with a variety of cutaneous, joint, cardiac, and nervous system signs, depending on the stage of the disease. Diagnosis of the infection is based primarily on clinical findings early in the disease and on a combination of clinical findings and serologic testing later in the disease process. The treatment of Lyme disease is based on the stage and severity of the disease.

References

1. Sigal LH. Academy of Medicine of New Jersey Lyme Disease Task Force. Lyme Disease in New Jersey: A practical guide for New Jersey Clinicians. (1993).
2. Bratton RL and Corey GR. Tick-Borne Disease. *American Family Physician.* 71(12):2323–2330. (2006).
3. Wormser GP, et al. The Clinical Assessment, Treatment, and Prevention of Lyme Disease, Human Granulocytic Anaplasmosis, and Babesiosis: Clinical Practice Guidelines by the Infectious Diseases Society of America. *Clinical Infectious Diseases.* 43:1089–1134. (2006).

Part V
Other Infectious Disease Topics

Chapter 16
Infective Endocarditis

Tina H. Degnan and Neil S. Skolnik

Introduction

Infective endocarditis (IE) was first recognized hundreds of years ago and remains a serious and sometimes fatal infection. Although it is still a relatively rare diagnosis, the incidence and severity of this disease has not decreased over the past several decades. IE remains a moving target both despite and because of numerous advances in medical care. Evolution in medicine has produced widely available antibiotics and, thus, newly resistant organisms. It has also produced procedures that are more invasive, indwelling catheters and devices, and, thus, more access and footholds for infective organisms; and more seriously ill and immunocompromised patients in hospitals who are more susceptible to serious infection. Chronic rheumatic heart disease, which was once the major risk factor for IE, is being replaced by new risk factors in the industrialized world, including intravenous drug use, valvular sclerosis of the elderly, and nosocomial exposures, such as hemodialysis. The microorganisms that cause endocarditis are also changing. *Staphylococcus aureus* is replacing *Streptococcus viridans* as the most common cause of IE. Oxacillin/methicillin resistance is common in nosocomial isolates of *S. aureus*, and vancomycin resistance has been seen in *S. aureus* as well as enterococcus species. This chapter describes the pathophysiology, presentation, diagnosis, treatment, complications, and antibiotic prophylaxis of this evolving disease, based on the most recent guidelines available from the American Heart Association (AHA).

Pathophysiology

Because transient bacteremia likely occurs with each daily toothbrushing and IE does not, the process by which the endocardium becomes infected must involve more than simple exposure to microbes in the blood. "Seeding" of an endocardial surface of the heart by microbes is a dynamic process in which microbial organisms, by virtue of their own binding proteins as well as host tissue factors, such as fibrin present on damaged or inflamed endothelial surfaces, adhere to exposed heart tissue[1].

N.S. Skolnik (ed.), *Essential Infectious Disease Topics for Primary Care.*
© Humana Press, Totowa, NJ

Adherent microbes trigger further tissue reaction, attracting and activating mono-cytes, which, in turn, produce cytokines and other factors, a cascade that finally results in the so-called vegetation of IE. A vegetation is composed of microbes, plate-lets, fibrin, and inflammatory cells, and adheres to the endocardium, insulating the microbes from host immune defenses and acting as a growing nidus of infection.[2] Given the pathogenesis of the vegetation, it is not surprising that organisms such as *S. aureus, Streptococcus* species, and enterococci that possess intrinsic surface adhes-ins and resist platelet-induced killing are the most common pathogens causing IE,[1] and that patients with mechanical or inflammatory endocardial lesions are their most frequent hosts.

Cases of IE are typically divided into four different categories based on primary host risk factor: native valve, prosthetic valve, intravenous drug use, and nosicomial. Although *S. aureus* now seems to be the most common cause of IE across all four categories,[3] stratification of patients into these categories remains useful in organ-izing clinical thinking regarding presentation and pathogens.

Native valve IE is associated with degenerative valve lesions and congenital heart disease (CHD). Rheumatic heart disease-related valvular scarring, once the classic risk factor for IE, is now rare in industrialized nations. It has been replaced by senile valve disease (common to our aging population) and the more controver-sial risk factor, mitral valve prolapse (MVP). MVP is a heritable condition that affects 2 to 4% of the population[1] and is the most common cardiac diagnosis in patients with IE.[2] It is very important to recognize, however, that this association is likely caused by the frequency of MVP in the general population rather than a sub-stantial risk of IE conferred by MVP.[2] Only patients with MVP *and* mitral regurgi-tation or thickened mitral leaflets seem to have an increased risk of IE, and their overall risk remains low.[4] In the past, guidelines supported antimicrobial prophy-laxis for patients with MVP plus valvular dysfunction.[3] However, patients with MVP—with or without evidence of valve dysfunction on echocardiogram—no longer require antimicrobial prophylaxis for dental procedures under the 2007 AHA guideline. Prophylaxis will be discussed in greater detail below.

According to different studies, prosthetic valve endocarditis (PVE) accounts for 1 to 5%[1] or up to 25%[2] of all IE cases and is further classified into "early" (within 2 months of valve replacement surgery) and "late" (>2 months after surgery). Most PVE occurs in the "early" category, is presumably acquired in the hospital, and results from infection with *S. aureus* or *S. epidermidis.*[1] According to some sources, late PVE cases occurring between 2 and 12 months after valve replacement surgery may be caused by either hospital- or community-acquired pathogens,[2] whereas PVE diagnosed longer than 12 months after surgery is caused by community-acquired organisms such as streptococci and the HACEK group (*Haemophilus* spp, *Actinobacillus actinomycetemcomitans, Cardiobacterium hominis, Eikenella corro-dens*, and *Kingella kingae*).[1] It is unclear whether it is mechanical or bioprosthetic valves that are more prone to PVE.

Not surprisingly, IE secondary to intravenous drug use affects a much younger population, with a median age of 30 to 40 years.[1] The tricuspid valve is most com-monly affected, in comparison to other categories of IE, which usually affect the left side of the heart. Mixed right- and left-sided IE is also seen in this population, and the vast majority of these patients have no preexisting valvular abnormalities. Pathogens arise from skin flora, and *S. aureus* is the predominant agent. In intravenous drug users (IVDUs) who are also HIV positive, risk of IE is increased over HIV-negative IVDUs only when the CD4 count is < 200 cells/µl.[1] HIV infection should prompt suspicion for more unusual etiologic organisms.

Nosocomial infection is responsible for a growing percentage of IE cases, and these infections carry a 50% mortality rate.[1] Rates of hospital-acquired *S. aureus* bacteremia are increasing, and *S. aureus* and other bacteria are rapidly gaining resistance to available antibiotics. Infections with methicillin/oxacillin-resistant *S. aureus* (MRSA/ORSA) and vancomycin-resistant enterococcus (VRE) are well known, and isolates of vancomycin-resistant *S. aureus* have been reported.[3] Indwelling catheters are the most common cause of *S. aureus* bacteremia leading to nosicomial IE, and cardiac devices, such as pacemakers and defibrillators, are other important sources. A minority of patients with nosicomial IE have predisposing valvular abnormalities. Hemodialysis patients account for an important subset of these cases, with a two to three times higher risk for IE than the general population or than those who receive peritoneal dialysis.[1]

Clinical Presentation

Clinical presentation of IE is highly variable, ranging from severe toxicity (acute endocarditis) to a more indolent illness (subacute endocarditis). Fever is the most common sign, but patients who are elderly, debilitated, or who have recently taken antibiotics may not mount a fever in response to IE and may present a diagnostic challenge. It is important to maintain a high index of suspicion for IE in any patient with unexplained fever in the setting of a prosthetic valve or valve disease, history of IVDU, recent major dental work or genitourinary procedure, cardiac surgery or implanted device, and in hospitalized or hemodialysis patients with indwelling venous catheters.

Patients with a more indolent presentation may complain of persistent, vague symptoms such as low-grade fever, chills, weight loss, night sweats, malaise, anorexia, and arthralgias. These symptoms may evolve over weeks to months, and such patients are more likely to have the classic extracardiac physical examination findings of IE thought to be immunologic (Osler nodes, Roth spots, hematuria) or vascular (Janeway lesions, splinter hemorrhages, palatal or conjunctival petechiae) phenomena. Osler nodes are tender subcutaneous nodules in the pads of fingers and toes; a Roth spot is a white spot on the retina surrounded by hemorrhage; hematuria is caused by glomerulonephritis; Janeway lesions are painless, erythematous macules usually found on the palms and soles; and splinter hemorrhages are linear lesions seen under fingernails and toenails that are red for 2 to 3 days and then appear brown.[2] Other extracardiac findings include pallor and splenomegaly.

Heart murmurs on physical exam in patients with IE are most often preexisting, but a new or changing murmur should always prompt concern. Other cardiac manifestations include signs of congestive heart failure (CHF) or new atrioventricular block. Patients may present with signs of septic embolism, such as stroke, septic arthritis, cellulitis, and pneumonia. Pulmonary symptoms may also be seen with right-sided or pacemaker lead endocarditis.

Laboratory abnormalities seen with IE include leukocytosis, anemia, elevated erythrocyte sedimentation rate and C-reactive protein, and microscopic hematuria. However, the cornerstones of diagnosis are blood cultures and echocardiography. Blood cultures (at least two sets, preferably drawn 12 hours apart, before initiation of antibiotics) and echocardiography should be urgently performed on all patients with suspected IE. Echocardiography is central not only to the diagnosis of IE but also to management, because identification of valvular dysfunction or cardiac abscess will prompt treatment that is more aggressive.

The question of whether to perform transthoracic echocardiography (TTE) versus transesophageal echocardiography (TEE) is addressed in detail in a recent AHA guideline.[4] TTE may be performed more rapidly and has a specificity of 98% but a sensitivity of at most 60 to 70% for vegetations. It is limited by body habitus and other factors that impact image quality. TEE is more invasive but has a sensitivity of 75 to 95% and specificity of 85 to 98%.[2] In general, the choice between TTE and TEE should be guided by the clinical scenario. Initial TTE is recommended for low-risk patients in whom clinical suspicion for IE is relatively low unless circumstances (e.g., chronic obstructive pulmonary disease, previous thoracic surgery, obesity) exist that would compromise image quality. If initial TTE is negative and suspicion for IE increases with clinical course, subsequent TEE should be performed; subsequent TEE is unlikely to alter management of a patient with a TTE positive for vegetation but who is deemed to be at low risk for complications. Initial TEE is recommended for all patients at high risk for IE (e.g., prosthetic valve, previous IE, CHD), in all cases with moderate to high clinical suspicion (e.g., S. aureus bacteremia, new heart block), and in all circumstances when imaging with TTE is difficult. When TEE is not immediately possible because of recent oral intake or other factors, TTE should be performed first. False-negative results may be secondary to small or embolized vegetations. False-positive results may occur with preexisting valvular pathology.

The complex task of incorporating risk factors, clinical presentation, and laboratory data to make the diagnosis of IE was addressed in 1994 with the publication of the Duke criteria.[5] This schema assigns weight to chosen diagnostic criteria to stratify patients into three categories: definite IE, possible IE, and diagnosis rejected. Although originally intended for research purposes, the Duke criteria have been studied and confirmed to have high sensitivity and specificity for the diagnosis of IE.[3] The Duke criteria as modified in 2000[6] are presented in Table 16.1. These criteria are composed of major and minor characteristics; stratification into the different categories is based on how many of these elements are present. As with most diagnostic tools, however, not every patient with the disease will fit the schema. Diagnosis of IE is difficult in situations in which blood cultures are negative secondary

Table 16.1 Modified Duke criteria for diagnosis of IE

Major criteria
1. Positive blood culture, defined as one of the following:
   Typical microorganisms from two separate blood cultures such as viridans streptococci,
   S. bovis, HACEK, or *S. aureus* OR enterococcus without primary focus
   Blood cultures persistently positive with typical organisms; i.e., at least two positive cultures
   drawn longer than 12 hours apart or all 3 or a majority of ≥4 separate cultures with first and
   last drawn ≥1 hour apart
   Single blood culture positive for *Coxiella burnetii*
2. Evidence of endocardial involvement as shown by positive echocardiogram; worsening/
   changing of preexisting murmur is not sufficient to meet this criterion

Minor criteria
1. Predisposing cardiac condition or IVDU
2. Temperature >38 °C
3. Vascular sequelae such as systemic emboli, Janeway lesions, conjunctival hemorrhage, intracranial hemorrhage, etc.
4. Immunologic sequelae such as Osler nodes, Roth spots, or glomerulonephritis
5. Positive blood culture that does not meet major criteria or serologic evidence of infection
   with typical microorganism

Definite IE
1. Pathologic criteria: presence of microorganisms proven by culture or histology of vegetation or cardiac abscess OR pathologic vegetation or abscess confirmed by histology showing
   active IE
2. Clinical criteria: 2 major criteria OR 1 major criterion and 3 minor criteria OR 5 minor
   criteria

Possible IE
1 major plus 1 minor criterion OR 3 minor criteria

Rejected diagnosis
Firm alternate diagnosis OR resolution of signs/symptoms with ≤4 days of antibiotic treatment OR
absence of pathologic evidence of IE at surgery/autopsy after ≤4 days of antibiotic treatment
OR insufficient criteria for possible IE as listed

to antibiotic use, atypical organisms, or other factors, or if echocardiography results
are inconclusive. In these cases, clinical judgment supersedes general diagnostic
criteria.

Treatment

Antibiotic treatment of IE is tailored to the causative organism and its susceptibility
profile. Specific antibiotic regimens are described in the AHA guidelines.[4]
Antibiotics must be administered intravenously or intramuscularly for a minimum
of 2 weeks (depending on organism and regimen); prosthetic valve IE requires
longer treatment than native valve IE caused by the same organism. In cases with
positive blood cultures, cultures should be re-drawn every 24 to 48 hours until
negative; duration of antibiotic treatment is counted beginning on the first day of
negative blood culture.

Surgical intervention should be considered immediately for IE patients with CHF, because surgical therapy greatly improves their mortality rate compared with medical therapy alone.[3] Other situations that may warrant cardiac surgery include persistence of positive blood cultures or worsening condition with medical therapy, fungal or aggressive/antibiotic-resistant bacterial IE, one or more embolic events during the first 2 weeks of antibiotics, and echocardiographic evidence of anterior mitral leaflet vegetation, vegetation > 10 mm, valvular perforation or rupture, or perivalvular extension.[3]

Anticoagulant or aspirin therapy for patients with IE has not been proven to reduce the risk of embolization and may increase the risk of intracerebral hemorrhage associated with central nervous system (CNS) emboli. Because of the possibility of surgical intervention in the course of IE, patients already on long-standing Coumadin therapy for prosthetic valves or other conditions should be changed to heparin therapy as soon as IE is diagnosed, and anticoagulation should be temporarily discontinued in those patients with evidence of CNS embolization and intracranial hemorrhage. According to some reports,[2] patients with *S. aureus* prosthetic valve IE are particularly susceptible to CNS hemorrhage, and suspension of anticoagulation during the acute phase of illness may be considered.

Complications

The mortality rate for IE varies depending on the causative organism, risk factors such as involvement of a prosthetic valve, comorbidities, and complications. Overall in-hospital mortality remains in the range of 16 to 25%[7] and usually results from CNS embolization or hemodynamic decompensation. Systemic embolization is a common complication of IE, occurring in 22 to 50% of cases.[3] The majority of these embolic events involve the CNS, with most emboli lodging in the middle cerebral artery; the lungs, coronary arteries, spleen, bowel, and extremities are other common sites. Splenic abscess is a rare complication of IE resulting from either septic embolus or bacterial seeding of a bland splenic infarct. Risk of embolization increases with size (> 10–15 mm) and mobility of vegetations. Location on the mitral valve has also been associated with greater risk in some reports; in general, however, it is difficult to determine a patient's individual risk for this complication. Because the risk of embolization is highest early in the course of antibiotic therapy and decreases dramatically after 2 to 3 weeks, if surgery is being considered for large vegetations, it should be performed early in the first week of treatment to have the most impact on embolic risk.

Perivalvular extension of infection occurs in up to 40% of native valve IE and is substantially more common in prosthetic valve IE, leading to an increased incidence of CHF, more surgical interventions, and increased mortality.[3] Heart block may result from extension into the membranous septum and atrioventricular node. Signs of extension other than heart block and CHF include persistent fever or bacteremia, embolus, or new murmur in a patient on adequate antibiotic therapy.

Development of CHF carries a grave prognosis and occurs most commonly with aortic valve involvement.[3] Decompensation may develop acutely or may slowly progress because of progressive valvular insufficiency or ventricular dysfunction. Patients with CHF should be urgently evaluated by a cardiac surgeon, because mortality is even higher without surgery.

Because of the possibility of severe complications, patients with IE should initially be stabilized and monitored carefully in the hospital. Although the risk of embolization wanes after 2 weeks of therapy, CHF may develop months after therapy has been completed. Patients who are allowed to complete parenteral antibiotics at home should be judged to be at low risk for complications and should be carefully monitored for signs of CHF and adverse drug reactions in the outpatient setting. TTE should be performed before completion of antibiotics to establish a new baseline for valvular anatomy and function.[3] Dental evaluation, rehabilitation for IVDU, and other risk factor modifications should be addressed. Patients should be educated regarding the signs of IE relapse, which most often occurs within 2 months of completing therapy; fevers and chills must be taken seriously and prompt blood cultures obtained before initiation of antibiotics.

Antibiotic Prophylaxis

As discussed above, transient bacteremia is common with activities of daily living such as eating and toothbrushing; only certain organisms are capable of causing IE; and susceptibility to IE-causing organisms depends on the presence of certain structural abnormalities of the heart or other predisposing conditions.[4, 8] Despite the frequency of transient bacteremia in the general population, IE is rare. The majority of cases are not attributable to dental or other invasive procedures; furthermore, no randomized, controlled trial has established that antibiotic prophylaxis is effective in preventing IE after any procedure that is known to produce bacteremia.[4, 8] For this reason, along with growing concern regarding unnecessary use of antibiotics in the face of increasing resistance, emphasis on IE prophylaxis in accepted guidelines began to grow increasingly controversial.[4, 9] The latest AHA guideline for IE prophylaxis was released in May 2007, and delineated an important shift in the clinical approach to IE prevention. The earlier 1997 guideline stratified patients into categories of high, moderate, and negligible risk based on potential outcome severity.[8] High-risk patients included those with both mechanical and bioprosthetic heart valves, previous IE, and complex CHD. The moderate-risk category included patients with most other uncorrected congenital cardiac malformations, hypertrophic cardiomyopathy, and acquired valvular dysfunction, including mitral valve prolapse with thickened leaflets or regurgitation. The negligible risk category for which prophylaxis was not recommended included patients with mitral valve prolapse without regurgitation, innocent heart murmurs, pacemakers/defibrillators, and history of surgical repairs of septal defects, coronary artery bypass graft (CABG), Kawasaki disease, or rheumatic fever without residual valve dysfunction. In addition, a long list of procedures for which prophylaxis was and was not required was included. These recommendations proved to be unwieldy in clinical practice.

In contrast, the 2007 guideline clearly states and supports that antibiotic prophylaxis has never been proven to prevent IE and that it should only be administered to the highest risk patients because of their increased potential morbidity and mortality from IE (Table 16.2).[4]

A summary of the 2007 AHA recommendations is as follows:

- Bacteremia leading to IE is much more likely to result from normal daily activities, such as chewing, than from dental or other procedures
- Improved oral hygiene should be emphasized over antibiotic prophylaxis
- Prophylaxis is not proven to prevent IE and should be reserved for patients with the following conditions because of increased morbidity and mortality from IE: prosthetic valve; previous IE; cardiac transplant *with valvulopathy*; or CHD including unrepaired cyanotic CHD, completely repaired CHD with prosthetic material placed by surgery or catheter *for the first 6 months after the procedure*, and repaired CHD with residual defects
- Patients with one of the conditions listed above should be given prophylaxis for dental procedures that perforate the oral mucosa or manipulate gingival tissue or the periapical region of teeth. Anesthetic injections through noninfected tissue, dental radiographs, placement or adjustment of orthodontic appliances, and shedding of teeth or bleeding from trauma to lips or mouth do not require antibiotics

Table 16.2 Cardiac conditions associated with the highest risk of adverse outcome from endocarditis for which prophylaxis for dental procedures is recommended[4]

Prosthetic cardiac valve

Previous IE

CHD including unrepaired cyanotic CHD, completely repaired CHD with prosthetic material placed by surgery or catheter *for the first 6 months after the procedure*, and repaired CHD with residual defects

Cardiac transplant recipients who develop cardiac valvulopathy

Table 16.3 Antibiotic regimens for IE prophylaxis in selected patients. All regimens are given as a single dose 30 to 60 minutes before the procedure

Route	Antibiotic	Adult dose	Child dose
Oral	Amoxicillin	2 g	50 mg/kg
Oral, penicillin allergic	Cephalexin OR	2 g	50 mg/kg
	Clindamycin OR	600 mg	20 mg/kg
	Azithromycin/ clarithromycin	500 mg	15 mg/kg
Parenteral (IM or IV)	Ampicillin OR	2 g	50 mg/kg
	Cefazolin or ceftriaxone	1 g	50 mg/kg
Parenteral (IM or IV), penicillin allergic	Cefazolin or ceftriaxone OR	1 g	50 mg/kg
	Clindamycin	600 mg	20 mg/kg

IM, intramuscular; IV, intravenous.

- Patients with MVP with or without regurgitation do not require prophylaxis
- Antibiotic prophylaxis should not be given before routine gastrointestinal and genitourinary procedures involving noninfected tissue for the sole purpose of preventing IE
- Antibiotic prophylaxis is not routinely recommended before broncoscopy unless it entails incision of respiratory tract mucosa
- It is reasonable to include an agent active against staphylococci and β-hemolytic streptococci for IE prophylaxis in the selected patients listed above before surgery on infected skin or other tissue

For the appropriate patients listed above, recommended antibiotic regimens are described in Table 16.3.

References

1. Moreillon, P. and Y.-A. Que. Infective Endocarditis. *Lancet*. 2004;363:139–149.
2. Mylonakis, E. and S.B. Calderwood. Infective Endocarditis in Adults. *New Engl J Med*. 2001;345:1318–1330.
3. Baddour, L.M. et al. AHA Scientific Statement. Infective Endocarditis: Diagnosis, Antimicrobial Therapy, and Management of Complications. *Circulation*. 2005;111: e394–e433.
4. Wilson, W. et al. Prevention of infective endocarditis. Guidelines from the American Heart Association. A guideline from the American Heart Association Rheumatic Fever, Endocarditis, and Kawasaki Disease Committee, Council on Cardiovascular Disease in the Young, and the Council on Clinical Cardiology, Council on Cardiovascular Surgery and Anesthesia, and the Quality of Care and Outcomes Research Interdisciplinary Working Group. *Circulation*. 2007; 115:1–19.
5. Durack, D.T. et al. Duke endocarditis service. New Criteria for Diagnosis of Infective Endocarditis: Utilization of Specific Echocardiographic Findings. *Am. J. Med*. 1994;96:200–209.
6. Li, J.S. et al. Proposed Modifications to the Duke Criteria for Clinical Diagnosis of Infective Endocarditis. *Clinical Infectious Diseases*. 2000;30:633–638.
7. Giessel, B.E., C.J. Koenig, and R.L. Blake, Jr. Management of Bacterial Endocarditis. *American Family Physician*. 2000;61:1725.
8. Habil, G. Management of Infective Endocarditis. *Heart*. 2006;92:124–130.
9. Dajani, A.S. et al. Prevention of Bacterial Endocarditis. Recommendations by the American Heart Association. *Circulation*. 1997;96:358–366.
10. Morris, A.M. and G.D. Webb. Antibiotics Before Dental Procedures for Endocarditis Prophylaxis: Back to the Future. *Heart*. 2001;86:3–4.

Suggested Reading

Millar, B.C., and J.E. Moore. Emerging Issues in Infective Endocarditis. *Emerging Infectious Diseases*. 2004;10:1110–1116.
Fowler, V.G. Jr. et al. *Staphylococcus aureus* Endocarditis. A Consequence of Medical Progress. *JAMA*. 2005;293:3012–3021.

Chapter 17
Meningitis

Anne T. Wiedemann

Introduction

Meningitis is defined as inflammation of the meninges, the tissue surrounding the brain and spinal cord. Despite advances in prevention and treatment, there are still one million cases of meningitis worldwide each year, leading to more than 200,000 deaths. In the United States, meningitis has an annual incidence of 2.5 cases/100,000 population. The mortality rate is 3 to 19% even with treatment, and up to 54% of survivors have some neurologic disability.

Three bacteria cause the majority of meningitis outside the neonatal period, *Streptococcus pneumoniae*, *Haemophilus influenza* type B (HIB), and *Neisseria meningitidis*, although numerous other bacteria, including *Streptococcus agalactiae*, *Escherichia coli*, *Listeria monocytogenes*, aerobic gram-negative bacilli, and *Staphylococcus aureus* have also been implicated (see Table 17.1).

The introduction of the conjugated HIB vaccine in 1987 has changed the epidemiology of bacterial meningitis is the United States. Before the vaccine, 1 in 200 children younger than 5 years of ago developed HIB meningitis or invasive disease and HIB was the causative agent in 70% of meningitis cases in this age group. Today, invasive disease from HIB has been virtually eradicated. *N. meningitidis* and *S. pneumoniae* now make up >80% of meningitis cases in the United States and the average age of meningitis has risen from 15 months to 25 years.

Pathophysiology

Few bacteria are able to penetrate the central nervous system (CNS) because of the effectiveness of the blood–brain barrier. Bacteria gain entry into the cerebrospinal fluid (CSF) through three major pathways. Colonization of nasopharynx with subsequent bacteremia and CNS invasion is the most common. Localized infection (from a urinary tract infection or endocarditis) that spreads to the CNS, or direct entry into the CNS from an otitis media, mastoid, or sinus infection, or after trauma, neurosurgery, or medical device placement, are the other routes of infection.

N.S. Skolnik (ed.), *Essential Infectious Disease Topics for Primary Care.*
© Humana Press, Totowa, NJ

Table 17.1 Age, most common pathogens, and antibiotic recommendations

Age	Common pathogens	Antibiotic choice
<1 month	Group B *Streptococcus,* *E. coli, L. monocytogenes, Klebsiella* species	Ampicillin plus cefotaxime or ampicillin plus gentamicin
1 month–2 years	*S. pneumoniae, N. meningitidis,* Group B *Streptococcus, H. influenzae, E. coli*	Vancomycin plus a third-generation (ceftriaxone, cefotaxime)
2–50 years	*N. meningitidis, S. pneumoniae*	Vancomycin plus a third-generation cephalosporin (ceftriaxone, cefotaxime)
>50 years	*S. pneumoniae, N. meningitidis, L. monocytogenes,* aerobic gram-negative bacilli	Vancomycin plus ampicillin plus a third-generation cephalosporin (ceftriaxone, cefotaxime)

Once in the CSF, bacterial multiply easily because of the relatively low concentrations of immunoglobulins. This rapid replication releases proinflammatory cytokines that stimulate the body's immune system. This leads to leukocyte invasion and increased blood–brain barrier permeability, which can result in cerebral edema, increased intracranial pressure, and neuronal damage. This inflammatory response has been implicated in the long-term neurologic sequelae of bacteria meningitis.

Clinical Presentation

In both children and adults, the presenting symptoms of meningitis are similar. Fever, stiff neck, and change in mental status are the classic triad of symptoms, although headache, vomiting, photophobia, and sore throat are also common. As the disease progresses, irritability, lethargy, delirium, and coma can develop. A large percentage of patients present with seizures or focal neurologic signs, such as cranial nerve palsies or hemiparesis. Joint pain, petechiae, and palpable purpura may also be present, especially with meningococcal infection. Waterhouse–Friderichsen syndrome, the development of hemorrhagic eruptions, and a shock-like state is virtually pathognomonic for meningococcal infection.

On physical exam, nuchal rigidity can be demonstrated by an inability to touch the chin to chest on either passive or active flexion. The Brudzinski and Kernig signs are classic tests to illustrate nuchal rigidity. The Brudzinski sign refers to spontaneous flexion of the hips with passive neck flexion, and the Kernig sign describes increased resistance to extension of the knees when the hips are flexed to 90 degrees.

Because of the risk of brainstem herniation from a lumbar puncture in a patient with a mass lesion, the Infectious Diseases Society of America (IDSA) recommends obtaining a computed tomography (CT) scan of the brain before lumbar puncture in immunocompromised patients (HIV infection, immunosuppressive therapy, or after transplant), patients with a history of CNS disease (stroke, mass, or focal infection), and patients with focal neurologic deficits, new onset seizure, papilledema, or abnormal levels of consciousness (Glasgow Coma Score <10). Lumbar puncture should also be performed with extreme caution in patients with a history of coagulopathy because of the increased risk of subarachnoid hemorrhage and subdural and epidural hematomas.

The definitive diagnosis of bacterial meningitis is made by examination of CSF. Gram stain, culture, and latex agglutination testing for specific bacterial antigen are the first priority. Gram stain can accurately identify the causative agent in 60 to 90% of patients, with a specificity of 97%. Bacterial antigen testing, although less sensitive, has also become an important tool for rapid identification of the organism. CSF polymerase chain reaction (PCR) is very helpful in cases of viral meningitis, but has not been proven useful for acute bacterial meningitis.

Cell counts, opening pressure, and glucose and protein tests also help distinguish bacterial meningitis from viral meningitis. With bacterial meningitis, the CSF often appears cloudy because of increased white blood cells, bacteria, and protein. Opening pressure on lumbar puncture is almost always elevated, generally in the range of 200 to 500 mmH$_2$O and CSF protein levels are also elevated. The CSF glucose level tends to be <40 mg/dL, with a CSF-to-serum glucose ratio of <0.4. Cell counts usually show more than 1,000 white blood cells, with >80% neutrophils, although white blood cell counts of <100 cells are not unheard of, and approximately 10% of patients with bacterial meningitis show lymphocyte predominance (>50% lymphocytes) in the CSF.

Differential Diagnosis

Aseptic or viral meningitis is most commonly confused with bacterial meningitis because the presenting symptoms are similar. Viral meningitis can only be distinguished from bacterial meningitis by lumbar puncture. With viral meningitis, on lumbar puncture, the opening pressure and glucose levels are usually normal, whereas protein levels are low and the Gram stain is negative. Although pleocytosis in the CSF is common with viral meningitis, there are usually fewer than 1,000 white blood cells and there is lymphocyte predominance. PCR for enterovirus, West Nile virus, herpes simplex virus (HSV), and Lyme disease should be sent if clinical suspicion is high for these pathogens. Viral meningitis is self-limiting and requires only supportive care with intravenous fluids and pain management.

Other important diagnoses to consider are subarachnoid hemorrhage, brain abscess, mass, and subdural empyema. CT scan before lumbar puncture will help distinguish many of these diagnoses.

Treatment

Successful treatment of meningitis requires rapid diagnosis and immediate antimicrobial therapy. Broad-spectrum antibiotics should be initiated as soon as possible and continued until culture and sensitivity results are known. At that point, antibiotic coverage can be modified. The IDSA recommends empiric therapy with vancomycin plus a third-generation cephalosporin (ceftriaxone or cefotaxime) to cover gram-positive and gram-negative organisms for patients ages 1 month to 50 years (see Table 17.1). If the patient is older than 50 years, has a history of trauma, recent neurosurgery, immunocompromised state, or alcohol abuse, the addition of ampicillin is recommended. There is no standard length of antibiotic therapy for meningitis. The length of treatment is dependent on the clinical course and on the isolated bacteria, but treatment should continue for a minimum of 7 days for *N. meningitides*, 7 to 10 days for *H. influenza*, and 10 to 14 days for *S. pneumoniae*.

Antibiotic treatment causes bacterial lysis, which adds to the inflammation in the subarachnoid space already begun by the host's immune response. This inflammation contributes to morbidity and mortality. Adjuvant treatment with an anti-inflammatory agent, such as intravenous dexamethasone, has been shown to decrease subarachnoid inflammation and subsequent unfavorable outcome by almost 10% in adults with pneumococcal meningitis, when given before or with the first dose of antibiotics. There has been no proof of improved outcome when the corticosteroids are given after antibiotic therapy has begun or with pathogens other than *S. pneumoniae*. Because the etiology of meningitis is usually unknown at presentation, all adults should receive 10 mg dexamethasone before or with the first dose of antibiotics and every 6 hours thereafter for 4 days. Some experts recommend discontinuing dexamethasone if Gram stain or culture does not support a diagnosis of pneumococcal meningitis.

Similar studies of the use of adjuvant dexamethasone in children have shown variable results. Children with HIB meningitis have shown a decrease in hearing loss with adjuvant corticosteroids, but controversy still exists over the use of dexamethasone in pneumococcal meningitis. At this point, the data are not sufficient to demonstrate a clear benefit with dexamethasone in pneumococcal meningitis, but the use of dexamethasone is not contraindicated. Therefore, current guidelines recommend the use of 0.15 mg/kg/dose dexamethasone every 6 hours in children with a high suspicion for HIB meningitis or patients with severe disease until the pathogen is properly identified.

Another issue surrounding the use of dexamethasone in the treatment of meningitis is its effect on vancomycin. Vancomycin has poor CSF penetration. It is only able to cross a damaged blood–brain barrier. It is thought that dexamethasone, by reducing inflammation of the CSF, decreases the permeability of the blood–brain barrier, and leads to decreased concentrations of vancomycin in the CSF. Therefore, vancomycin should never be administered as a single agent, but combined with a third-generation cephalosporin.

Further supportive therapies include respiratory isolation for at least 24 hours, especially in suspected meningococcal disease; antipyretic agents; adequate oxygenation, including intubation and airway management as needed; prevention of hypoglycemia; close monitoring for neurologic sequelae; and anticonvulsants when necessary. Because of a risk of hyponatremia with bacterial meningitis, fluid restriction has been recommended in the past. Studies in both adults and children have shown no improvement in outcome with salt restriction and, as a result, intravenous fluids are routinely used with the goal being a normovolemic state. Some physicians recommend elevation of the head of the bed to decrease intracranial pressure.

Secondary attack rates for household or close contacts to those infected with *N. meningitidis* are 3 to 4 per 1,000; 500 to 800 times higher than for the general population. Because these rates are so high, chemoprophylaxis is recommended for close contacts of infected patients. There are three recommended agents for prophylaxis against *N. meningitides*—rifampin, ceftriaxone, and ciprofloxacin. Oral rifampin is the drug of choice for prophylaxis and should be administered every 12 hours for 2 days at 10 mg/kg/dose in children older than 1 month, 5 mg/kg/dose in infants younger than 1 month, and 600 mg/dose in adults. Alternatively, a single intramuscular dose of 125 mg ceftriaxone for children younger than 15 years of age or 250 mg in those older than 15 years or a single oral dose of 500 mg ciprofloxacin can be used. Ciprofloxacin is not approved for the use in children or pregnant women.

Repeat lumbar puncture is not routinely recommended in patients who have responded to initial therapy to prove CSF sterilization. However, repeat lumbar puncture is essential in patients without clinical improvement in 48 hours. This is particularly important in patients with pneumococcal meningitis and a question of penicillin or cephalosporin resistance, especially if adjuvant dexamethasone was used.

Outcome and Complications

The prognosis and outcome with bacterial meningitis is multifactorial, depending on causative organism, age of patient, severity of symptoms at presentation, and time to treatment. Risk factors for unfavorable outcome include advanced age, presence of otitis or sinusitis, impaired consciousness, systemic compromise, and infection with *S. pneumoniae*.

Systemic circulatory problems are a dreaded complication of meningitis and are associated with poor outcome. Profound shock, disseminated intravascular coagulation, and gangrene of the extremities can be seen with meningococcal infection.

Herniation as a result of increased intracranial herniation is another disastrous complication of meningitis. Airway protection and mannitol can be used to decrease intracranial pressure, but, despite these measures, herniation has been reported in approximately 5% of meningitis cases.

Although the rate of meningitis has steadily decreased in the past decade, the infection still results in high morbidity and mortality. Pneumococcal meningitis has a case fatality of 20% whereas *N. meningitidis* and *H. influenza* have lower mortality rates of 10% and 5%, respectively. Approximately 15% of survivors have long-term sequelae including seizures, hearing loss, memory impairment, gait disturbances, and learning and behavioral problems in the pediatric population.

Additional Information

The introduction of the HIB vaccine has changed the face of bacterial meningitis in the developed world. As the use of *N. meningitides* vaccines for 11-year-old children and *S. pneumoniae* vaccinations for children younger than 2 years of age and adults older than 65 years become more widespread, we expect to see further declines in meningitis cases in the United States. With these changes in immunity, other organisms that currently account for a small number of meningitis cases will likely make up a larger percentage of annual cases and the average age of patients with meningitis will no doubt continue to rise.

Despite these advances, bacterial meningitis remains a significant cause of morbidity and mortality. HIB meningitis is still a major cause of disease in developing nations. Access to effective antibacterials and vaccinations is limited and must be addressed. Along with this, the problem of antimicrobial resistance, seen now with *S. pneumoniae*, continues to evolve. The development of new and effective antibiotics is imperative, and healthcare providers must detect the emergence of new resistant strains. The role of corticosteroids as adjuvant therapy must also be evaluated in further depth to help dispel the controversy surrounding it and provide clear-cut recommendations for its use. Timely diagnosis and treatment of meningitis is essential.

Suggested Reading

1. Tunkel AR, Harman, BJ, Kaplan SL, et al. Practice guidelines for the management of bacterial meningitis. Clin Infect Dis, 2004;39:1367–1384.
2. Van de Beek, D. Community-acquired bacterial meningitis in adults. N Engl J Med, 2006 Jan 5; Vol 354 (1), 44–53.
3. Van de Beek D. Clinical features and prognostic factors in adults with bacterial meningitis. N Engl J Med, 2004 Oct 28; Vol 351 (18), 1846–1859.
4. Yogev R. Bacterial meningitis in children: critical review of current concepts. Drugs, 2005; Vol 4 (4), 1097–1112.
5. Saez-Llorens X. Bacterial meningitis in children. Lancet, 2003 Jun 21; Vol 361 (9375), 2139–2148.
6. Negrini, B. Cerebrospinal fluid findings in aseptic versus bacterial meningitis. Pediatrics, 2000 Feb; Vol 105 (2), 316–319.
7. Kasper, Braunwald, Fauci, et al. *Harrison's Principles of Internal Medicine 16th Edition*. New York: McGraw Hill, 2005;2471–2477.

Chapter 18
Urinary Tract Infections

Jennifer Neria and Matthew Mintz

Introduction

Urinary tract infections (UTIs) are among the most common illnesses presenting to the primary care physician's office. In the United States in 2000, 8.27 million physicians' office and outpatient hospital visits were made by patients aged 20 years or older with a primary diagnosis of UTI.[3] Almost 83% of those patients were women.[3] Between 1988 and 1994, roughly 53% of women and almost 14% of men aged 20 years or older reported having had at least one UTI.[3] UTI is not only a common illness, but a costly one. The cost of evaluation and treatment of patients with UTIs in 2000 totaled approximately $3.5 billion.[3] Furthermore, UTIs affect both sexes and span all age groups, making them important infections to recognize and appropriately manage. If not diagnosed and treated appropriately, UTIs can lead to serious sequelae, especially in high-risk populations such as children and pregnant women. UTIs present with a range of symptoms, which can be correlated with the location and severity of infection within the urinary tract (Table 18.1). Healthy women ordinarily have uncomplicated UTIs, whereas patients with functional or structural abnormalities of the urinary tract have complicated UTIs. In addition, men, pregnant women, children, and patients in institutionalized settings, such as the elderly, are described as having complicated UTIs (Table 18.2).This chapter details the different types of UTIs, the important differential diagnoses, and the unique presentation and management by age group and/or comorbidity.

Pathophysiology

The most common causative organisms are *Escherichia coli*, which is responsible for approximately 80% of UTIs, *Staphylococcus saprophyticus*, which constitutes approximately 20%, and a variety of *Enterococci*.[7] The same pathogens typically afflict men and women, with the exception of *S. saprophyticus*, which is primarily a cause of UTIs in young sexually active women.[2,8] In complicated UTIs, additional organisms can be the cause of infection, including *Proteus, Pseudomonas,*

N.S. Skolnik (ed.), *Essential Infectious Disease Topics for Primary Care.*
© Humana Press, Totowa, NJ

Table 18.1 Definition and symptoms of UTIs

	Definition and symptoms
Cystitis	Bladder infection (lower UTI) Any combination of the following: • Dysuria • Increased urinary frequency • Suprapubic pain • Hematuria
Pyelonephritis	Upper UTI Any combination of the following: • Flank pain • Fever • Nausea/vomiting • With or without symptoms of cystitis
Urosepsis	Sepsis attributable to a UTI • May present with renal failure or frank sepsis • Clinical evidence of UTI, and $\geq$ 2 of the following[4]: 1. Temperature $\geq$ 38 °C or $\leq$ 36 °C 2. Heart rate $\geq$ 90 beats per minute 3. Respiratory rate $\geq$ 20 breaths per minute, or $PaCO_2 \leq$ 32 mmHg 4. White blood cell count $\geq$ 12,000 cells/mm³, $\leq$ 4,000 cells/mm³, or $\geq$ 10% band forms

Table 18.2 Patients with complicated UTI

Complicated UTI
Structural or functional abnormalities of the urinary tract system
Neurological disease
Diabetes mellitus
Sickle cell disease
Immunocompromised states
Multi-drug resistant causative organisms
Recent genitourinary instrumentation (e.g., Foley catheterization)
Recent history of urologic surgery
All pregnant women
All men with UTI
Elderly, especially if in nursing homes or hospital

Klebsiella, Serratia, and *Providencia* species.[8] The unique etiologies of each type of UTI will affect treatment strategies and antibiotic selection.

UTIs are most often caused by local spread of fecal flora from the perianal area to the genitourethral area, where organisms ascend via the urethra into the urinary tract. Bacterial adherence allows a pathogen to accomplish this ascent. For example, when the bacterial membrane and fimbriae make contact with the uroepithelial cell, adhesins on the bacteria irreversibly attach to receptors on the uroepithelial cell membrane.[9] Sexual intercourse further promotes this local migration of organisms, and is the most common cause of UTIs in young sexually active women. In addition, UTIs can be the result of hematogenous spread in a bacteremic patient, and, in these cases, additional pathogens, such as *Staphylococcus aureus*, should be suspected. In addition to sexual activity, other predisposing factors for developing UTIs include poor bladder evacuation, urinary retention, use of anticholinergic medications, intrinsic obstruction of the urinary tract caused by nephrolithiasis, and extrinsic obstruction of the urinary tract caused by an enlarged prostate. Certain comorbidities can further increase the risk of developing UTIs and can lead to more significant complications. For example, in diabetes mellitus, glucose can spill into the urine and lead to greater bacterial growth and increased risk of UTIs. This can be associated with perinephric abscesses and can increase a diabetic patient's risk of papillary necrosis.[5] UTIs in patients with sickle cell disease can lead to papillary necrosis.[5]

Women are more susceptible to developing UTIs than men, with sexual intercourse as a major risk factor. Shorter urethras provide a shorter distance for causative organisms to migrate into the urinary tract, and moist perineal areas foster colonization of the introitus. In addition, spermicides can modify the normal vaginal environment and further predispose women to UTIs. Important risk factors include recent sexual intercourse, history of UTI, and the use of a diaphragm and spermicide.[1,2]

Pregnant women have additional susceptibilities, which can be attributed to the effects of progesterone during pregnancy. These normal changes include smooth muscle relaxation leading to ureteral dilation and decreased ureteral peristalsis, as well as increased bladder volume.[5,10] These changes allow bacteria to ascend from the bladder to the kidneys with greater ease, thus, placing pregnant women at greater risk of developing pyelonephritis.[10]

Men, on the other hand, are less prone to developing UTIs. This is because of longer urethras, drier periurethral areas that may be less prone to bacterial colonization, and prostatic fluid that contains antibacterial properties.[8] Because UTIs are much less common in men, when they do occur, the clinician should be alert to possible unidentified causes, and the infection should be considered complicated. Possible contributing comorbidities include anatomic or functional abnormalities of the urinary tract, acute or chronic prostatitis, and HIV infection. Other risk factors for men include benign prostatic hypertrophy (BPH), genitourinary instrumentation, uncircumcised penis, homosexuality, and sex with an infected female partner.[8]

Clinical Presentation

History

The presenting complaints of UTIs are similar, regardless of a patient's age or sex. They include dysuria, urinary urgency, increased urinary frequency, suprapubic pain, and hematuria. These symptoms suggest cystitis, or infection of the bladder.

When a patient presents with fever, unilateral or bilateral flank pain, and/or nausea and vomiting, with or without the symptoms of cystitis, the clinician should suspect involvement of the upper urinary tract, referred to as pyelonephritis. Pyelonephritis requires management that is more aggressive and incurs risk of more serious complications.

A history of previous UTIs should be elicited from all patients, including children, because recurrent infections may indicate a need for further workup or urologic consultation. A family or personal history of renal cell carcinoma or its variants are helpful when neoplasm is among the differential diagnoses. Additionally, it is important to inquire about the presence of constitutional symptoms, such as unintentional weight loss, night sweats, fever, and malaise when considering neoplasm as a cause of UTIs.

Women

In women, because symptoms of UTIs, vaginal infections, and sexually transmitted illnesses (STIs) can overlap, it is important to elicit additional history and a review of systems. This should include inquiry regarding new sexual partners, use of barrier contraception, and any history of STIs. It is important to note that UTIs can coexist with other genitourinary illness, therefore, UTI should remain in the differential even when other diagnoses are made.

Men

In men, symptoms of UTI should be distinguished from those of prostatitis. Prostatitis typically presents with pelvic or perineal pain, dysuria, pain during ejaculation, fever, and/or flu-like symptoms, such as malaise and myalgias. Chronic prostatitis should be suspected in men with recurrent UTIs.[8,11] Furthermore, men with HIV infection, both homosexual and heterosexual, are at greater risk of prostatitis.[11] Similar to women, sexually active men should also be asked about symptoms of urethritis or STIs, such as urethral discharge and genital ulcers. Cultures for *Chlamydia trachomatis* and *Neisseria gonorrheae* should be carried out when STI is suspected.

Children

In children, the diagnosis of UTI, as well as the distinction between cystitis and pyelonephritis, is more difficult than in adults because symptoms in children can be more nonspecific. Further confounding the diagnosis is the fact that symptoms like fever can be indicative of other concomitant illness, such as otitis media or other diseases that commonly afflict children. Children who present with fever with no obvious source should also be evaluated for UTI. Other signs and symptoms that may suggest UTI include increased fussiness, failure to thrive in infants, and complaints of dysuria in older children. Interestingly, in younger children, diarrhea, vomiting, poor feeding, and foul-smelling urine have not been shown to predict UTI.[12,13] Older children, on the other hand, can present with more common UTI symptoms, such as dysuria, suprapubic pain, and/or hematuria. Children with abnormalities such as vesicoureteral reflux (VUR), who have suffered recurrent UTIs, may present with secondary complications, such as hypertension and renal insufficiency. Inquiring about urine output can also be important in the assessment of UTI in children. Questions about voiding habits may be helpful if physical examination and laboratory findings are negative, because voiding dysfunction can be among the differential diagnoses in children. Finally, immunization history is also pertinent to the pediatric history for possible UTI.

Physical Examination

Physical examination should include vital signs, with special focus on temperature and blood pressure. Elevated blood pressure may be found in children with VUR who have had recurrent UTIs, and it can be a physical examination finding in renal cell carcinoma as well. Measuring the patient's weight and comparing it with previous records may be appropriate if unintentional weight loss was revealed on history. An abdominal examination should check for signs suggesting other etiologies, such as cholecystitis, appendicitis, or pancreatitis. The clinician should also examine for any palpable masses. Costovertebral angle (CVA) tenderness should be elicited, gently tapping at these areas bilaterally, and noting that palpation rather than vibration may not adequately elicit true tenderness. Additional components of the physical examination for specific subgroups follow.

Women

Because UTI and vaginal infections can have overlapping symptoms, in women who also complain of vaginal discharge, vaginal odor, dyspareunia, and/or pruritus, a pelvic examination should be performed. The pelvic examination should pay particular attention to any vaginal discharge, odor, ulcerations, appearance of the cervix, and any cervical motion tenderness, which could suggest pelvic inflammatory disease (PID).

Men

A digital rectal examination (DRE) is indicated in all men with symptoms of UTI or prostatitis to help distinguish between the two diseases. Given that UTI is less common in men, prostatitis should be high on the differential diagnosis.

In acute prostatitis, DRE typically reveals a boggy and exquisitely tender prostate gland. DRE should be done gently, not only because the prostate is so tender, but also because vigorous palpation of the prostate in prostatitis can cause bacteremia.[11] Although DRE findings can be similar in chronic prostatitis, they can also reveal no abnormalities. When chronic prostatitis is suspected, prostate massage should be used to collect prostatic secretions for culture and diagnosis.

Children

Physical examination is similar for children, such as checking vital signs and evaluating for CVA tenderness. It should also include examination of the genitourethral area, looking for concomitant infections, trauma, and other causes of the child's symptoms, including vulvovaginitis, vaginal foreign bodies, and STIs or sexual abuse.

Diagnosis

Although the differential diagnosis can be very long and varied (Table 18.3), clinical presentation is often sufficient to diagnose UTI, especially in healthy sexually active women. Nonetheless, urine dipstick is typically used to confirm the diagnosis. The urine sample should be a mid-stream "clean-catch" specimen, with patients cleansing the urethral area with three single antibacterial wipes and then collecting the urine mid-stream in a designated sterile container. These precautions aim at reducing contamination of the specimen. The standard definition of a positive urine culture is at least 10^5 colony-forming units (CFU)/ml of urine.[14] However, if fecal contamination can be excluded, or an otherwise healthy nonpregnant woman presents with acute UTI symptoms with pyuria, a colony count criteria of at least 10^2 CFU/ml can be sufficient to confirm UTI.[14] In pregnancy, this lower colony count threshold of at least 10^2 CFU/ml is used in diagnosing acute cystitis when typical symptoms are present.

A positive urine dipstick includes the presence of leukocyte esterase, indicating pyuria, and/or nitrites, which indicates the presence of nitrate-reducing bacteria, such as *Enterococci, S. saprophyticus*, and *Acinetobacter*. Leukocyte esterase is 75 to 96% sensitive and 94 to 98% specific for detecting 10^5 CFU/ml of urine.[2,3,7] Occasionally, the urine specimen will reveal red blood cells, but this is not necessary for a urine dipstick or urinalysis to be positive for UTI.

If the urine is negative for leukocyte esterase, white blood cells, or nitrites, but the patient's symptoms are highly suggestive of a UTI, microscopic urinalysis and

Table 18.3 Differential diagnosis

Differential diagnosis
• Acute or chronic prostatitis
• Appendicitis (may present with fever, pyuria, and abdominal pain[13])
• Cholecystitis (especially if complaints of right upper quadrant (RUQ) pain)
• Group A streptococcal infection (may present with fever, pyuria, and abdominal pain[13])
• HIV infection
• Kawasaki disease (may present with fever, abdominal pain, and pyuria[13])
• Nephrolithiasis
• Noninfectious inflammation
• Pancreatitis (especially if complaints of RUQ pain radiating to the back)
• Prune belly syndrome
• Renal cell carcinoma
• STIs (e.g., *Chlamydia trachomatis, Neisseria gonorrheae*, PID, etc.)
• Structural abnormalities of the urinary tract system
• Trauma
• Vaginal foreign body
• VUR
• Voiding dysfunction (in children)

urine culture are indicated, given that the urine dipstick is likely a false negative result.[14] Occasionally, clinicians may choose to send urine for microscopic urinalysis, culture, and sensitivity even with a positive urinalysis, to support and further define the results of the in-office urine dipstick. Urine culture is particularly valuable in the event that the patient does not respond appropriately to empiric antibiotic treatment. If the urine culture is also negative, tests for *Chlamydia trachomatis* and *Neisseria gonorrheae* are warranted, as are investigations for other etiologies of the patient's symptoms. Furthermore, in all cases of complicated UTIs, a urine culture should be performed.

All women of childbearing age should also have a pregnancy test performed. The result is important in guiding management of UTIs in these circumstances, including the choice of antibiotics. Cervical cultures for *Chlamydia trachomatis* and *Neisseria gonorrheae* should also be performed if vaginitis, cervicitis, or PID are suspected.

Because the diagnosis of UTI is primarily a clinical diagnosis and the treatment of UTI is usually successful, imaging tests are usually not indicated. However, in certain circumstances, imaging studies, such as renal ultrasound or computed tomography (CT) scanning, are appropriate workup, such as when the diagnosis is uncertain, if the patient is critically ill or immunocompromised, or in patients with pyelonephritis not improving after 3 days of appropriate treatment. In addition, if a neoplasm is suspected based on family history, complaints, or physical examination, an imaging workup is essential.

Pregnant Women

All pregnant women should have a urinalysis and urine culture performed at their first prenatal visit, to screen for asymptomatic bacteriuria, along with cervical cultures for *Chlamydia trachomatis* and *Neisseria gonorrheae*. Because urine dipstick and other rapid screening tools in this population have shown to be less sensitive and specific compared with urine culture, they should not be used.[10] Recurrent UTIs are common during pregnancy, and prophylactic antibiotics are indicated when this occurs (see below, in "Treatment"). Test of cure with urine culture should be performed 1 week after antibiotic treatment is completed, and monthly screening should be performed thereafter until delivery.[10] Also of note is that when Group B *Streptococcus* (GBS) is identified within a urine culture during pregnancy, GBS testing is not necessary at 32 to 36 weeks, because the patient is automatically considered to be GBS colonized based on the positive urine culture.

Men

As with women, a mid-stream clean-catch urine specimen should be collected for urine dipstick, urine microscopy, and urine culture. Asymptomatic bacteriuria in men is defined by the standard colony count criteria of at least 10^5 CFU/ml of clean-catch urine.[8] However, acute cystitis in men is diagnosed with a colony count of at least 10^4 CFU/ml of clean-catch urine.[8] Because UTIs are uncommon in men and can suggest a functional or anatomic abnormality of the urinary tract system, acute or chronic prostatitis, or another comorbidity, all UTIs in men should be considered complicated. As such, a urine culture should be performed. Prostatitis is highly suggested when a patient has appropriate signs and symptoms with an elevated serum prostate-specific antigen (PSA) level.[11] Chronic prostatitis can be diagnosed with positive cultures and elevated leukocyte count of expressed prostatic secretions. Because men are less likely to develop UTIs, renal ultrasound or CT scanning should be considered in any aged male presenting with UTIs, especially with pyelonephritis.[15]

Children

Because symptoms in children can be nonspecific, laboratory testing is required to confirm the diagnosis. Urine culture is indicated when there is high suspicion of UTI, positive leukocyte esterase or nitrites on urine dipstick, or the child presents with cloudy urine.[12] Because urine dipstick is less sensitive in children, even a negative result requires urine culture.[13] The standard colony count criteria of at least 10^5 CFU/ml is used for children if a clean-catch urine specimen is obtained. Occasionally bladder catheterization may be needed, given that it is more challenging to collect a proper clean-catch urine sample from children.[13] The colony count criteria for a urine sample obtained by bladder catheterization is at least 50,000 CFU/ml.

Although there is limited evidence supporting the value of imaging in young children to prevent renal scarring and other complications of UTI, imaging studies can be performed to identify anatomic abnormalities. Renal ultrasound is a sensible imaging modality because it is noninvasive and can identify gross abnormalities of the urinary tract, including megaureter, renal abscess, and obstruction. However, many of these abnormalities can be detected on prenatal ultrasound. In addition, renal ultrasound in children is not very effective at identifying conditions such as VUR. VUR occurs when urine flows pathologically from the bladder into the upper urinary tract. It is one of the most common causes of UTI in children and is a significant risk factor for renal scarring. It is most common in children up to 2 years of age, and is significantly more common in girls than in boys.[16] It is best diagnosed with voiding cystourethrogram (VCUG), rather than renal ultrasound. If diagnosed, it should be treated medically or surgically to prevent pyelonephritis and renal scarring.[17]

Although evidence is limited, recommendations regarding imaging in children include renal ultrasound and VCUG in: 1) UTI in febrile children younger than age 5 years, 2) males at any age with their first UTI, 3) girls younger than age 3 years with their first UTI, and 4) children with recurrent UTIs.[13] However, if prenatal ultrasound was performed at 30 to 32 weeks gestation, renal ultrasound in symptomatic children is generally unnecessary. An additional indication for renal ultrasound, as well as repeat urine culture, is if the child does not show improvement after 48 hours of antibiotic treatment.[12,13]

Treatment

Treatment options are summarized in Table 18.4

Asymptomatic Bacteriuria

Asymptomatic bacteriuria is defined as a positive urine culture in a patient without symptoms. More specifically, it is defined as a colony count of at least 10^5 CFU/ml of urine on two consecutive clean-catch urine specimens. No benefit has been found in routinely screening for or treating bacteriuria in asymptomatic, healthy individuals. Asymptomatic bacteriuria is often transient.[18] There are certain exceptions that do require screening and treatment if bacteriuria is present. These include: 1) all pregnant women, 2) men before transurethral resection of the prostate (TURP), and 3) men before any urologic procedure that may cause mucosal bleeding.[8,18] In addition, some practitioners support screening and treatment of young children with VUR and patients with struvite stones, although, in the latter case, stone extraction is the preferred treatment.[18] Asymptomatic men, diabetic patients, patients with spinal cord injury, and elderly patients do not require treatment or monitoring of asymptomatic bacteriuria.[6,18]

In pregnancy, asymptomatic bacteriuria significantly increases a woman's risk of preterm labor, low birth weight, and perinatal mortality;[10] therefore, it should be

Table 18.4 Summary of antibiotic treatment options

Subgroup		Antibiotic regimen options
Pregnant women	Asymptomatic bacteriuria	• 50 mg nitrofurantoin orally four times daily for 3–7 days • 3 g fosfomycin orally as a single dose • 100 mg cefpodoxime proxetil orally every 12 hours for 3–7 days • 500 mg sulfisoxazole orally three times daily for 3–7 days • 500 mg amoxicillin orally three times daily for 3–7 days • 500 mg amoxicillin–clavulanate orally twice daily for 3–7 days
	Recurrent asymptomatic bacteriuria (*prophylaxis*)	• 50–100 mg nitrofurantoin orally at bedtime or postcoitally • 250–500 mg cephalexin orally at bedtime or postcoitally
	Acute cystitis (*considered complicated*)	• 500 mg amoxicillin orally twice daily, or 250 mg orally three times daily for 3–7 days • 100 mg nitrofurantoin orally twice daily for 3–7 days • 500 mg cephalexin orally twice daily for 3–7 days
Uncomplicated UTI	Healthy nonpregnant women	• 160/800 mg TMP-SMX orally twice daily for 3 days • 250 mg ciprofloxacin orally twice daily for 3 days • 500 mg ciprofloxacin XR orally daily for 3 days • 100 mg nitrofurantoin orally twice daily for 7–10 days
	Postmenopausal women	• 160/800 mg TMP-SMX orally twice daily for 7 days • 250 mg ciprofloxacin orally twice daily for 7 days • 100 mg nitrofurantoin orally twice daily for 7 days
	Recurrent uncomplicated cystitis[23] (*prophylaxis*)	• 40/200 mg TMP-SMX orally postcoitally • 40/200 mg TMP-SMX orally daily for 6 months • 50–100 mg nitrofurantoin orally daily for 6 months • 200 mg norfloxacin orally daily for 6 months • 250 mg cephalexin orally daily for 6 months • 100 mg trimethoprim orally daily for 6 months

(continued)

Table 18.4 (continued)

Subgroup		Antibiotic regimen options
Complicated UTI		• 500 mg ciprofloxacin orally twice daily for 7–14 days • 1 g ciprofloxacin XR orally daily for 7–14 days • 500 mg levofloxacin orally daily for 7–14 days
Pyelonephritis (*outpatient*)		• 500 mg ciprofloxacin orally twice daily for 7–14 days • 1 g ciprofloxacin XR orally daily for 7–14 days • 500 mg levofloxacin orally daily for 7–14 days
Men	Any UTI (*all are considered complicated*)	• 500 mg ciprofloxacin orally twice daily for 7–14 days • 1 g ciprofloxacin XR orally daily for 7–14 days • 250–500 mg levofloxacin orally daily for 7–14 days
	Acute prostatitis	• 500 mg ciprofloxacin orally every 12 hours for 4–6 weeks • 500 mg levofloxacin orally daily for 4–6 weeks • 1 double-strength TMP-SMX tablet orally every 12 hours for 4–6 weeks • *Staphylococcal* infection: 500 mg cephalexin orally every 6 hours for 4–6 weeks
	Chronic prostatitis[11]	• 500 mg ciprofloxacin orally every 12 hours for 6–12 weeks • 500 mg levofloxacin orally daily for 6–12 weeks

Children[25,26]		• 8 mg/kg/day TMP-SMX every 6 hours for 7–14 days
		  ○ Contraindicated in children younger than 2 months old
		• 5–7 mg/kg/day nitrofurantoin every 6 hours for 7–14 days
		  ○ Not a good choice for pyelonephritis
		• Cephalosporin (e.g., 25–50 mg/kg/day cephalexin every 6 hours) for 7–14 days
		  ○ No *Enterococcus* or *Pseudomonas* coverage

treated. Antibiotic choices include nitrofurantoin, fosfomycin, cefpodoxime proxetil, sulfisoxazole, amoxicillin, and amoxicillin–clavulanate. Fluoroquinolones are avoided in pregnancy because of the possibility that they may cause enthesopathy or other tendon- or bone-related damage in the fetus. Because there is increased resistance to sulfisoxazole and amoxicillin, sensitivities should be obtained before beginning these antibiotics. Use of sulfonamides at term can theoretically increase the risk of kernicterus in the newborn, but they are not associated with birth defects when used earlier in pregnancy. Use of nitrofurantoin should be avoided at term because of the theoretical risk of hemolytic disease in the newborn, a particular concern in glucose-6-phosphate-dehydrogenase (G6PD) deficiency.[10]

When asymptomatic bacteriuria recurs during pregnancy despite two or more courses of treatment, it should be treated with either daily or postcoital prophylactic antibiotics (see Table 18.4).

Uncomplicated UTI

Because the history often leads to appropriate diagnosis and successful treatment of UTIs, recent evidence has shown that telephone triage by a nurse and prescription treatment are an appropriate option for suspected uncomplicated UTIs in healthy nonpregnant women without vaginal symptoms.[7,19,20] This approach has led to both decreased cost and increased satisfaction among these patients.[7] If telephone triage and treatment is done, explicit instruction must be made to these patients to contact the primary care office if symptoms worsen or do not improve within 2 to 3 days of treatment.[20]

Trimethoprim–sulfamethoxazole (TMP-SMX), ciprofloxacin, and nitrofurantoin are appropriate first-line choices for the treatment of uncomplicated UTIs in nonpregnant women. Earlier recommendations were for 7 to 10 days of therapy, however, studies that are more recent show that shorter courses can be effective. Advantages include decreased cost and increased compliance, but may yield lower cure rates, especially if the infection is higher in the urinary tract.[4] Single-dose therapy cure rates range from 65 to 100%, but studies have show that 3-day treatment yields are superior to 1-day regimens.[21] The Infectious Diseases Society of America recommends using 3 days of therapy with standard doses for treatment of uncomplicated UTIs in women.

Resistance of *E. coli* to TMP-SMX is increasing in the United States.[2,7] TMP-SMX is typically effective at treating *S. saprophyticus*. Older fluoroquinolones, such as ciprofloxacin, are still effective at treating UTIs, with resistance well under 5%.[2] The resistance rate to ampicillin is >20% in many areas of the country, making it a less effective antibiotic choice for UTIs. For uncomplicated UTI in postmenopausal women, evidence supports the use of antibiotic treatment for 7 days instead of 3 days because there is greater treatment failure with the shorter antibiotic regimen.[7]

In addition to antibiotic treatment, patients with severe dysuria can also be prescribed phenazopyridine 200 mg orally every 8 hours for urinary tract analgesia to help their symptoms. Although immediate postcoital urination may help prevent the ascent of pathogens leading to UTI, there are no studies yet that support this.[22] In addition, recent studies have shown that drinking cranberry juice is not effective at preventing or treating UTI.[7] However, because these two approaches are generally safe and well tolerated, it is not unreasonable to allow patients to follow these practices if they wish, in addition to proper medical treatment when needed.

Recurrent UTI is defined as at least two episodes within a 6-month period, or at least three episodes in a 12-month period.[22,23] Recurrent uncomplicated cystitis is not uncommon and does not necessarily suggest an anatomic abnormality or other illness. However, suspicion should arise for such abnormalities if a patient fails to improve with appropriate antibiotic treatment. Such circumstances warrant repeat urine culture and may include imaging studies. Prophylactic antibiotics can be highly effective at preventing recurrent uncomplicated cystitis.[22] Further studies are needed for alternative regimens, such as once weekly dosing.

Complicated UTI

Complicated UTIs are best treated with a fluoroquinolone, especially given the increasing resistance of *E. coli* to TMP-SMX. The newer moxifloxacin should not be used to treat UTIs because it does not achieve adequate concentrations in the urine.[24]

Pyelonephritis in an otherwise healthy nonpregnant woman can be managed on an outpatient basis, provided that the patient has uncomplicated pyelonephritis, and there are no concerns regarding treatment compliance or reliable follow-up. However, as with any patient with UTI, patients should be hospitalized if they are unable to tolerate oral intake; have high fever, persistent nausea, and vomiting, or other signs of severe illness; there is uncertainty regarding the diagnosis; or there are concerns regarding patient compliance and follow-up. If managed on an outpatient basis, patients with pyelonephritis should be contacted 2 to 3 days after they initiate antibiotic therapy to ensure that they are responding to treatment. Concurrently with antibiotic treatment, patients who suffer severe dysuria can also take 200 mg phenazopyridine orally every 8 hours for urinary tract analgesia for symptomatic relief.

Pregnant Women

UTI in pregnancy is typically considered complicated, given the increased risks associated with infection, which include preterm birth, low birth weight, and perinatal mortality.

Fluoroquinolones should be avoided during pregnancy, and nitrofurantoin should not be used at term.

Because pregnant women are at greater risk of developing pyelonephritis and consequently more serious complications, pregnant patients with pyelonephritis should be hospitalized and treated with intravenous antibiotics until the patient is afebrile for at least 24 hours and demonstrating symptomatic improvement. Severe pyelonephritis can lead to acute respiratory distress syndrome (ARDS), acute renal failure with suppurative pyelonephritis and microabscesses, or sepsis.[10]

Men

If there is acute urinary retention, the initial step in treatment is to evacuate the urinary bladder with Foley catheterization to prevent sequelae such as hydronephrosis. However, this is contraindicated in acute prostatitis because of acute inflammation of the urethra, as well as when there is evidence of blood at the urethral meatus. Suprapubic catheterization may be used in this circumstance. Because UTIs in men are uncommon and, therefore, considered complicated, the duration of antibiotic treatment should be at least 7 days. Fluoroquinolones are the recommended antibiotic. Nitrofurantoin and β-lactams should not be used in men because these do not reliably achieve adequate tissue concentrations and are ineffective if the patient has occult prostatitis.[8]

For acute prostatitis, patients should be prescribed nonsteroidal anti-inflammatory drugs (NSAIDs) for analgesia and anti-inflammatory effects, provided that they do not have renal disease or a history of peptic ulcer disease. Because the prostate has a barrier between its stroma and microcirculation, adequate penetration by antibiotics is a concern. However, because inflammation in acute prostatitis results in increased permeability of this barrier, this is not as much of a concern as it is in chronic prostatitis. Nonetheless, prolonged antibiotic therapy is therefore indicated, specifically for 4–6 weeks, even if urine culture is negative sooner. Improvement in dysuria and fever should be expected in 2–6 days after initiation of treatment.[11] Selection of empiric antibiotic should be guided by Gram stain results of the patient's prostatic fluid. A fluoroquinolone or TMP-SMX is effective treatment, provided that the patient is not so sick to require hospitalization and intravenous antibiotics. *Staphylococcal* infection can be treated with a cephalosporin. Complications of acute prostatitis include prostatic abscess, sepsis, extension of the infection to the spine, and epididymitis.[11] Due to bacterial lysis, septic shock can occur at the beginning of antibiotic therapy for acute prostatitis, so the patient should be monitored closely.

Unlike acute prostatitis, the duration of antibiotic therapy in chronic prostatitis should be longer, about 6–12 weeks, because of the intact barrier between the prostatic stroma and its microcirculation. A fluoroquinolone is the recommended treatment for chronic prostatitis.[11] Other antibiotics are ineffective at treating chronic prostatitis.

Children

Empiric treatment of UTI should be avoided in young children, given that symptoms are often non-specific in this population and may actually indicate some other illness.[13] For children ≥ 2-months-old, outpatient treatment of UTI is acceptable as long as there is reliable follow-up.[24] However, as with all populations, inpatient management is indicated if a child is unable to tolerate oral intake; has a high fever, persistent nausea and vomiting, or other signs of severe illness; there is uncertainty about the diagnosis; or there are concerns about patient compliance and follow-up. Outpatient antibiotic treatment in children should last 7–14 days.[25,26] Similar to pregnancy, the safety of fluoroquinolones in children has not been established. Complications of UTI in this population can include hypertension, renal scarring, or decreased renal function.[3,13] VUR can lead to recurrent pyelonephritis and renal scarring.[12]

Follow-Up

All patients should experience symptomatic improvement within 24 to 48 hours of initiation of antibiotic treatment. If there is no improvement within 72 hours, if the patient continues to have persistent fever, or if symptoms improve but then recur within 2 weeks, further testing should be done and a urologic consultation may be considered.[24] Further testing would include repeat urine culture and imaging studies, such as renal ultrasound or CT scan to exclude structural or other abnormalities.[8] Complicated pyelonephritis should be followed with urine culture 1 to 2 weeks after treatment is completed.[24] Furthermore, recurrent pyelonephritis should be investigated further, because this can indicate more serious illness and can lead to more severe complications compared with recurrent cystitis. Pregnant women with asymptomatic bacteriuria should have a follow-up urine culture performed 1 week after treatment is finished. Further follow-up urine cultures should be done monthly thereafter until delivery.[10] Conversely, follow-up urine culture is generally unnecessary in nonpregnant women who are asymptomatic after treatment for uncomplicated cystitis.[2,24]

References

1. Hooten TM, Scholes D, Hughes JP, Winter C, Roberts PL, Stapleton AE, Stergachis A, Stamm WE. (1996, August 15). "A prospective study of risk factors for symptomatic urinary tract infection in young women." *N Engl J Med*, 335(7), 468–474.
2. Hooten TM, Stamm WE. (2006). "Acute cystitis in women." In: *UpToDate*, Rose, BD (Ed), *UpToDate*, Waltham, MA.
3. National Kidney and Urologic Diseases Information Clearinghouse. "Urinary Tract Infections (UTIs)." Retrieved July 25, 2006, from http://kidney.niddk.nih.gov/kudiseases/pubs/kustats/index.htm#11.
4. Sobel JD, Kaye D. (2005). "Chapter 66: Urinary Tract Infections." In Mandell GL, Bennett JE (Eds.), *Mandell, Douglas, and Bennett's Principles and Practice of Infectious Disease* (6th edition). Philadelphia, PA: Elsevier, Inc.
5. Shoff WH, et al. (2006, June 19). "Pyelonephritis, Acute." Retrieved July 5, 2006, from http://www.emedicine.com/MED/topic2843.htm.
6. Weintrob AC, Sexton DJ. (2006). "Asymptomatic Bacteriuria in Patients with Diabetes Mellitus." In: *UpToDate*, Rose, BD (Ed), *UpToDate*, Waltham, MA.
7. Mehnert-Kay SA. (2005, August 1). "Diagnosis and Management of Uncomplicated Urinary Tract Infections [Electronic version]." *American Family Physician*, 72(3), 451–456.
8. Hooton TM, Stamm WE. (2006). "Acute Cystitis and Asymptomatic Bacteriuria in Men." In: *UpToDate*, Rose, BD (Ed), *UpToDate*, Waltham, MA.
9. Meyrier A, Zaleznik DF. (2006). "Bacterial Adherence and Other Virulence Factors for Urinary Tract Infection." In: *UpToDate*, Rose, BD (Ed), *UpToDate*, Waltham, MA.
10. Hooton TM, Stamm WE. (2006). "Urinary Tract Infections and Asymptomatic Bacteriuria in Pregnancy." In: *UpToDate*, Rose, BD (Ed), *UpToDate*, Waltham, MA.

11. Meyrier A, Fekete T. (2006). "Acute and Chronic Bacterial Prostatitis." In: *UpToDate*, Rose, BD (Ed), *UpToDate*, Waltham, MA.
12. Alper BS, Curry SH. (2005, December 15). "Urinary Tract Infection in Children [Electronic version]." *American Family Physician*, 72(12), 2483–2488.
13. Shaikh N, Hoberman A. (2006). "Clinical Features and Diagnosis of Urinary Tract Infections in Children." In: *UpToDate*, Rose, BD (Ed), *UpToDate*, Waltham, MA.
14. Meyrier A, Zaleznik DF. (2006). "Urine Sampling and Culture in the Diagnosis of Urinary Tract Infection in Adults." In: *UpToDate*, Rose, BD (Ed), *UpToDate*, Waltham, MA.
15. Hooton TM, Stamm WE. (2006). "Indications for Radiologic Evaluation in Acute Pyelonephritis." In: *UpToDate*, Rose, BD (Ed), *UpToDate*, Waltham, MA.
16. McLorie G, Herrin JT. (2006). "Clinical Manifestations and Diagnosis of Vesicoureteral Reflux." In: *UpToDate*, Rose, BD (Ed), *UpToDate*, Waltham, MA.
17. McLorie G, Herrin JT. (2006). "Management of Vesicoureteral Reflux." In: *UpToDate*, Rose, BD (Ed), *UpToDate*, Waltham, MA.
18. Fekete T, Hooton TM. (2006). "Approach to the Patient with Asymptomatic Bacteriuria." In: *UpToDate*, Rose, BD (Ed), *UpToDate*, Waltham, MA.
19. Kripke C. (2005, December 1). "Cochrane Briefs: Duration of Therapy for Women with Uncomplicated UTI [Electronic version]." *American Family Physician*, 72(11). Retrieved July 3, 2006, from www.aafp.org/afp/20051201/cochrane.html.
20. National Guideline Clearinghouse. (2006, July 3). "Uncomplicated Urinary Tract Infection in Women." Retrieved July 4, 2006, from www.guidelines.gov/summary/summary.aspx?doc_id=5570&nbr=003767 &string=UTI#s23.
21. Warren JW, Abrutyn E, Hebel JR, et al (1999): Guidelines for antimicrobial treatment of uncomplicated acute bacterial cystitis and acute pyelonephritis in women. Infectious Diseases Society of America (IDSA). *Clin Infect Dis*. 29, 745–758
22. Hooton TM, Stamm WE. (2006.) "Recurrent Urinary Tract Infection in Women." In: *UpToDate*, Rose, BD (Ed), *UpToDate*, Waltham, MA.
23. Schooff M, Hill K. (2005) "Cochrane for Clinicians: Antibiotics for Recurrent Urinary Tract Infections." *American Family Physician*, 71(7), 1301.
24. Hooton TM, Stamm WE. (2006). "Acute Pyelonephritis: Symptoms; Diagnosis; and Treatment." In: *UpToDate*, Rose, BD (Ed), *UpToDate*, Waltham, MA.
25. Shaikh N, Hoberman A. (2006). "Management, Prognosis, and Prevention of Urinary Tract Infections in Children." In: *UpToDate*, Rose, BD (Ed), *UpToDate*, Waltham, MA.
26. Layton KL. (2003, June). "Diagnosis and Management of Pediatric Urinary Tract Infections." *Clinics in Family Practice*, 5(2), 367–383.

Chapter 19
Adult Immunizations

John Russell and Ross H. Albert

Introduction

Tens of thousands of American adults die each year because of diseases that could have been prevented by vaccination. The centers for disease control and prevention (CDC) adult vaccination schedule gives clear guidance for appropriate evidence-based approach to adult vaccination.

The average life span in the United States has increased by 30 years during the 20th century. Much of this gain is attributable to improvements in the treatment and prevention of infectious diseases. The lowering in mortality from many infectious diseases is directly linked to the use of vaccines. However, although public attention is focused on the immunization of children, adult immunization receives little attention. Mortality statistics suggest that our immunization focus should be broadened to include adults. Although several hundred children die in the United States each year as a result of vaccine-preventable infections, 25,000 to 30,000 adults die annually because of illnesses that could have been prevented by immunization.

A new immunization schedule for adults, including recommendations for patients with medical conditions, was published in October of 2006 by the Advisory Committee on Immunization Practices (ACIP) through the CDC and is available at: http://www.cdc.gov/mmwr/preview/mmwrhtml/mm5540-Immunizational.htm. It should be integrated into the fabric of the adult routine healthcare visit (See Fig. 19.1).

Hepatitis B

The annual incidence of new hepatitis B virus (HBV) infections has decreased from an estimated 232,000 to an estimated 51,000 from 1990 to 2005. The largest decrease was among children and adolescents, for whom the HBV vaccine has become standard of care. Among adults, however, lower vaccination rates, notably among those at highest risk, accounts for a less significant decrease in infection rates. Approximately 1.25 million Americans are chronic carriers of the HBV, which leads to an increased risk of developing hepatocellular carcinoma, chronic liver failure, or death. Overall, approximately 4.9% of the population has been infected with HBV.

N.S. Skolnik (ed.), *Essential Infectious Disease Topics for Primary Care.*
© Humana Press, Totowa, NJ

Recommended Adult Immunization Schedule, by Vaccine and Age Group
UNITED STATES • OCTOBER 2006–SEPTEMBER 2007

Vaccine ▼ Age group ▶	19–49 years	50–64 years	≥65 years
Tetanus, diphtheria, pertussis (Td/Tdap)[1],*	1-dose Td booster every 10 yrs		
	Substitute 1 dose of Tdap for Td		
Human papillomavirus (HPV)[2]	3 doses (females)		
Measles, mumps, rubella (MMR)[3],*	1 or 2 doses	1 dose	
Varicella[4],*	2 doses (0, 4–8 wks)	2 doses (0, 4–8 wks)	
Influenza[5],*	1 dose annually	1 dose annually	
Pneumococcal (polysaccharide)[6,7]	1–2 doses		1 dose
Hepatitis A[8],*	2 doses (0, 6–12 mos, or 0, 6–18 mos)		
Hepatitis B[9],*	3 doses (0, 1–2, 4–6 mos)		
Meningococcal[10]	1 or more doses		

*Covered by the Vaccine Injury Compensation Program. NOTE: These recommendations must be read with the footnotes (see reverse).

| | For all persons in this category who meet the age requirements and who lack evidence of immunity (e.g., lack documentation of vaccination or have no evidence of prior infection) | | Recommended if some other risk factor is present (e.g., on the basis of medical, occupational, lifestyle, or other indications) |

Fig. 19.1 Recommended adult immunization schedule, by vaccine and age group.

Current recommendations state that all newborns and adolescents should be vaccinated against HBV. Additionally, other high-risk groups that need vaccination have been identified in the adult population. These groups can be divided based on medical indications, occupational indications, behavioral indications, and other specific cases.

- *Medical indications*: Patients with end-stage renal disease, including those requiring hemodialysis; patients being evaluated or treated for a sexually transmitted disease, including HIV, or any client of an STD or HIV clinic; patients with chronic liver disease; and patients requiring clotting factor concentrates.
- *Occupational indications*: Healthcare workers and public safety workers who may be exposed to body fluids, and clients and staff of patients with developmental disabilities.
- *Behavioral indications*: Sexually active patients with more than one partner in the previous 6 months; patients currently or recently using intravenous drugs; and men who have sex with men.
- *Other indications*: Household contacts and sex partners of patients with hepatitis B infection; international travelers to nations with high rates of hepatitis B infection; and any patient requesting hepatitis B protection.

The HBV vaccine is a recombinant surface protein used to induce antibodies to the virus' surface antigens. The vaccine is given in three intramuscular doses, with 1 month separating the first and second immunizations and at least 5 months separating the second and third immunizations. These immunizations can be given simultaneously with other vaccines. If the series of immunizations is interrupted, the next shot dose should be given as soon as possible—the sequence does not need to be reinitiated. There is no risk of contracting the disease from the vaccine because the vaccine contains only the surface protein of the virus; thus, the vaccine can be used safely during pregnancy.

Postvaccination testing is generally unnecessary, however, it may be considered in patients at high occupational risk of exposure to the virus and in patients undergoing hemodialysis or with immunodeficiencies. Testing should occur 1 to 6 months after completion of the vaccine series. In patients who do not demonstrate immunity, 15 to 25% will respond to one additional dose of the vaccine, and 30 to 50% will respond to a repeated vaccine series. Also of note is that in immunocompromised patients or those undergoing hemodialysis, larger doses of HBV vaccine are usually required to induce immunity. Current recommendations suggest that testing for protective antibody levels be performed yearly. A booster dose of vaccine should be given to patients whose antibody titers are < 10 mIU/ml.[1]

Hepatitis A

Infection with hepatitis A virus (HAV) is associated with substantial morbidity—10 to 20% of patients infected require hospitalization. In 2004, an estimated 24,000 new HAV infections occurred, a decrease from an estimated 93,000 in 2001, and from approximately 270,000 in the 1980s, before vaccination implementation. Approximately 31% of the population has been infected with HAV at some point. Most infections occur in community-wide outbreaks, with 12 to 26% attributable to household or sexual contacts. Although infected adults can become acutely ill, it is important to note that infection in children (the majority of HAV cases) is typically asymptomatic.

The current recommendations for the HAV vaccine include routine vaccination of all children in the United States. This is a change from previous recommendations, in which the only recommended vaccination is for states or communities thought to have a high incidence (more than 20 cases per 100,000 people) of HAV infection.

For those aged 18 years and older who have not been vaccinated, the two-injection vaccine series can be given, with doses separated by 6 to 12 months. Protective antibody levels are present approximately 4 weeks after the first dose of vaccine in 94 to 99% of patients. The vaccine can safely and effectively be given with other vaccines. The safety of the vaccine in pregnancy has not been adequately evaluated. A combination vaccine that provides protection against HAV and HBV is now available, as well.

The CDC recommends vaccination of all adults considered to be at increased risk for exposure to HAV, including the following:

- *Medical indications*: Patients with chronic liver disease; patients receiving clotting factor concentrates.
- *Behavioral indications*: Men who have sex with men; illicit drug users.

- *Occupational indications*: People working with hepatitis A in a research laboratory and with animals infected with the virus.
- *Other indications*: Travelers to areas with high rates of hepatitis A infection; any patient requesting hepatitis A protection.[2]

Measles, Mumps, and Rubella

Efforts to immunize children with the measles, mumps, and rubella (MMR) vaccination as part of the routine immunization schedule during the last three decades have virtually eliminated these diseases in the United States. However, recent outbreaks of these infections in the USA demonstrate that the vaccination effort must continue. Unvaccinated children and adults at risk for these diseases should be identified and vaccinated.

In general, patients born before 1957 can be considered immune to MMR. They are also considered immune if they have documented vaccination, a history of previous infection, or serologic evidence of immunity. People without adequate evidence of immunity should undergo immunization with the MMR vaccine.

The MMR vaccine series is a two-shot regimen, with doses separated by at least 28 days. The vaccine is a comprised of live attenuated MMR viruses.

The immunization is generally well tolerated, with some associated fever, transient rash, and lymphadenopathy in a small percentage of recipients. There is also an increased risk for rare but serious events such as anaphylaxis, thrombocytopenia, febrile seizures, and acute arthritis associated with the immunization. No evidence suggests a causal relationship between the MMR vaccine and vasculitis, otitis media, conjunctivitis, optic neuritis, ocular palsies, psychiatric or developmental disorders, or Guillain-Barré syndrome (GBS).

Contraindications to vaccination include pregnancy, severe illness, and a history of anaphylactic reactions to neomycin or other components of the vaccine. In susceptible women, pregnancy should be excluded before providing MMR vaccination, and pregnancy should be avoided for 4 weeks after immunization. Patients who have recently received immunoglobulin should also avoid the vaccine. Immunocompromised patients should also not be given the MMR vaccine. This includes patients with leukemia, lymphoma, malignancy, or those receiving chemotherapy, radiation, or high doses of corticosteroids. Immunodeficiency caused by HIV is also a contraindication to immunization.

One special population with respect to the MMR vaccine is women who could become pregnant. Screening of women of childbearing age for immunity to rubella could prevent complications in pregnancy and in the subsequent childhood period. Rubella infection during pregnancy increases the risk of miscarriage, stillbirth, and fetal anomalies. Congenital rubella syndrome (CRS) includes auditory, ophthalmic, cardiac, and neurologic anomalies in fetuses born to women who are infected with rubella during pregnancy. An estimated 20 to 25% of infants born to mothers infected during the first 20 weeks of gestation will display some degree of CRS.

An estimated 85% infected within the first 8 weeks of gestation demonstrate some effect by age 4 years. Because of the above complications, the American College of Obstetrics and Gynecology (ACOG) currently recommends that all pregnant women be screened for rubella immunity with each pregnancy.[3]

Varicella and Zoster

The varicella zoster virus is the causative agent of both *varicella simplex* (chicken-pox) and *herpes zoster* (shingles). The virus is a member of the herpes virus family, which can cause acute infection but can also lay dormant in nerve cells for decades before reemerging again to cause overt disease. Typically, infection with varicella causes mild symptoms in children, but illness that is more significant in adults. In addition to the typical vesicular skin rash, the disease can be complicated by central nervous system (CNS) disease, pneumonia, and secondary bacterial skin infections. Pregnant women and their unborn children are also at high risk of complications caused by varicella infection.

Approximately 25% of people develop zoster during their lifetime, and there are approximately one million cases of shingles per year. The risk of developing shingles increases significantly at approximately 50 years old. Shingles is associated with significant morbidity because of acute pain during episodes as well as chronic pain caused by post-herpetic neuralgia. The rationale behind vaccination against zoster is that repeated exposure to varicella has been found to be boost immunity to varicella, which naturally wanes as people age. Vaccination would, in theory, accomplish the same end, which is becoming more critical because childhood vaccination is indirectly diminishing the reexposure of the elderly to the natural virus.

Varicella

Vaccination against varicella is now a standard component of the childhood immunization schedule in the United States, in part to prevent transmission of the virus from children to susceptible adults. The vaccination was initially given as a one-time injection at 1 year of age, but new CDC recommendations suggest that a second pediatric dose be given at age 4 to 6 years old.

The varicella vaccine is also recommended for teenagers and adults with no history of varicella infection. A documented history of varicella infection or positive serologic testing negates the need for this immunization. Because a large proportion of patients with no recollection of chickenpox have been found to have serologic evidence of previous illness, serologic testing may be a cost-effective way to reduce the number of immunizations given. The vaccine is currently recommended for adults at high risk who lack a history of varicella, including nonpregnant women of childbearing age, healthcare workers, teachers, military personnel, and residents and staff of institutional settings.

The varicella vaccine is a live, attenuated virus. The vaccine is given in two doses separated by at least 4 weeks. The most common side effect caused by the vaccine is local skin reactions. Approximately 20% of recipients have localized erythema and tenderness. A maculopapular rash develops in 1 to 3% of patients at the vaccination site. A generalized rash, with an average of five lesions, occurs in 1 to 6% of those who receive the vaccine, and 10% of adult recipients experience a fever. The vaccine can be given simultaneously with the MMR vaccine, if desired. Because this is a live vaccine, immunosuppression and pregnancy are contraindications to immunization. Patients receiving blood products, including varicella immune globulin, should delay immunization for 3 to 11 months.[4]

Zoster

A newly approved vaccine targeted at the prevention of herpes zoster was approved by the FDA in the fall of 2006. Preliminary studies showed that immunization of more than 38,000 patients aged 60 years and older reduced the incidence of herpes zoster by more than 50% during the next 3 years. The vaccine also led to modest reductions in pain and duration of zoster when it did occur. The study also analyzed the incidence of post-herpetic pain, a serious consequence that follows outbreaks of herpes zoster. Post-herpetic neuralgia was reduced by two thirds in the vaccinated group of the study.

The herpes zoster vaccine is a single dose immunization of a live attenuated varicella virus. The concentration of virus is more than 10 times that of the traditional varicella vaccine, therefore the two vaccines are not interchangeable. The vaccine is approved for patients older than the age of 60 years. It is contraindicated in patients with immunodeficiency or pregnancy. The immunization is not approved to treat zoster infection nor post-herpetic neuralgia.[5,6]

Human Papillomaviruses

Cervical cancer is the second most common malignancy in women, and accounts for more than 3,700 deaths annually in the United States. Infection with certain human papillomaviruses (HPV) can lead to cancer of the cervix, as well as of the anus, vagina, vulva, penis, and mouth. HPV types 16 and 18 are associated with 50 and 20% of all cervical cancers, respectively. HPV 6 and 11 are associated with approximately 80% of all genital warts.

Clinical trials of a quadrivalent HPV vaccine containing type-specific L1 capsid proteins from HPV 6, 11, 16, and 18 were performed to assess the efficacy of the vaccine in generation of an antibody response and prevention of various endpoints.

Five years of trials have shown that the vaccine is well tolerated, and generates an effective and lasting antibody response. The vaccine seems effective at preventing persistent HPV infection, genital warts, and cervical intraepithelial neoplasia (CIN) and adenocarcinoma when compared with placebo.

The quadrivalent HPV 6, 11, 16, 18 L1 virus-like particle vaccine has been approved by the FDA in 2006 for the prevention of cervical cancer caused by these viruses. The vaccine is approved for women aged 9 to 26 years old. The ACIP and ACOG recommend a three-dose vaccination schedule, with the initial dose followed by doses at 2 and 6 months later. According to the CDC, the recommended age for vaccination is 11 to 12 years old, with vaccine able to be given as young as age 9 years. It is recommended that adolescents and adults 13 to 26 years who have not been vaccinated for HPV received catch-up vaccination. It is important to note that vaccination does not change the recommendations for routine cervical cancer screening. The vaccine will likely be given at age 11 to 12 years old in the pediatric population, along with the tetanus toxid plus diphtheria antigen with pertussis antigen (Tdap) booster. If the series of immunizations is interrupted, the next shot dose should be given as soon as possible—the sequence does not need to be reinitiated. There is no data available to support the use of the vaccine in men or in women older than the age of 26 years, although trials are currently being carried out to assess efficacy of the vaccine in these groups.[7-11]

Pneumococcal Vaccine

Streptococcus pneumoniae is one of the most common causes of serious bacterial infections in the United States. An estimated 175,000 cases of pneumococcal pneumonia, 50,000 cases of pneumococcal bacteremia, and 3,000 to 6,000 cases of pneumococcal meningitis occur annually. Pneumococcal disease causes an estimated 3,400 deaths each year in senior citizens older than the age of 65 years.

The purified polysaccharide vaccine (PPV23) contains antigen from 23 types of pneumococcal bacteria, which cause 88% of invasive pneumococcal disease. The vaccine is 60 to 70% effective overall in the prevention of invasive pneumococcal disease, although it may be less effective in those with underlying serious illnesses. Antibody levels decrease over 5 to 10 years, but the nature of the relationship between antibody levels and the degree of protection is unclear.

Published evidence confirms that the pneumococcal vaccine provides excellent protection against bacteremia in older adults, although other strategies may be necessary to combat nonbacteremic pneumonia. The use of the pneumococcal conjugate vaccine (PCV7) in children might decrease the rate of resistant strains of pneumococcal bacteremia in adults.[12,13]

The vaccine is indicated for all adults older than 65 years, as well as any person older than 2 years with chronic illnesses (excluding asthma), immunosuppression, HIV infection, sickle cell anemia, or splenic dysfunction. Persons with chronic disease include patients with chronic cardiovascular disease (e.g., congestive heart failure [CHF] or cardiomyopathies), chronic pulmonary disease (e.g., chronic obstructive pulmonary disease [COPD] or emphysema, but not asthma), diabetes mellitus, alcoholism, chronic liver disease (cirrhosis), or cerebrospinal fluid (CSF) leaks. In addition, persons aged 2 to 64 years who are living in environments or social settings in which the risk for invasive pneumococcal disease or its complications is increased (e.g., Alaskan Natives and certain American Indian populations) should be vaccinated. A one-time revaccination is indicated for those vaccinated before age 65 years or for members of the highest-risk groups who were vaccinated more than 5 years earlier (asplenic or immunosuppressed patients or those with renal failure or who have had an organ transplant). The pneumococcal vaccine is administered intramuscularly or subcutaneously with 25 µg of each antigen per dose. The most common adverse reactions are pain, swelling, and erythema that occur at the site of injection in 30 to 50% of vaccinees. These are self-limited and require no treatment. Local reactions are more common with revaccination. More systemic symptoms of fever and myalgias occur in approximately 1% of vaccine recipients. The vaccine is contraindicated in those with a moderate to severe acute illness and in those who have an allergic reaction to the vaccine's components or who experienced previous adverse reactions to the vaccine. It may be administered simultaneously with the influenza vaccine but at another anatomic site.

Approximately 60% of American adults aged 65 years and older have ever received the pneumococcal vaccine. Rates are lower in younger adults with chronic illnesses. National health objectives for 2010 include increasing the pneumococcal vaccination rate in elderly adults to more than 90%. To meet this goal, physicians need to seize opportunities in outpatient and inpatient settings. Studies have shown that 65% of those with severe pneumococcal disease had been hospitalized, and yet not vaccinated, within the past 3 to 5 years. With an increase in pneumococcal resistance to penicillin, it makes more sense than ever to try to prevent the diseases that are less responsive to antibiotics.[14]

Influenza Vaccine

Each year, influenza epidemics cause the deaths of at least 20,000 to 40,000 Americans, most of them elderly or ill with a chronic disease. Influenza and pneumonia together are the sixth leading cause of death overall in the United States and the number one cause of death from infectious disease.

Because of antigenic drift in the virus and waning immunity in the vaccine recipient, the vaccine needs to be given each fall. The inactivated vaccine usually includes two type A strains of influenza and one strain of type B. The exact composition of the influenza vaccine is based on strains prevalent at the end of the preceding flu season and outbreaks in other parts of the world. The effectiveness of the vaccine is partly based on the similarity of the vaccine to circulating strains. A new antigenic strain can result from antigenic shift, which leads to worldwide pandemics, the last of which occurred between 1968 and 1969.

The vaccine is a split virus that is given via the intramuscular route. Vaccination programs typically begin in mid-October. Immunity begins approximately 2 weeks after vaccination. The overall efficacy is 70 to 90% in those younger than 65 years and 30 to 40% in frail elderly persons. Nonetheless, the vaccine is 80% effective in reducing death from complications of influenza among elderly patients.

The influenza vaccine is indicated for all patients older than 50 years, any patient with chronic cardiopulmonary illnesses, including asthma, and patients with other chronic medical problems, such as immunosuppression, renal disease, and diabetes. It is also recommended for anyone who resides with a high-risk person. Other candidates include pregnant women who are beyond 20 weeks' gestation during the flu season, all residents of long-term care facilities, and healthcare workers. A study conducted in 2000 showed that only 38% of healthcare workers were immunized. Studies have shown that employees are often the source of influenza spread in long-term care facilities.

Local soreness at the immunization site occurs in approximately 20% of recipients. Systemic symptoms occur in < 1% of recipients, most often after the first influenza vaccination. Some patients may need reassurance that the vaccine does not cause the flu. In 1976, an increased number of cases of GBS occurred in patients who had received the vaccine, and patients with a history of GBS should not receive the influenza vaccine. Immunization is deferred until recovery in persons with moderate to severe acute illnesses. Patients with an egg allergy should be excluded from vaccination in most circumstances. Our national health goals for 2010 target a 90% yearly influenza vaccination rate.

A nasally inhaled, live-attenuated influenza vaccine (LAIV) is now available. This product, which has been approved by the FDA for use in persons aged 5 to 49 years, may be more acceptable to patients, thereby increasing immunization rates. In adults, studies have shown an efficacy statistically the same as the injectable influenza vaccine. It cannot be used in asthmatic patients, pregnant women, diabetic patients, or any other group that falls in a high-risk group for influenza. Similar to the injectable flu vaccine, it cannot be used in those with egg allergy. The rate of infection of close contacts of those that receive the LAIV is 0.6 to 2.4%. Therefore, those with contact with patients with severely weakened immune (e.g., patients receiving stem cell transplants) systems should not receive the LAIV. Those in contact with patients with diabetes, HIV, or asthmatic patients taking steroids can receive this vaccine.[15]

Tetanus, Diphtheria, and Pertussis

Pertussis an acute respiratory infection caused by the fastidious coccobacillus, *Bordetella pertussis*. It is the cause of "whooping cough" in children. It has been part of routine childhood immunization since the 1940s. It was originally thought that natural infection gave lifetime immunity. It has been found that natural infection only confers 15 years of immunity and the Diphtheria Tetanus acellular Pertussis (DTaP) given at 4 to 5 years of age only confers 6 years of immunity. It has been suggested that this waning immunity is reflected in 800,000 to 3.2 million cases annually in the USA. Because of this increase in the incidence in pertussis, the ACIP in 2006 recommended to change the adolescent Td (tetanus toxid plus diphtheria antigen) to the Tdap (the Td with pertussis antigen). Later in the same year, they recommended that all adult tetanus booster up to 65 years of age be changed from The Tdap differs from the DTap, given in the first 7 years of life, by having less diptheria and pertussis antigen as represented by lower case lettering. The recommendations also urged those with close contact to newborns, such as parents, grandparents, and healthcare workers be given the Tdap to decrease the chance of transmission to vulnerable newborns. The vaccine can be given in intervals as short as 2 years to those in close contact with newborns. The Tdap is category C, although pregnant women were excluded from prelicensure trials. Breastfeeding mothers can receive the Tdap immediately in the postpartum period.

Clostridium tetani is a slender, gram-positive, anaerobic rod that is sensitive to heat and cannot survive in oxygen. However, the bacteria produce a terminal spore that survives antiseptics and even autoclaving. The spores are ubiquitous and are often found in soil and in the intestines of farm animals. In the anaerobic environment of a contaminated wound, the spores germinate and produce the endotoxin tetanospasmin, which spreads via blood and lymph. Tetanospasmin opposes inhibitory impulses, leading to muscle spasm, seizures, and autonomic dysfunction. Significant morbidity and mortality, including laryngospasm, aspiration, and death, are associated with tetanus.

Proper use of the tetanus vaccine has substantially decreased the incidence of tetanus during the past several years. In 2001, only 27 cases of tetanus occurred in the United States, and the mortality rate has declined to 10%. Worldwide, more than 270,000 people die of tetanus each year, however.

The vaccine is a formaldehyde-treated toxin available in several forms. The adult tetanus vaccine is available as Td, in which the tetanus toxoid is combined with the diphtheria antigen. The difference between adult and pediatric forms of the vaccine is that the pediatric composition contains 3 to 4 times more diphtheria vaccine. Td is recommended for use in all people older than age 65 years.

For an adult who has never received the primary vaccine series, three vaccinations are given, with 1 month separating the first two doses and 6 to 12 months separating the second and third dose. The first vaccine would be the Tdap followed by two doses of Td. After the primary vaccination series, antitoxin levels diminish over time, requiring the use of booster doses to maintain immunity. Some people demonstrate lifelong protective antitoxin levels. In others, antitoxin levels are no longer protective after 10 years. A small percentage of people require boosters every 5 years because protective antitoxin levels diminish much more quickly.

Tetanus prevention includes booster vaccination and thorough wound cleansing. Routine tetanus booster vaccination should be administered every 10 years. A patient who has received the primary vaccine and has a clean, minor wound should receive a booster tetanus dose if more than 10 years have elapsed since the previous dose. In contrast, a patient with a large, contaminated wound, especially an animal bite, needs a booster tetanus dose if more than 5 years have elapsed since the previous dose. Almost all cases of clinical tetanus occur in people who have either never received the vaccine or have not had a booster dose within 10 years.

The vaccine has few side effects. The most common are erythema, induration, and pain at the injection site. An exaggerated Arthus-like reaction can occur after vaccination with Td, and this reaction is characterized by extensive, painful swelling and induration from the shoulder to the elbow 2 to 8 hours after dosing. This reaction often occurs in patients who have received frequent booster vaccination and, therefore, have higher serum antitoxin levels. This reaction is not an absolute contraindication to further vaccination, but routine booster doses should not be given more frequently than every 10 years.[16]

Meningococcal Vaccine

Each year, 1,400 to 2,800 cases of meningococcal disease occur in the United States. Of these, 98% are sporadic, but an increase in localized outbreaks has been observed during the past 15 years. In 2000, the ACIP recommended the MSPV4 for all dormitory-living college freshmen. In 2005, the ACIP changed the recommendations to state that all children at age 11 years receive the MCV4 because of a significant incidence of meningococcal disease in children from 15 to 17 years. Others that might be candidates for meningococcal vaccination include those with certain complement deficiencies, anatomic and functional asplenia, and travelers to the area of sub-Saharan Africa known as the "meningitis belt."

Meningococcal disease presents as bacteremia or acute meningitis and is characterized by a 10% fatality rate and a 10% rate of severe morbidity, including hearing loss, neurologic disease, and limb loss. The disease is caused by serogroups A, B, C, Y, and W-135. The proportion of meningococcal cases caused by serogroup Y increased from 2% during 1989 to 1991 to 37% during 1997 to 2002. Serogroups B, C, and Y are the major causes of meningococcal disease in the United States, each being responsible for approximately one third of cases. The proportion of cases caused by each serogroup varies by age group. Among infants aged younger than 1 year, >50% of cases are caused by serogroup B, for which no vaccine is licensed or available in the United States. Of all cases of meningococcal disease among persons aged at least 11 years, 75% are caused by serogroups (C, Y, or W-135) that are included in vaccines available in the United States.

There are now two different meningococcal vaccines available; a polysaccharide and a conjugate vaccine. MPSV4 is a tetravalent meningococcal polysaccharide vaccine (Menomune-A,C,Y,W-135). It has been used for many years in the military and in mass immunizations. MPSV4 is administered subcutaneously as a single 0.5-mL dose to persons aged older than 2 years. At this point, it is the preferred vaccine for those 2 to 10 years and those older than 55 years at high risk for meningococcal disease. Studies have shown waning immunity after 3 years. Revaccination might be indicated for persons previously vaccinated with MPSV4 who remain at increased risk for infection (e.g., persons residing in areas in which disease is epidemic), particularly children who were first vaccinated at age younger than 4 years. Such children should be considered for revaccination after 2 to 3 years if they remain at increased risk. Although the need for revaccination among adults and older children after receiving MPSV4 has not been determined, if indications still exist for vaccination, revaccination might be considered after 5 years.

MCV4 is a tetravalent meningococcal conjugate vaccine (Menactra) that was licensed for use in the United States in January 2005. It is administered as a single subcutaneous dose of 0.5 ml containing serogroups A, C, Y, and W-135. It is indicated as the preferred vaccine for those from 11 to 55 years. The advantages of conjugate vaccines are longer-lasting immunity, herd protection, and elimination of nasal carriage. At this point, it is not clear how long the immunity from the MCV4 administration lasts, but the pre-adolescent visit should cover the increase risk seen in those same children as college freshmen.

Both vaccines are safe and well tolerated. Approximately 5% of patients have local reactions, and severe reactions occur in only 0.1/100,000 vaccine doses. There is a slightly higher incidence of local reactions in the MCV4 versus the MPSV4. Both vaccines can be administered with any other vaccine.[17]

Conclusion

Vaccines are an important part of public health and are one of the cornerstones of preventive medicine. They save lives, as well as healthcare expenditures. A review of vaccination status should be part of every health maintenance visit.

References

1. Centers for Disease Control and Prevention. A Comprehensive Immunization Strategy to Eliminate Transmission of Hepatitis B Virus Infection in the United States Recommendations of the Advisory Committee on Immunization Practices (ACIP) Part II: Immunization of Adults. MMWR. 2006;55(No. RR-16).
2. Centers for Disease Control and Prevention. Prevention of Hepatitis A through active or passive immunization: recommendations of the Advisory Committee on Immunization Practices (ACIP). MMWR. 2006;55:(No. RR-7).
3. Centers for Disease Control and Prevention. Measles, Mumps, and Rubella—Vaccine Use and Strategies for Elimination of Measles, Rubella, and Congenital Rubella Syndrome and Control of Mumps: Recommendations of the Advisory Committee on Immunization Practices (ACIP). MMWR. 1998;47(No. RR-8).
4. ACIP Provisional Recommendations for Prevention of Varicella. CDC. Released June, 2006.
5. Oxman MN, Levin MJ, Johnson GR, et al. "A vaccine to prevent herpes zoster and postherpetic neuralgia in older adults." N Engl J Med. 2005;352:2271–2284.
6. Oxman MN, et al. The Shingles Prevention Study Group. "A vaccine to prevent herpes zoster and postherpetic neuralgia in older adults." N Engl J Med. 2005;253(22):2271–2284.

7. American Cancer Society. Detailed Guide: Cervical Cancer—What Are the Key Statistics About Cervical Cancer? 2006. Available at: http://www.cancer.org/docroot/CRI/content/CRI_2_4_1X_What_are_the_key_statistics_for_cervical_cancer_8.asp?sitearea=.

8. Clifford GM, et al. Worldwide distribution of human papillomavirus types in cytologically normal women in the International Agency for Research on Cancer HPV prevalence surveys: a pooled analysis. Lancet. Sep 17–23, 2005;366(9490):991–998.

9. Munoz N, et al. Against which human papillomavirus types shall we vaccinate and screen? The international perspective. Int J Cancer. Aug 20, 2004;111(2):278–285.

10. Villa LL, et al. Immunologic responses following administration of a vaccine targeting HPV types 6, 11, 16, and 18. Vaccine. 2006;24:5571.

11. Villa LL, et al. High sustained efficacy of a prophylactic quadrivalent human papillomavirus types 6/11/16/18 L1 virus-like particle vaccine through 5 years of follow-up. Br J Cancer. Dec 4, 2006;95(11):1459–1466.

12. Jackson LA, Neuzil KM, Yu O, et al. Effectiveness of pneumococcal polysaccharide vaccine in older adults. N Engl J Med. 2003;348:1747–1755.

13. Kyaw MH, Lynfield R, Schaffner W, et al. Effect of introduction of the pneumococcal conjugate vaccine on drug-resistant Streptococcus pneumoniae. N Engl J Med. 2006; 354:1455–1463.

14. Prevention of Pneumococcal Disease: Recommendations of the Advisory Committee on Immunization Practices (ACIP). MMWR. April 4, 1997;46(RR-08):1–24.

15. Prevention and Control of Influenza: Recommendations of the Advisory Committee on Immunization Practices (ACIP). MMWR. July 28, 2006;55(RR10):1–42.

16. Preventing Tetanus, Diphtheria, and Pertussis Among Adults: Use of Tetanus Toxoid, Reduced Diphtheria Toxoid and Acellular Pertussis Vaccines. MMWR. Dec 15, 2006; 55(RR-17):1–33.

17. Prevention and Control of Meningococcal Disease: Recommendations of the Advisory Committee on Immunization Practices (ACIP). MMWR. May 27, 2005;54(RR07):1–21.

Chapter 20
Clinical Ethics and Infectious Disease in Family Medicine

Janet Fleetwood

Introduction

Although much of the literature in medical ethics focuses on high profile ethical issues such as genetic engineering, cloning, or multiorgan transplants, family physicians regularly encounter less dramatic ethical issues that affect the daily lives of real people. "Clinical ethics," a branch of medical ethics that examines ethical issues in the physician–patient relationship, considers the questions that face physicians in day-to-day practice. Patients with infectious diseases pose particularly challenging ethical questions for physicians; questions that require familiarity with ethics, law, and public health to resolve. In this chapter, we look at two such cases and apply a practical method for bioethical analysis.

Most bioethical analysis relies on the use of three basic principles. They include Respect for Persons, Beneficence, and Justice. Although some ethicists prefer virtue-based ethics, feminist ethics, or religiously grounded methods, principalism remains the prevalent American system of bioethical analysis.[1,2]

The Principle of Respect for Persons entails respecting the choices of people who can articulate reasoned decisions. It also requires that individuals who cannot make their own decisions be protected. Sometimes the Principle of Respect for Persons is described as the "Principle of Autonomy," although such a narrow characterization omits the duty to protect those who are unable to make their own, reasoned choices. This principle underlies many foundational concepts in medicine, such as informed consent.

The second principle, the Principle of Beneficence, encompasses both the obligation to help patients and the basic obligation to do no harm. It advises physicians to consider each intervention as a possible source of harm as well as benefit, and to help the patient determine their relative weight. In combination with the Principle of Respect for Persons, the Principle of Beneficence encourages helping patients to make their own rational choices that are consistent with what the patient believes is in his or her best interest.

The last principle, the Principle of Justice, entails distributing benefits fairly. The Principle of Justice does not specify what counts as "fair" but does require that physicians only consider relevant characteristics when making decisions regarding distributing benefits and burdens among competing claimants.

N.S. Skolnik (ed.), *Essential Infectious Disease Topics for Primary Care.*
© Humana Press, Totowa, NJ

Although ethical principles serve as a useful framework for bioethical decision making, there is no clear priority among them. Most bioethicists assert the general primacy of Respect for Persons and the inherent value of autonomy, yet often the well-being of others may seem to take priority. Therefore, in addition to the principles, we need an organized framework for bioethical decision making; a framework that this chapter delineates.

Doesn't the Law Resolve Most Bioethical Issues?

Many physicians see the law as both a sword and a shield. As a sword, the law can cut to the very soul of a physician, alleging that actions taken with diligence, skill, and good intent were done negligently or carelessly. This is the essence of a malpractice lawsuit, where the plaintiff's goal is to show that the physician did not perform in the way most reasonable physicians would. As a shield, physicians hope adhering to the law will protect them from liability—an assumption that many physicians will readily assert is naïve at best. Although knowledge of case law, statutes, and regulations are important, the law frequently does not provide the level of protection physicians expect. Moreover, although the law may set forth a minimally acceptable standard of behavior, often the intricacies of a specific situation make application of the law complex and unclear. Finally, sometimes two legally permissible actions are in conflict, leading the physician bereft of real guidance. In short, being informed about the law is necessary, but not sufficient, for the practice of good medicine.

Won't Professional Oaths and Codes Solve Ethical Issues?

Many oaths, codes, or professional statements, such as those from the Hippocratic writings, those put forth by the American Medical Association, or those from the American Academy of Family Physicians, can be useful guidelines. However, often codes address general issues but are difficult to apply to specific situations. For example, the Hippocratic Oath omits any discussion of informed consent— clearly an essential element of medical ethics today. In addition, oaths and codes do not allow much consideration of the specific patient's values, religion, or cultural beliefs. Although oaths and codes can provide a useful starting point, like the law, they cannot fully resolve ethical issues.

A Framework: Case Analysis in Clinical Ethics

Early in medical school, physicians in training are taught how to "present patients" by describing the patient's chief complaint, history of the present illness, medical history, family and social history, physical findings, and laboratory and test data. Physicians can approach ethical decision making in an analogous way. Although there is no simple "cookbook" approach to ethical decision making, any more than there is a "cookbook" in clinical medicine, an organized framework can help one work through a complex ethical dilemma. The four boxes in Table 20.1 provide a composite approach, drawn from several models in the literature, which parallels the process used in clinical medicine and summarizes the key steps to recognize, analyze, and resolve issues in clinical ethics.[3] Although the four steps to ethical analysis do not always go in a step-wise order, they are a useful starting point for the hypothetical scenarios encountered by Dr. Morgan, a family medicine physician in a small private practice.

Table 20.1 Four steps for analyzing ethical issues in patient care

Assessment in clinical medicine	Ethical analysis in clinical medicine
1. Data Collection (history and physical) • Present chief complaint • History of present illness • Past medical history • Family history • Social history • Physical findings • Diagnostic test data (e.g. lab data, imaging studies)	1. Information Collection (issue and analysis) • Relationship of chief complaint to ethical issue • History of ethical issue, especially whether it has been dealt with in the past for this patient • Decisional capacity of patient • Patient preferences about *who* decides and *how* they decide • Competing interests (family, hospital, staff, physicians, public health implications, third party payer, society)
2. Differential Diagnosis	2. Ethical Evaluation • Apply ethical principles to help identify sources of conflict • Consider options for resolution, consulting expert sources (journals, texts, consultants, ethical guidelines and codes, law, ethics committee) • Collaborate with patient, other decision makers, and outside stakeholders (if any) to negotiate a resolution
3. Initiate Therapy • Implement decision • Assess outcomes for clinical effectiveness	3. Initiate Ethical Approach • Implement decision • Assess outcome for consistency with patient's goals and values as well as good medical care
4. Review and Evaluate	4. Review & Evaluate Ethics • Evaluate decisions by asking, "Would I make the same decision again today?" and "Am I willing to have my decision publicly scrutinized, for example, if it appeared in the press?" • Reflect on decisions as circumstances change and new facts develop • Consider whether preventive ethics could have helped avoid the situation • Examine whether it is possible to prevent a similar event by taking proactive steps now.

Case 1: No Harm in Asking

Cheryl Lewis, a 27-year-old preschool teacher, has been Dr. Morgan's patient for 3 years. She is in generally good health and, like today, usually comes in only for routine checkups and follow-up of her mild eczema. Since graduating from the local university five years ago, Ms. Lewis has worked in Chinatown in a Head Start childcare program. Ms. Lewis is concerned about her exposure to many children in the course of her workday, thinks that some of her children may be at future risk for bird flu from newly arrived relatives and friends from China, and is worried about transmission. She is worried about catching the flu from one child and then inadvertently spreading it to the many children in her class. She also reminds Dr. Morgan that she is financially supporting her husband and their 2-year-old daughter while her husband is in graduate school, and that she cannot afford to miss work. She tells Dr. Morgan that she "doesn't want to be a victim or a vector" and asks Dr. Morgan for a prescription for Tamiflu "to keep on hand, just in case." Does Dr. Morgan have an obligation to grant her request?

Step 1: Information Collection

Ms. Lewis is requesting a prescription for a drug that is not indicated, but which she hopes to stockpile, and which is in very short supply. Dr. Morgan realizes that Ms. Lewis has never made a request for treatment that was not indicated in the past. Her reasons now seem like reasonable ones; she is exposed to many children during her workday, those children may possibly be exposed to people who have recently been to places where the bird flu has been found; she does not want to spread bird flu; and she is concerned about the financial, physical, and emotional impact influenza would have on herself and her family. She clearly has decisional capacity, and is basing her request on information she has obtained from the popular press. Of course, third-party interests and public health concerns make her request particularly problematic, therefore, although one may initially feel sympathetic to her concerns, an ethical analysis demands more careful scrutiny.

Step 2: Ethical Evaluation

This is a classic example in which the three principles of medical ethics conflict. Although the Principle of Respect for Persons generally requires that physicians uphold patient choices, part of the physician's role is to discuss the range of *medically appropriate* treatments. In implementing the Principle of Beneficence, physicians must use their best clinical judgment regarding the risks and benefits of a possible treatment. Finally, physicians have an obligation to apply the Principle of Justice fairly. Examining each principle in turn and examining how it applies to the case will help illuminate an ethically justifiable course of action.

Ms. Lewis is exercising her right to request a treatment that she perceives could be beneficial to her. Like the right to give or withhold consent for a procedure, many patients think that they have the right to request specific medications or interventions. In 1914, Justice Benjamin Cardozo, wrote, "Every human being of adult years and sound mind has a right to determine what shall be done with his own body,"[4] setting forth our early concept of informed consent, which has been a central tenet in American bioethics ever since. If we apply the principles of Respect for Persons and Beneficence, we realize both that individuals have a right to determine what happens to their own bodies and that there is widespread agreement that the best person to assess the patient's best interests is the patient, because the patient is most familiar with his or her own responsibilities, goals, and values. It might seem that if we allow that Ms. Lewis can refuse interventions that she feels are overly burdensome, we should similarly respect her right to request interventions that she thinks will be beneficial. Don't physicians have an obligation to provide benefit for their patients and respect their autonomous decisions? Yet what about the simultaneous obligation to justice and to ensure that those people in society that most need the bird flu drug will be able to obtain it? Does Dr. Morgan have a public health obligation in addition to an obligation to Ms. Lewis?

This problem is ethically analogous to cases in which patients request antibiotics for viral infections or magnetic resonance imaging (MRI) scans for back sprains. In short, physicians are not obligated to honor requests for treatments, procedures, or tests that are not beneficial or even necessary.[5] Physicians are obligated to practice evidence-based, scientific medicine, and recognize that there needs to be clear benefit to a patient before any level of risk is warranted.

This is a classic case in which the Principle of Justice conflicts with what the patient thinks is in her best interest. In essence, the physician is being asked to ration a benefit that is in short supply. The need to ration healthcare is not new; 8 of the 11 childhood vaccines have been in short supply in recent years[6] and there have been intermittent shortages of a wide range of drugs. Moreover, personal stockpiling is ethically problematic. The Infectious Diseases Society of American and the Society for Healthcare Epidemiology of America have stated that personal stockpiling will deplete the limited available supplies, making fewer drugs available for priority groups.[7] Moreover, it could lead to inappropriate use and wastage, and could even foster antiviral drug resistance. Finally, they point out the issues of fair allocation, showing that those who choose not to hoard the drug or cannot afford to stockpile will have less access to the drug in the case of an epidemic. Dr. Morgan needs to consult the National Vaccine Advisory Committee and the Advisory Committee on Immunization Practices[8] to review the prioritization plan and see where Ms. Lewis fits in the triage scheme.

These facts necessitate collaborative decision making with Ms. Lewis. First, Dr. Morgan should reassure Ms. Lewis that, ordinarily, the doctor would accede to her request for a treatment or procedure that was low risk and offered potential benefit, and that the doctor would treat all patients that make such a request the same way. Then Dr. Morgan needs to inform Ms. Lewis about the complexities of her request. She must understand her current medical status and the purpose, risks, benefits, costs, alternatives, and probability of success of Tamiflu (oseltamivir), insofar as that information is known. She needs an accurate understanding of the likelihood that she will catch bird flu given our current knowledge about transmissibility. She needs to understand that we do not yet know whether Tamiflu will be the drug of choice if there were a human outbreak, or how effective it will be. She needs to understand that the public health recommendations are designed to help everyone in society and how important that is in the case of an actual outbreak. Finally, she needs a clear recommendation based on Dr. Morgan's clinical judgment and experience that is consistent with current public health recommendations.

Dr. Morgan should explain these factors to Ms. Lewis, give Ms. Lewis information regarding illness prevention (such as careful hand washing techniques and cough etiquette for herself and her young students), alert her to the news reports about fraudulent sale of counterfeit Tamiflu, educate her about the early symptoms of bird flu, and offer to see her in the office promptly if she should experience any of the symptoms. She needs to be made aware that many people travel to parts of the world with various infectious agents, and that it is problematic to target a group of neighborhood children as possible vectors of disease when there is no evidence to support that. The physician could also stress that if everyone *refuses* to stockpile, there might be sufficient Tamiflu for those who are affected or most likely to be exposed. By reassuring Ms. Lewis that she is not currently in a targeted, high-risk occupation, and that, should an outbreak develop, Dr. Morgan will assist her, the physician can simultaneously meet the obligation of beneficence and protection of public health.

Step 3: Initiate Ethical Approach

Ms. Lewis may be very unhappy with Dr. Morgan's response. However, she might feel differently if, for example, her child and husband were affected and there was no more Tamiflu available because it had been stockpiled by healthy adults like her. By appealing to her basic values and sense of fairness, it might be possible to change her perspective. It is possible that the patient will, nevertheless, seek Tamiflu elsewhere or simply seek another physician, but those choices are beyond Dr. Morgan's control.

Step 4: Review and Evaluate

There are several criteria for determining whether this action is ethically justifiable. First, the physician should decide whether he or she would make the same decision again.

The physician should ask whether having the decision scrutinized by colleagues or even the public would be acceptable. The physician should consider whether he or she will treat all patients making a similar request the same way, and should determine, in advance, if he or she will make exceptions to the public health recommendations. If the doctor is satisfied that Ms. Lewis' autonomy and best interests were balanced with public health issues, then the decision is ethically justified.

Case 2: What We Don't Know Can Hurt Us

Christine Jones is a 19-year-old new patient who arrived in Dr. Morgan's office with her 3-month-old daughter, Devin. She explains that they recently relocated from another state after she severed her relationship with the baby's 29-year-old father, Charles Foster, who owns a popular nightclub. She has no health records for herself or the baby with her, but has provided the staff with permission and the address of her former family physician who cared for both her and baby Devin, so that the staff can obtain their health records. Ms. Jones now lives with her sister, her brother-in-law, and her sister's two children. She complains of 3 weeks of flu-like symptoms and fatigue "more than you'd expect with a new baby." The baby appears small for her age but otherwise well.

Dr. Morgan takes Ms. Jones' history. She says her pregnancy and vaginal delivery were normal, and that, until recently, her health has been good. She gained 25 pounds with the pregnancy and she happily reports that she has lost 40 pounds since the baby's birth, saying that she is "even skinnier" now than before she became pregnant. She wonders aloud if that is because of breast feeding. She says she has always been healthy until the last several weeks, when she developed occasional fevers, fatigue, cough, and sore throat. She eventually tells you that reason she severed her relationship with Charles was because of his intravenous drug use. She seems very embarrassed and reveals that she knew he had been a "recreational drug user" for a while but that things spiraled out of control during the last year. She was shocked when he was arrested for possession of crack cocaine just before the baby's birth. She delivered the baby and promptly moved in with her sister. She explains that, although her sister knows about Charles' arrest, her brother-in-law is a police officer and does not know the reason for her separation. She explains that with a new baby and no job, she had nowhere else to go and thought it best to conceal the truth.

Dr. Morgan asks Ms. Jones about birth control and safe sex, and she tells the doctor that she is sure she is "safe" because she has not had sex in a long time. She goes on to say that she and Charles used no birth control for the last year because she was already pregnant.

The doctor proceeds with the physical exam and notices slightly swollen lymph glands. Between the unusual weight loss, fatigue, swollen glands, and risk factors, Dr. Morgan advises Ms. Jones that she should have several tests, including a throat culture and blood tests. Dr. Morgan inquires whether she was offered an HIV test during her pregnancy and at delivery. Ms. Jones says that she was offered both times and both times chose to "opt out." She says that she was not concerned about HIV because Charles is not the type to share needles or hang around crack houses. Dr. Morgan expresses concern and advises her that she needs an HIV test. She becomes agitated and refuses the test. She points out that Charles is not sick, so there really is no reason to think she would have HIV. Besides, she says, they did not have sex during the last 2 months of her pregnancy, so she has not had sex in 5 months. Dr. Morgan then suggests testing baby Devin for HIV and Ms. Jones adamantly refuses, stating "there's nothing wrong with my beautiful baby!" She quickly packs up and prepares to leave the office. What, if anything, is Dr. Morgan's ethical obligation to Ms. Jones, baby Devin, and Charles?

Step 1: Information Collection

It is often puzzling when a patient refuses to have a test that will elicit information that is key to the patient's personal health and well-being, and, in this case, the health of a child. Although Ms. Jones came in for treatment for her fatigue and other symptoms, there are two patients involved. Especially because one of those patients is a child, the physician needs to try to ensure that both receive the medical care that is clinically and ethically appropriate.

The first task is to determine why Ms. Jones has refused, and is continuing to refuse, the test for herself and also her baby. She clearly has the mental capacity to make the decision for herself and her child. She wants to be the sole decision maker in this case, and does not want to involve the baby's father. However, there are issues regarding protecting the child, as well as potential public health issues regarding whom Ms. Jones might unknowingly expose to HIV in the future.

At the outset, the physician should help Ms. Jones separate the decision for herself from the decision for little Devin. The doctor should emphasize the need for prompt testing and treatment for both, and Ms. Jones' obligation to do what is best for Devin even if it is not best for her. Dr. Morgan can be most effective by separating out the decisions and working with Ms. Jones to examine the risks and benefits of each.

Initially, Ms. Jones needs information regarding the purpose, risks, benefits, and alternatives of the test, and the likelihood that the results will be accurate. She needs to know about the safeguards for confidentiality of the results, what kinds of protections are available, and the value of prompt treatment. She needs to understand the impact of continued breastfeeding if she is positive for HIV and that she should stop breastfeeding to minimize the chance of transmission. Current data shows that mother-to-child transmission can be prevented almost entirely with antiretroviral prophylaxis, elective cesarean section and refraining from breastfeeding.[9] Although she cannot change the past, stopping breastfeeding would be an important step now. Finally, she needs to know about safe sex and the prevention of HIV and sexually transmitted diseases (STDs).

The physician needs to explore Ms. Jones' fears and determine why she is refusing the test. Does she doubt the value of the test? Does she have misunderstandings about the value or risks of available treatments? Is it simply fear of the blood test itself? More likely, it is fear of positive results and ramifications of that finding; a much more complex issue.

A similar conversation needs to occur pertaining to testing of baby Devin. Ms. Jones needs to know the risks, benefits, alternatives to, and accuracy of the test, and the physician needs to explore her concerns regarding the test results. It needs to be clear to Ms. Jones that her primary obligation is to protect the health of her child and that, although it may be difficult for her to deal with positive test results should that occur, she has a duty to obtain the best healthcare possible for the baby, and that giving permission for the HIV test is essential toward that goal. Obviously, Ms. Jones could refuse to give permission for treatment that is of limited or questionable benefit or is highly risky, but, in this case, the test is clearly of benefit and of little risk. In cases in which parents refuse to give permission for their children's treatment, for example on religious grounds, the courts often step in to protect the child, reasoning that the child is too young to make the choice. As a widely quoted court ruling has stated, although "parents may be free to become martyrs themselves" they are not similarly free to "make martyrs of their children."[10] Given the doctor's strong suspicion that Ms. Jones is positive for HIV now and was likely positive for HIV during delivery, Dr. Morgan should involve social service and possibly seek court mandated testing for this child.

One thing the physician should *not* do is perform a "surrogate" CD4 test to indirectly ascertain HIV status. Although this information might be available as part of the other routine testing, it would be unethical for the doctor to elicit this information solely for the purpose of circumventing her refusal of the HIV test. Such surreptitious testing violates the law as well as basic tenets of ethics, which clearly require complete disclosure before testing for HIV occurs.

Of course, even if Ms. Jones eventually agrees to the test, the ethical issues do not end. If the test is positive, there are treatment issues. Will Ms. Jones consent to treatment for herself? Will she give permission for treatment for Devin?

Step 2: Ethical Evaluation

How can the physician fulfill the ethical obligations to Ms. Jones, Devin, and Charles? Whether or not Ms. Jones agrees to the test and treatment, she needs social support. Some might argue that, if her test is positive, the state has an interest in ensuring that she gets prompt treatment because she is the primary caregiver for the baby. In any case, the physician should provide resources or referrals for her and her child. A support group could help her comes to terms with the need for testing and prompt treatment, if necessary, and give her the tools for discussing the issues with her sister and brother-in-law. If she declines a support group, she might agree to see a social worker or a clergyperson of the appropriate faith.

The Principle of Respect for Persons allows Ms. Jones to refuse the test for herself. If she persists in refusing, the physician should stress to her the need to stop breastfeeding for prompt treatment and urge her to practice safe sex. Should she agree to test but refuse treatment, the Principle of Respect for Persons also supports that choice.

However, the Principle of Respect for Persons also requires protecting those who cannot protect themselves. Combined with the Principle of Beneficence, the two principles direct the physician to intervene in behalf of the baby. Ms. Devin should be strongly encouraged have Devin tested. She should be told that the baby's small size could be related to HIV and that Devin could also be susceptible to infections. Moreover, if the baby tests positive, the physician or social service agency may have to intervene to ensure prompt, continuous, consistent treatment. Clearly, testing and treatment are in the child's best interest because HIV is serious, likely, and treatable—or perhaps even preventable—in this case. Although Ms. Jones may be psychologically harmed when her choice is overridden, and may subsequently lose trust in the healthcare profession, the potential life-threatening costs to the child far outweigh the anger and betrayal Ms. Jones may feel.

The physician's ethical obligations to Charles are limited and depend on whether or not Ms. Jones ultimately agrees to be tested and has a positive result. Charles is an adult, so does not need the level of protection that baby Devin does. If Ms. Jones continues to refuse testing, the physician can only encourage her to notify Charles that he should be tested himself. If she is tested and has a positive test result, however, state laws determine whether or not there is a legal obligation to warn a partner. Sometimes the health department carries out partner notification, enabling the physician to fulfill the obligation simply by reporting the cases. In some states, the health department does not perform partner notification and only uses the data for epidemiologic purposes. Moreover, sometimes the law only protects physicians who warn individuals who are at *future* risk of infection, not those who may have been infected in the past. Thus, the physician needs to understand the law in that jurisdiction to fulfill the legal requirements. In addition, the doctor must analyze any additional ethical obligation by assessing the likelihood, severity, and preventability of the harm. Although the law may set a minimum standard of behavior and give guidelines for how to notify a contact if the physician so chooses, the ethical decision regarding whether or not to notify the contact may fall squarely on the physician despite public health requirements to report for epidemiologic purposes.

Although Ms. Jones is the only one that Dr. Morgan can easily communicate with, there are three people directly involved in this case; Ms. Jones, Charles, and baby Devin. Ms. Jones needs to realize that her scope of authority is absolute over decisions for herself, more limited over decisions regarding Devin, and sharply circumscribed when it comes to notifying Charles.

Step 3: Initiate Ethical Approach

Dr. Morgan needs to elicit Ms. Jones' fears, which turn on her concern regarding isolation and banishment from her sister's home if her brother-in-law, a police officer, discovers that her boyfriend uses illegal drugs. The physician needs to be clear with Ms. Jones regarding the ethical, legal, and public health obligations while working with her to explore her values and goals. Dr. Morgan should keep the "door open" for Ms. Jones to return at any time should she change her mind and desire testing, and offer counseling and support for her regardless of her decision about her own health.

As for the child, however, Dr. Morgan should be more assertive in obtaining Ms. Jones' permission and even seek social service or court intervention, if necessary. Dr. Morgan can also negotiate with Ms. Jones toward a compromise, such as stopping breastfeeding immediately while agreeing to return for Devin's testing in 3 days, which would give Ms. Jones time to adjust and perhaps get the emotional support of her sister. Obviously, if Ms. Jones did not return for the follow-up appointment with Devin, the physician could then involve social services.

Step 4: Review and Evaluate Ethics

Ms. Jones is an adult with the ability to make her own decisions, and an HIV test cannot be mandated for her. However, protection of the vulnerable child is another matter and the physician should intervene. Dr. Morgan need only think about the repercussions of not testing the baby and initiating prompt treatment if the test is positive. Moreover, Dr. Morgan would undoubtedly feel inadequate as a physician if the choice not to intervene became widely known. Although a decision to override parental choice is undeniably damaging to the physician–patient relationship, the greater concern is the life and health of the child.

Summary

These two cases illustrate several of the ethical issues family medicine physicians encounter in practice. The steps for analyzing ethical issues in clinical care can enable physicians to recognize, analyze, and choose legally sound and ethically justifiable solutions. Although not always easy or straightforward, a comprehensive analysis using basic ethical principles can help physicians move through ethical quagmires with a sense of organization and purpose.

References

1. Jonsen AR, Siegler M, Winslade WJ, Eds. Clinical Ethics: A Practical Approach to Ethical Decisions in Clinical Medicine, 5th ed. New York, NY: McGraw Hill, 2002:1–12.
2. Lo B. Resolving Ethical Dilemmas: A Guide for Clinicians. 3rd edition. Philadelphia, PA: Lippincott Williams and Wilkins, 2005:1–16.

 3. Fleetwood J, Kassutto Z, Lipsky MS. Clinical Ethics in Family Medicine. FP Essentials, Edition No. 302, AAFP Home Study, Leawood, Kan: American Academy of Family Physicians, July 2004.
 4. Schloendorff v. Society of New York Hospital, 211 N.Y. 125, 129–130, 105 N.E. 92, 93 (1914).
 5. Brett AS, Zuger A. "The run on Tamiflu—should physicians prescribe on demand?," N Engl J Med. December 22, 2005;353:2636–2637.
 6. Couzin J. "Ethicists to guide rationing of flu vaccine. (Infectious Diseases)." Science. Nov 5, 2004; 306.5698:960(2).
 7. Joint Position Statement of the Infectious Diseases Society of America and Society for Healthcare Epidemiology of America on Antiviral Stockpiling for Influenza Preparedness. Approved October 31, 2005.
 8. Temte JL. "Preparing for an Influenza Pandemic: Vaccine Prioritization", Family Practice Management, January 2006. Downloadable at www.aafp.org.fpm.
 9. Thorne C, Newell ML. "Treatment options for the prevention of mother-to-child transmission of HIV." Curr Opin Investig Drugs. 2005;6(8):804–811.
10. Prince v. Massachusetts. 321 U.S. 158 (1944).

Index

Printed in the United States of America